Cochlear Implants

Second Edition

Susan B. Waltzman, PhD
New York University School of Medicine
New York, New York

J. Thomas Roland Jr., MD
Department of Otolaryngology
New York University School of Medicine
New York, New York

Thieme Medical Publishers
New York • Stuttgart

Thieme Medical Publishers, Inc.
333 Seventh Ave.
New York, NY 10001

Associate Editor: Owen Zurhellen
Production Editor: The Egerton Group, Ltd.
Vice President, Production and Electronic Publishing: Anne T. Vinnicombe
Sales Director: Ross Lumpkin
Associate Marketing Director: Verena Diem
Chief Financial Officer: Peter van Woerden
President: Brian D. Scanlan
Compositor: Techset Composition Limited
Printer: Everbest Printing Co.

Library of Congress Cataloging-in-Publication Data is available from the publisher.

Important note: Medical knowledge is ever-changing. As new research and clinical experience broaden our knowledge, changes in treatment and drug therapy may be required. The authors and editors of the material herein have consulted sources believed to be reliable in their efforts to provide information that is complete and in accord with the standards accepted at the time of publication. However, in view of the possibility of human error by the authors, editors, or publisher of the work herein or changes in medical knowledge, neither the authors, editors, or publisher, nor any other party who has been involved in the preparation of this work, warrants that the information contained herein is in every respect accurate or complete, and they are not responsible for any errors or omissions or for the results obtained from use of such information. Readers are encouraged to confirm the information contained herein with other sources. For example, readers are advised to check the product information sheet included in the package of each drug they plan to administer to be certain that the information contained in this publication is accurate and that changes have not been made in the recommended dose or in the contraindications for administration. This recommendation is of particular importance in connection with new or infrequently used drugs.

Some of the product names, patents, and registered designs referred to in this book are in fact registered trademarks or proprietary names even though specific reference to this fact is not always made in the text. Therefore, the appearance of a name without designation as proprietary is not to be construed as a representation by the publisher that it is in the public domain.

Printed in the United States of America

5 4 3 2 1

TMP ISBN 0-86577-987-2
GTV ISBN 3 13 127531 6
GTV ISBN 978-3 13 117452 9
US ISBN 978-1-58890-413-3

Contents

Preface

We are delighted to present the second edition of *Cochlear Implants*. Due to the hard work of the many contributors, the first edition became a comprehensive reference text for clinicians, researchers, and students alike, and served to offer all others interested in cochlear implants a wide scope of information. This current edition is intended to build on that success. Many of the original contributors have updated their chapters to provide recent and relevant material on implant design and processing, medical/surgical aspects, evaluation, programming, outcomes in children and adults, and poststimulation care. In an effort to broaden and update the scope of the book, more experts have contributed new chapters in several areas, including historical foundations, genetics, sound processing, binaural hearing, and electroacoustic stimulation.

Careful readers will notice that the reference format of the individual chapters varies between American Medical Association (AMA) and American Phonetics Association (APA) style. This is deliberate, and indicative of the interdisciplinary nature of this book, with contributions from otolaryngologists, audiologists, and numerous others. All have done an outstanding job of incorporating recent data and current thinking to present a wide and balanced perspective providing a framework for the understanding of future developments.

The broad scope of this book equips clinicians, researchers, students, and others interested in the field with an understanding not only of the concepts related to implantation but of the recipients who benefit. And, most importantly, it provides knowledge and tools that will ultimately enhance the benefits to implant users.

Susan B. Waltzman
J. Thomas Roland Jr.

List of Contributors

Paul J. Abbas, PhD
Department of Speech Pathology
    and Audiology
University of Iowa
Iowa City, Iowa

Sue M. Archbold, MPhil
The Ear Foundation
Nottingham
United Kingdom

Carolyn J. Brown, PhD
Department of Speech Pathology
    and Audiology
University of Iowa
Iowa City, Iowa

Steven B. Chin, PhD
Department of Otolaryngology
Indiana University
    School of Medicine
Indianapolis, Indiana

Noel L. Cohen, MD
New York University
    Cochlear Implant Center
New York, New York

Michael F. Dorman, PhD
Department of Speech and
    Hearing Science
Arizona State University
Tempe, Arizona

Ward R. Drennan, PhD
V. M. Bloedel Hearing Research
    Center
University of Washington
Seattle, Washington

Rosemarie A. Drous, MEd, Cert AVT
New York University
    Cochlear Implant Center
New York, New York

Camille C. Dunn, PhD
University of Iowa
Iowa City, Iowa

Marc D. Eisen, MD, PhD
Department of Otolaryngology
ORL
Philadelphia, Pennsylvania

Christine P. Etler, MA
Department of Otolaryngology
University of Iowa
Iowa City, Iowa

James B. Fallon, PhD
Bionic Ear Institute
East Melbourne
Victoria, Australia

Andrew J. Fishman, MD
Department of Otolaryngology,
New York University
    School of Medicine,
New York
Department of Otolaryngology
Head and Neck Surgery and
    Neurosurgery
Amrita Institute of Medical Sciences
Kochi, Kerala, India

Bruce J. Gantz, MD
Department of Otolaryngology
University of Iowa
Iowa City, Iowa

Kate E. Gfeller, PhD
Department of Speech Pathology
    and Audiology
University of Iowa
Iowa City, Iowa

John G. Golfinos, MD
Department of Neurosurgery
New York University
    School of Medicine
New York, New York

Roy A. Holliday, MD
Department of Radiology
New York Eye and Ear Infirmary
New York, New York

Tina C. Huang, MD
Department of Otolaryngology
New York University
    School of Medicine
New York, New York

Anil Kumar Lalwani, MD
Department of Otolaryngology
New York University
    School of Medicine
New York, New York

Enrique A. Lopez-Poveda, PhD
Laboratory of Neurobiology
    of Hearing
Instituto de Neurociencias
    de Castilla y León
Universidad de Salamanca
Salamanca, Spain

Noah E. Meltzer, MD
Center for Hearing and Balance
Department of Otolaryngology
Johns Hopkins University
Baltimore, Maryland

William G. Noble, PhD
School of Psychology
University of New England
Armidale, Australia

Andrew K. Patel, MD
Division of Otolaryngology – Head
    and Neck Surgery
University of California – San Diego
San Diego, California

**Amy McConkey Robbins,
    MS, CCC-Sp**
Communication Consulting Services
Indianapolis, Indiana

J. Thomas Roland Jr., MD
Department of Otolaryngology
New York University
    School of Medicine
New York, New York

Jay T. Rubinstein, MD, PhD
V. M. Bloedel Hearing
    Research Center
University of Washington
Seattle, Washington

David K. Ryugo, PhD
Center for Hearing and Balance
Johns Hopkins University
    School of Medicine
Baltimore, Maryland

Reinhold Schatzer, PhD
Christian Doppler Laboratory
    for Active Implantable Systems
University of Innsbruck
Innsbruck, Austria

William H. Shapiro, MA
New York University
Cochlear Implant Center
New York, New York

Robert K. Shepherd, PhD
The Bionic Ear Institute
East Melbourne
Victoria, Australia

Anthony J. Spahr, PhD
Department of Speech and
    Hearing Science
Arizona State University
Tempe, Arizona

Eric G. St. Clair, MD
Resident in Neurosurgery
New York University
    School of Medicine
New York, New York

Mario A. Svirsky, PhD
New York University
    School of Medicine
New York, New York

Christopher W. Turner, PhD
Department of Speech Pathology
    and Audiology
University of Iowa
Iowa City, Iowa

Richard S. Tyler, PhD
University of Iowa Hospital
Iowa City, Iowa

Susan B. Waltzman, PhD
New York University
    School of Medicine
New York, New York

Blake S. Wilson, BS
Research Triangle Institute
Research Triangle Park
North Carolina

Shelley A. Witt, MA, CCC-A
University of Iowa
    Hospitals and Clinics
Iowa City, Iowa

William Yost, PhD
Loyola University
Chicago, Illinois

Teresa A. Zwolan, PhD
University of Michigan
    Hearing Rehabilitation Center
Ann Arbor, Michigan

Acknowledgments

As with the first edition, this book has truly been a cooperative effort. First, we would like to thank the contributors, all experts in their respective areas, who provided outstanding chapters that required little editing. We feel privileged and proud to have had the opportunity to work with them. Second, it has been a pleasure to work with Esther Gumpert and Owen Zurhellen at Thieme Medical Publishers. They have been incredibly supportive and patient, and their guidance, hard work, and gentle personalities have brought this book to fruition. And, finally, we wish to thank our friends and colleagues at the New York University Cochlear Implant Center: our achievements are in a large part due to their labor-intensive efforts, dedication, and commitment to the patients and field of cochlear implants. It is an honor and pleasure for us to be associated with them.

Susan B. Waltzman
J. Thomas Roland Jr.

1

History of the Cochlear Implant

Marc D. Eisen

The cochlear implant has created a paradigm shift in the treatment of sensorineural hearing loss. It has had great impact in the brief time it has been available. In less than four decades, the cochlear implant progressed from the first attempts to elicit hearing via direct electrical stimulation of the auditory nerve to a commercially available device that has restored varying degrees of hearing to tens of thousands of deaf patients. Several themes that pervade the implant's history are widely applicable to the development of other neural prostheses. For one, the implant's development was truly an interdisciplinary effort. Significant contributions came from members of fields as diverse as engineering, otology, audiology, auditory neurophysiology, psychoacoustics, and industry. The interaction among these players was not always harmonious, but the strife yielded synthesis and progress.

Another theme is the courage of a few clinicians to risk their reputations and eschew scientific dogma in the hope of helping the patients that sought their care. Lastly is the theme of patients being willing to take substantial risks in serving as research subjects, sometimes without any promise of individual medical gain. This chapter does not aim to be exhaustive in mentioning each and every contributor or contribution that occurred during the implant's early development. Rather, it discusses in depth a selection of events and characters that—with the aid of the "retrospectroscope"—exemplify these themes and demonstrate a progression of events leading toward a device that allows the patient who has lost all hearing to regain the ability to converse on the telephone, and one that allows the deaf child to develop near-normal speech production and understanding.

The story of the implant's development is parsed into several periods. The first began in 1957 and continued throughout the 1960s. This was the period of pioneering and experimentation. The second period in the 1970s was a time of feasibility study, exploring whether the implant safely stimulated the auditory pathway and elicited useful hearing. The third period led to the development of a commercially viable multielectrode cochlear prosthesis.

◆ Precursors

Several discoveries made during the first half of the 20th century were not directly related to electrical stimulation of the cochlear nerve, but were influential on the early development of the cochlear implant and therefore warrant mention. These include Homer Dudley's work on the synthesis of speech and his "vocoder," Glenn Wever and his discovery of the cochlear microphonic, and S. S. Stevens and coworkers' description of electrophonic hearing.

The Vocoder

Homer Dudley was a researcher at the Bell Telephone Laboratories in New York. He described and demonstrated in 1939 a real-time voice synthesizer that produced intelligible speech using circuitry designed to extract the fundamental frequency of speech, the intensity of its spectral components, and its overall power. The spectral components were extracted with a series of 10 band-pass filters covering the frequency range of speech.[1] He named the synthesizer the "vocoder," a compressed version of "coding the voice."

The operating principles of the vocoder for condensing speech into its principal components formed the basis of early speech processing schemes for multichannel cochlear implants.

The Cochlear Microphonic

In 1930, Wever and Bray[2] recorded and described the electrical potentials in the cochlea that faithfully reproduced the sound stimulus. This phenomenon became known as the "Wever–Bray effect." The source of these measured potentials was initially incorrectly assumed to represent auditory nerve discharges. This theory of the origin of these potentials would be equivalent to the "telephone" theory of hearing, referring to the analog representation of the voice carried along the "cable" of the auditory nerve as it would along the wires of a telephone line. In truth, what Wever and Bray were recording was not a response of the cochlear nerve, but the cochlear microphonic produced by the outer hair cells in the cochlea. Regardless of the ultimate dismissal of the telephone theory of hearing, it inspired several of the earliest pioneers of the cochlear implant.

Electrophonic Hearing

S. S. Stevens[3] and his colleagues classically described in the 1930s the mechanism by which the cochlear elements respond to electrical stimulation to produce hearing. This mechanism was coined "electrophonic hearing." We now know that electrophonic hearing results from the mechanical oscillation of the basilar membrane in response to voltage changes. The primary tenet of their description was the requirement that the cochlea be intact. Prior to 1957, efforts to stimulate hearing electrically were performed on subjects with at least partially functioning cochleae. In these subjects, therefore, responses could be accounted for by electrophonic hearing rather than direct nerve stimulation. Furthermore, the earliest cochlear implant efforts had the burden of proving that they were directly stimulating the cochlear nerve rather than eliciting electrophonic hearing.

◆ Pioneers (1957 to 1973): André Djourno and Charles Eyriès

Although numerous attempts to treat deafness with electricity have been reported over the past several centuries,[4] the first reported direct stimulation of the cochlear nerve for the purpose of generating hearing appeared as recently as 1957 with the work of André Djourno and Charles Eyriès. Despite the revolutionary impact that the cochlear implant has had on all auditory disciplines, these beginnings in Paris received little attention.

André Djourno (1904–1996) received degrees in both science and medicine, yet he devoted his career to science. His early endeavors were studying the electrophysiology of the frog peripheral nerve.[5,6] He then ventured into more medical applications of electricity. Several of Djourno's earlier innovations reflected his inventiveness: a device to measure the pulse continuously,[7] high-frequency electrical stimulation to remove metal fragments from bones,[8] and the use of electroencephalography (EEG) to study narcolepsy.[9] Perhaps the most prescient development from this period was artificial respiration utilizing direct phrenic nerve stimulation.[10] Although this innovation did not reach widespread clinical implementation, it demonstrated Djourno's interest in neural prostheses.

Djourno focused the next phase of his career on fabricating and testing implantable induction coils to be used for "telestimulation," or stimulation through inductive coupling without wires. Djourno assembled these induction coils himself and called them "microbobinages," as the coils wound with wire resembled small spools of thread (**Fig. 1–1**). Both the active coil and the ground electrode were implanted under the skin of an animal, and stimulation was *trans*cutaneous (rather than *per*cutaneous). The implantable coils were first used to stimulate the sciatic nerve and thus trigger a jump behavior in rabbits. Djourno studied numerous aspects of telestimulation, including electrode biocompatibility (he described using one of the first bioresistant resins, *araldite*, for example, to coat the electrodes[11]). He addressed the effect of stimulus frequency on muscle contraction, and he found that with higher

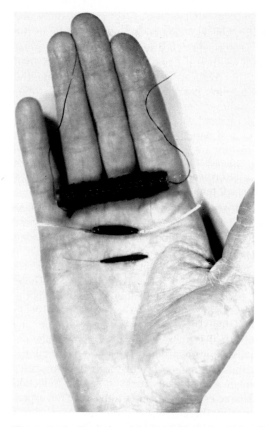

Figure 1–1 Example of implantable induction coils ("microbobinages") assembled by Djourno in his laboratory. Induction coils like the ones shown here were used in various applications, including the stimulation of the auditory pathway. The hand holding the coils gives perspective to the implant's size. (Courtesy of John Q. Adams Center for the History of Otolaryngology–Head and Neck Surgery, Alexandria, VA.)

frequency stimuli, muscles would not contract, whereas with lower frequency stimuli muscle contraction was painful. Djourno found the "right" stimulus frequency between 400 and 500 Hz. Because this frequency was within the speech range, he began to use the analog signal of his own voice as the telestimulating stimulus.[12] Triggering a nerve with his voice may well have contributed to the idea of stimulating the cochlear nerve to restore hearing.

Djourno also addressed the safety of repetitive stimulation on tissue, demonstrating that the sciatic nerve from an implanted rabbit, when examined histologically and grossly, showed no changes after 2 years of repetitive stimulation.[13] Throughout this time Djourno revealed little interest in hearing. He recognized, however, the potential of using the microbobinages to stimulate the auditory system, as he and Kayser noted the possibility of "treating deafness" as a potential application in a 1954 publication.[12]

Charles Eyriès (1908–1996) completed his training in otolaryngology in Paris in the early 1940s. Clinically, Eyriès earned early recognition for his description of a procedure to treat *ozena*, or atrophic rhinitis, by placing implants underneath the nasal mucosa to decrease the caliber of the nasal passages.[14] This procedure became known in the French literature as the "Eyriès operation." Eyriès was named chief of otorhinolaryngology and head and neck surgery at L'Institut Prophylactique in 1953, which has since been renamed L'Institut Arthur Vernes. Although primarily a clinician, he had research interests in neuroanatomy and embryology of the facial nerve, and he wrote about surgical facial nerve repairs.[15] Eyriès had shown little interest in hearing at this point in his career and had never worked with Djourno, although he knew of Djourno because both he and Djourno had laboratories in the medical school associated with the hospital.

As the local expert on facial nerve repairs, Eyriès was asked in February 1957 to provide a consultation for a rather unfortunate patient—a 57-year-old man who suffered from large bilateral cholesteatomas. A right-sided temporal bone resection was performed 5 days prior to the consultation and an extensive left temporal bone resection was performed several years earlier. Both procedures involved ablation of the labyrinth and facial nerve sectioning. As a result, the patient was left with bilateral deafness and bilateral facial nerve paralysis. Eyriès was consulted to consider a facial nerve graft for reanimation.[16]

On examination, Eyriès found that the caliber of the patient's remaining nerve was too small to support a local nerve transfer. Eyriès therefore embarked on a search for appropriate graft material. He went to the medical school seeking cadaverous material, where he met Djourno, who offered to help and suggested stimulating hearing at the same time. Although Eyriès was primarily interested in his patient's facial reanimation, he agreed to implant an electrode into the patient at the time of surgery. Eyriès' justification for agreeing to the implantation was that the cavity was already exposed and the patient had nothing to lose in having the extra procedure.[16] From Djourno's standpoint, the patient was deaf and begging to escape from the silence that haunted him, and Djourno was fascinated by the opportunity to telestimulate the auditory system.[17]

The procedure took place on February 25, 1957. Eyriès performed the right-sided facial nerve graft using fetal sciatic nerve as the graft material, which purportedly proved to be successful. At the time of surgery, the proximal cochlear nerve stump was found to be significantly shredded. Djourno and Eyriès chose to seat the active electrode into the remaining stump and place the induction coil into the temporalis muscle. A postoperative lateral skull film confirmed its placement (**Fig. 1–2**).

Some testing was done intraoperatively. The stimulus waveforms included bursts of a 100-Hz impulse signal administered 15 to 20 times per minute, low-frequency alternating current, and the analog signal of words spoken into a microphone. The patient described detecting auditory sensations. Several qualitative observations were made: the patient's discrimination of intensity was good, frequency discrimination was poor, and no speech recognition was evident. The patient underwent an extensive postoperative rehabilitation with the implant under the guidance of the speech therapist. Over the ensuing months more complex stimuli were administered, and the patient was able to differentiate between higher frequency (described as "silk ripping") and lower frequency (described as "burlap tearing") stimulation. He appreciated environmental noises and several words, but could not understand speech. The publication that resulted from this work is the seminal citation for direct cochlear nerve stimulation.[18]

Several months later, during testing, the electrode suddenly ceased to function. Djourno and Eyriès brought the patient to the operating room to investigate. They found that a solder joint connecting the wires to the ground electrode embedded into the temporalis muscle had broken, and the implant was replaced. The second implant, however, suffered the same fate. Eyriès held Djourno

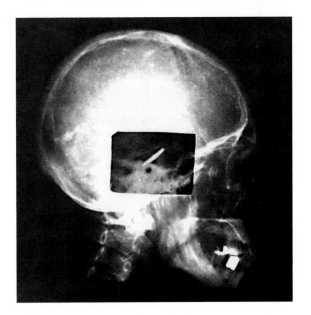

Figure 1–2 Lateral skull film of Djourno and Eyriès' first implant following surgery. The coil has been embedded in the temporalis muscle, whereas the electrodes were placed near the remaining stump of the cochlear nerve. (Courtesy of John Q. Adams Center for the History of Otolaryngology–Head and Neck Surgery, Alexandria, VA.)

responsible for the broken electrodes and refused to perform a third implantation.[19] The falling out between the two men over this problem was the end of Eyriès involvement in the project. After this event, he and Djourno rarely conversed for the rest of their lives.

This was not quite the end of the story for Djourno, however. He went on to address several aspects of hearing applicable to electrical stimulation. For one, he examined the oscillographic representation of spoken words in an effort to give deaf patients a visual representation of speech that they could use for biofeedback when learning to speak.[20] After the first implant effort, a colleague approached Djourno to enter into a business venture to develop the implant. The colleague proposed that in exchange for an exclusive arrangement on the project, he would provide Djourno with the financial and engineering support of industry.[17] Djourno was always an academic idealist, and he did not believe in profiting from his discoveries. Furthermore he detested industry and would have no part in granting exclusivity. As a matter of principle, Djourno chose to do another implant with a different otolaryngologist, Roger Maspétiol.[17] This second patient, deafened from streptomycin ototoxicity, was implanted with an electrode near the promontory, rather than within the temporal bone. The patient showed little enthusiasm for her device, and she was lost to follow-up only a few months after it was implanted. Djourno subsequently lost funding for further implant work.[21] This signaled the end of Djourno's participation in developing an auditory prosthesis.

The legacy of the Djourno and Eyriès work was sustained despite the abrupt departure of the two men. Claude-Henri Chouard, who was a student in Eyriès' laboratory working on the facial nerve, resumed work on the cochlear implant several years later. Chouard[22] was instrumental in developing one of the first functional multichannel implants, and he credits Charles Eyriès as his major source of inspiration.

Although Djourno and Eyriès' implantation on February 25, 1957 is typically credited as the first cochlear implant, a closer evaluation of the patient's anatomy raises the question of whether the cochlear nerve or the auditory brainstem was stimulated by the implanted electrodes, as wallerian degeneration may have destroyed the cochlear ganglion cells.[23] Whether Djourno and Eyriès stimulated the cochlear nerve or the cochlear nucleus should not overshadow the significance of their work. Electrical methods to treat deafness had been described by numerous practitioners for almost 200 years prior to 1957, beginning with the classic work of Alessandro Volta in the late 18th century.[4] These previous efforts, however, were either aimed at treating deafness with therapeutic electrical stimulation, or they were examples of electrophonic hearing.

◆ Early Developments in America

Dissemination of the work of Djourno and Eyriès was slow to arrive in America. This is likely attributable to the fact that their publication appeared only in the French medical literature. Additionally, of the pair, the more likely to present his work among clinicians was Eyriès, as he was an otolaryngologist. Eyriès' demonstrated little enthusiasm for the project, however, and his interest was short lived. Djourno was a physiologist rather than a clinician, making interaction between him and American otolaryngologists less likely despite his continued interest. Word of their work reached William House in California serendipitously when his patient brought a summary of the Djourno and Eyriès work written in English to him sometime around 1959.[24] The piece was optimistic regarding electrical stimulation to replace hearing, and House was inspired.

Los Angeles

William House was a dentist-turned-otologist who began working with his brother Howard House at the Otologic Medical Group in Los Angeles upon completion of his residency in 1956. Early in his career he had already made significant contributions to otology and neurotology, including the facial recess approach. He was working at the time on the middle fossa approach to the internal auditory canal in collaboration with John Doyle, a neurosurgeon who also practiced at St. Vincent's Hospital in Los Angeles.[25] House and Doyle first sought to record the cochlear nerve response to sound when the nerve was exposed during the middle fossa approach for vestibular neurectomy as a treatment for Meniere's disease. Specifically, they sought to record the nerve output associated with tinnitus.[26] They relied on Doyle's brother, James Doyle, an electrical engineer, to address the technical challenge of recording such signals intraoperatively. The nerve output was recorded, but no tinnitus was observed. Successful recordings of sound-induced potentials from the cochlear nerve, however, inspired stimulating the nerve with similar waveforms to restore hearing.

House and Doyle first attempted electrical stimulation to elicit hearing during stapes surgery by placing a needle electrode on the promontory or into the open oval window. An ear speculum inserted into the external auditory canal served as a ground lead. With square wave stimuli, patients reported hearing the stimulus without discomfort, dizziness, or facial nerve stimulation. These responses were sufficient to encourage House and Doyle to implant a patient with a hard-wire device. The first willing subject was a 40-year-old man with severe otosclerosis and deafness. Promontory stimulation of the right ear on January 5, 1961, revealed consistent responses. On January 9, therefore, a gold wire electrode was inserted under local anesthesia through a postauricular approach into the round window. The wire was brought out through the postauricular skin.[27] The patient reported hearing the electrical stimuli, but he had poor loudness tolerance. Several weeks later the wire was removed.

A second patient was also implanted in January 1961. The woman had deafness, tinnitus, and vertigo associated with congenital syphilis, and she was brought to the operating room for a vestibular neurectomy through the middle fossa approach. During the procedure, a single gold wire electrode was placed through the middle fossa approach into scala tympani at the basal part of the cochlea. The wire was brought out through a skin incision. The patient described hearing the square wave stimulation upon waking from anesthesia. Over the ensuing days, the current intensity required to elicit a response increased. For fear of infection or edema, the wire was removed.

With the first patient's encouraging responses, and with the hope of producing discrimination of higher frequencies, House and Doyle decided to reimplant him with a five-wire-electrode array inserted through the mastoid facial recess and round window. The electrode array was attached to a more permanent electrode induction system seated in the skull. Over a several-week testing period, the patient's intensity requirement increased and his post-auricular skin began to swell. This device was also removed for risk of infection. Worries of biocompatibility of materials ensued.

The theoretical basis for the multiple electrode design was to spread high-frequency stimuli among spatially separated electrodes. By stimulating different subpopulations of auditory nerve fibers at rates slower than their refractory period, they thought, summation among the subpopulations would purportedly yield an overall high-frequency response along the whole nerve. This implant design and its theoretical basis became the foundation for an early cochlear implant patent application submitted by James Doyle and Earle Ballantyne in 1961. The patent was not granted until 1969.[28] Despite being founded on what has since been shown to be an erroneous theory of electrical stimulation, the patent was ironically prescient in its statement that a 16-channel unit would be necessary for implant patients to be able to converse on the telephone.

Word of the two implanted patients reached the lay press. The brief articles were overly optimistic in their descriptions of an "artificial ear," going so far as to announce that "surgical implantation of a transistorized device designed to restore hearing of deaf persons is scheduled within 30 days."[29] The effect of the lay press publications were calls from deaf patients to Drs. House and Doyle seeking a cure for their deafness, as well as investors seeking to cash in on emerging medical technology. Dr. House recognized the danger in such publicity, and broadcasting of the implant work became an area of considerable strife between the Doyles and House. Disagreement over how aggressive to proceed with the implant, given the initial bio-incompatibility problems, opened an irreparable rift between House and the Doyles that brought an end to their collaboration. House had a very busy otologic practice, and implant development took a low priority for several years to follow. The Doyles, on the other hand, continued to experiment, implanting numerous subjects. They collaborated with the Los Angeles otolaryngologist Frederick Turnbull, whose office was used for most of the testing. They reported their results in local[30] and national[31] forums, reporting optimistically that electrical stimulation could yield speech perception, but not offering systematic testing or analysis. The Doyles ceased their investigations in 1968 due to a lack of research funding.[26]

Stanford University

F. Blair Simmons had worked as a research associate in the laboratory of S. S. Stevens at Harvard as a medical student and then with Robert Galambos at the Walter Reed Institute prior to his residency in otolaryngology at Stanford University. Simmons was an assistant professor in Stanford's Division of Otolaryngology in 1962 for less than a month before he was presented with an unexpected opportunity to stimulate the cochlear nerve intraoperatively. The patient was an 18-year-old who had developed a recurrence of a cerebellar ependymoma that manifested itself as mild hearing loss. Exploratory craniotomy under local anesthesia was planned, and the cochlear nerve would be exposed during the procedure. Prior to surgery, Simmons discussed stimulating the patient's cochlear nerve electrically. The patient agreed to the intraoperative testing and to a preoperative auditory training session. During the awake craniotomy, the patient was asked to describe what he heard when a bipolar electrode was used to stimulate the exposed cochlear nerve with 100-μs square wave pulses. The patient described auditory sensations and was able to discriminate stimulation frequencies up to 1 kHz.[32]

Simmons's first implanted device was then placed 2 years later, in 1964. This second subject was a 60-year-old man who had been unilaterally deaf for several years, and whose better hearing ear became deaf. He also suffered from retinitis pigmentosum and had associated severe sight disability. Despite being made fully aware that implantation would likely fail and very likely yield no useful hearing, the subject agreed to undergo the implantation. Local anesthesia was used, and the promontory exposed through a postauricular transmeatal approach and elevation of a tympanomeatal flap. A 2-mm cochleostomy and then subsequent 0.1-mm drill hole into the modiolus were performed. A partial mastoidectomy was also performed, and the middle ear entered anterior to the facial nerve by removing the incus. A six-electrode array was placed through the mastoid opening into the epitympanum and then through both the cochleostomy and the modiolar opening to a depth of 3 to 4 mm. The electrodes were attached to a plug that was then secured to the mastoid cortex. Psychoacoustic testing was performed both at Stanford and at Bell Laboratories in New Jersey.[33] Unfortunately, the combination of disabilities made psychophysical testing very challenging. Simmons's conclusions from these experiences were pessimistic regarding the future of implantation. He estimated the likelihood that electrical stimulation of the auditory nerve could ever provide a clinically useful means of communication to be "considerably less than 5%."[34] Human implantation at Stanford was postponed until further animal testing could prove its utility.

House Resumes Work

With the advancements in pacemakers and ventriculoperitoneal shunts in the late 1960s, William House resumed an interest in cochlear implantation with more confidence in the safety and efficacy of indwelling devices (**Fig. 1–3**). House was working with a talented engineer named Jack Urban, a collaboration best known for several influential developments in neurotologic instruments. House and Urban aggressively pursued implanting their single-channel device in human patients. As much as any other parameter, the durability and safety of the device was on House's

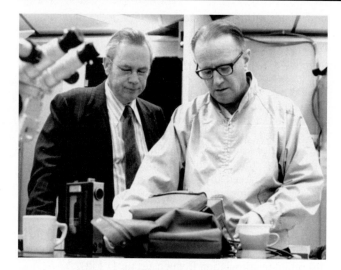

Figure 1–3 William House (left) and Robin Michelson (right) collaborating in the early 1970s. (Courtesy of John Q. Adams Center for the History of Otolaryngology–Head and Neck Surgery.)

mind with this group of patients. Of several patients implanted in 1969, one required having his implant removed due to tissue rejection, and another was lost to follow-up. A third patient, however, was Charles Graser, who became a long-term experimental subject. In Graser, House found that stimulation levels and results remained stable over the course of years. This gave credence to the safety of electrical stimulation.

Charles Graser was deaf for 10 years from ototoxicity. Postimplantation, he worked intensely as a research subject, and continued to do so enthusiastically for many years. Many of the observations and modifications that House and Urban reported in the 1960s were based on testing only of Graser. For instance, one of the surprising findings from work with Graser was that a 16,000-Hz carrier frequency signal helped him appreciate higher frequencies, and amplitude-modulating the carrier with the acoustic signal generally sounded the best. This signal processor strategy became standard on the House/3M (St. Paul, MN) cochlear implant. Reporting of these early results was primarily by testimonial experiences of the individual subjects rather than systematic study. Another important outcome of these early studies was abandoning the multiple electrode systems for the single-wire electrode.[35]

San Francisco

Robin Michelson (**Fig. 1–3**) was an otolaryngologist in private practice in the 1960s in Redwood City, California. He was the grandson of the Nobel Prize–winning physicist Albert Michelson. Robin Michelson's inspiration for cochlear implantation came from seeing a patient, T. I. Moseley, who had severe tinnitus and otosclerosis. Michelson had sought to monitor the cochlear microphonic during a stapedectomy as a means of immediate feedback, since he performed the procedure under local anesthesia. Moseley, an engineer, agreed to build him a high-gain amplifier with an earpiece

that Michelson could use in the operating room. Michelson placed an electrode against the round window. Feedback from the amplifier elicited the sensation of sound for the patient that he was subsequently able to pitch match.[36]

Michelson, like House, originally subscribed to the telephone theory of hearing: that the cochlea presented the auditory nerve with the analog electrical signal of the auditory stimulus, and that all that was required to restore hearing was to stimulate the auditory nerve with a similar signal. In an attempt to demonstrate that electrical stimulation of the auditory nerve elicited auditory responses, he implanted an electrode into the cat cochlea and measured the cochlear microphonic in the opposite ear. He found that electrical stimulation suppressed the contralateral cochlear microphonic similarly to acoustic stimuli. He concluded that electrical stimulation was therefore carried along auditory pathways.[37] Although Michelson was likely demonstrating electrophonic hearing rather than direct auditory nerve electrical stimulation, this result inspired him to implant a human volunteer with hearing loss.

Michelson's first implant was a single-channel device implanted into a congenitally deaf woman. Testing after implantation revealed that she obtained auditory sensations from stimulation, and that pitch perception was possible for stimulus frequencies less than ~600 Hz. More interesting to Michelson, however, was that the subject could differentiate a square wave from a sine wave stimulus.[36] Michelson interpreted this to indicate that the fine structure of the electrical stimulus could be conveyed along auditory pathways. The gold wire electrode hardened several days postoperatively, broke from the rest of the implant, and needed to be removed. Several additional patients received fully implantable single-channel devices, and this preliminary work was presented to the American Academy of Ophthalmology and Otolaryngology in October 1970, and then a follow-up study presented at the 1971 meeting of the American Otological Society. The patients had pitch perception based on stimulus frequency and could recognize speech stimuli but had no word understanding. All implanted patients lost whatever residual hearing they had prior to implantation.[38]

It was around this time that Francis Sooy visited Michelson in Redwood City and saw his work in progress with implantation. Sooy was the chairman of the nascent Department of Otolaryngology from the University of California at San Francisco (UCSF), and this interaction with Michelson confirmed his belief in the potential of cochlear implantation. He persuaded Michelson to join the faculty at UCSF and bring his implant investigations to the university. Sooy also believed that the successful development of the cochlear implant required a university-based scientific foundation. Aside from recruiting Michelson, Sooy then recruited Michael Merzenich from the University of Wisconsin. Merzenich was a young neurophysiologist whose interest was mapping the inferior colliculus. Merzenich joined the UCSF faculty and began working on recordings from the inferior colliculus for several months before meeting with Michelson about the cochlear implant. Merzenich was initially quite skeptical about the merits of the implants and showed little interest in joining efforts toward its development. After seeing a few patients on a documentary film created by the otolaryngology resident C. Robert Pettit, however, Merzenich became convinced of its potential.[39] The collaboration between Michelson, a clinical pioneer, and Merzenich, a talented basic scientist with a solid foundation in neurophysiology, was masterminded by Frank Sooy and was an indispensable element in the development of the UCSF cochlear implant program.

One of the first studies Merzenich performed was recording the response properties of single units in the cat inferior colliculus in response to both sound stimulation from one ear and electrical stimulation from the other ear of implanted cats. He showed that the inferior colliculus neurons responded similarly to electrical and sound stimuli, but that the tuning curves for electrical stimulation were very flat and showed little tuning. Additionally, the responses from animals with ototoxin-induced hair cell destruction showed the same responses to electrical stimuli as untreated cochlea. This was the first definitive demonstration that auditory sensation with implants arose from direct stimulation of the auditory nerve rather than electrophonic effects. Responses in the cat were then compared with psychoacoustic measures in the human implanted subjects using the same electrical stimuli in both groups. The conclusions from this work were that with single electrode devices, periodicity pitch up to ~600 Hz is possible, but no place coding of frequency is possible. Thus to convey complex sounds such as speech, multiple electrode arrays would be necessary.[40] This work was presented to the American Otological Society at the 1973 annual meeting in St. Louis, and it marks the beginning of the race toward development of a multichannel cochlear implant.

◆ Controversies and Doubts

The year 1973 represents a crossroads in the cochlear implant's development. Until this time, cochlear implantation would have been considered, at best, an idea with potential to help some deaf people sometime in the future, and at worst as a dangerous experimental procedure promising nothing better than vibrotactile information. Simmons had downplayed the potential of implants and abandoned human implantation. The only clinicians performing human implants, House and Michelson, were surgeons far from the mainstream and whose funding was from private sources. In order for the implant development to proceed, implants would need to be granted legitimacy as a valid research pursuit with National Institutes of Health (NIH) funding and demonstrate broad-based clinical application. The following section highlights events in the 1970s that accomplished both.

National Institutes of Health

The NIH itself was partly responsible for giving scientific legitimacy to the cochlear implant. In 1970 a Neural Prosthesis Program was established within the National Institute of Neurological Diseases aimed at promoting extramural research on neural prostheses primarily by capitalizing on the contract mechanism of the NIH.[41] Initially the program

did not focus on an auditory prothesis, but rather on developing a visual prosthesis for the blind, and the first contracts focused on this goal. In addition to awarding contracts, the Neural Prosthesis Program under the guidance of F. Terry Hambrecht initiated and maintained an annual Neural Prosthesis Workshop. The workshop brought together a multidisciplinary group of contractors and consultants to the NIH campus to discuss research findings, delineate important problems, and develop strategies for the development of neural prostheses. At the third workshop in January 1973, auditory prostheses first commanded a significant part of the agenda. Participants included Michelson, Merzenich, and Simmons. Both Merzenich and Simmons also obtained extramural NIH funding for their implant-related research by this time.[41]

Early Cochlear Implant Meetings

Several meetings over the next several years pitted the implant pioneers against the otology/hearing science establishment. These symposia began to bring cochlear implantation into the limelight, often resulting in considerable controversy. Between 1971 and 1973 significant work removed doubts that the auditory nerve could be stimulated directly with the implant. Concerns that the prominent oto-scientists expressed toward the implant therefore shifted and coalesced during meetings in 1973 and 1974 of the Otological Society, the First International Conference on Electrical Stimulation in San Francisco, and the Third Workshop of the Neural Prosthesis Program. These concerns and their rationale are as follows:

Concern: Remaining nerve fiber population in deafness is not sufficient to support tonotopic stimulation of the nerve. This was based on the finding of Hal Schuknecht and coworkers that only a minority of temporal bones examined demonstrated more than two thirds of the normal population of cochlear ganglion cells.[42] Additionally, Nelson Y. S. Kiang, a neurophysiologist at the Massachusetts Institute of Technology (MIT) who had defined how single auditory nerve units respond to sound in cat, led a vehement opposition to human cochlear implantation. His point of view was that cochlear implants with the current design could never produce speech understanding or "useful hearing" because electrical stimuli could not convey the complex auditory stimuli that the cochlea provided.[43] Implanting humans with devices that offered little more than improved lip reading, he thought, could not be considered "prudent."

Concern: Electrical stimulation could convey sounds out of the speech frequency range. Cochlear damage in deafness is typically in its basal half, where high-frequency stimuli are transduced. The electrodes described at the time extended only into the proximal basal part of the cochlea. Therefore, if the place principle were utilized, electrical stimulation would only yield sound frequencies higher than the speech range.[44]

Concern: The dynamic range of loudness with electrical stimulation would be too narrow to convey useful sound information. Although loudness grows with sound intensity in the cochlea over a range of nearly 100 dB, the intensity range with electrical stimulation is only ~6 dB, which would severely limit loudness discrimination. The dynamic range of the firing of cochlear nerve fibers of the cat in response to both electrical and acoustic stimulation revealed a similar finding—that the dynamic range in response to sound is 20 to 40 dB, and to electrical stimuli 4 dB.[43]

Concern: Intracochlear manipulation that would occur with cochlear implantation would result in significant damage to the cochlea; anything that disturbs scala media would cause degeneration of the remaining sensory fibers. This concern arose from studies of Schuknecht[45] showing that one aspect of cochlear pathology was auditory nerve fiber degeneration. Why, then, perform an invasive procedure like the cochlear implant when an externally worn device such as a vibrotactile stimulator could be used to the same end?

These concerns did not dissuade the core group of implant developers from proceeding onward, yet a strong aura of doubt surrounded the cochlear implant. At the forefront of cochlear implant support, however, was Francis Sooy. Sooy was responsible for assembling the implant devotees in October 1974 with the support of the NIH to evaluate the progress and define the research goals for the implant, and to establish guidelines for patient selection and implantation protocols. Two important decisions were made at this meeting. First, criteria for implantation were delimited: full informed consent that the procedure is experimental; no useful hearing in either ear; only those patients able and willing to participate in psychophysical testing; otherwise healthy patients; and finally, adults only. Second, a consensus decision was made to stop implanting all single-channel devices until an objective evaluation of the patients already implanted could be performed.[46] The NIH took the lead in this objective evaluation with a call for applications for a formal objective evaluation of the single-channel recipients. The future of implant development rested on this objective evaluation, as a finding that the implant had limited utility may have curtailed allocation of further resources from the Neural Prosthesis Program. The contract to perform the objective assessment was awarded in June 1975 to a team from the University of Pittsburgh led by Robert Bilger.

The Bilger Report

Thirteen adult single-channel implant subjects, 11 implanted by House and two by Michelson, were flown to Pittsburgh for a week-long testing session to take part in the study. The subjects underwent extensive audiological, psycho-acoustic, and vestibular testing. Several of the results were not surprising: Subjects could not understand speech with the implant alone, but the implant helped the patients' lipreading scores. Also not surprising was the finding that the subjects' quality of life was aided by the implant. A surprising finding, however, was that the subjects' speech *production* was significantly aided by their implants. The investigators concluded from the study that single-channel implants helped deaf patients. Although this conclusion may not seem profound, it was the first objective, scientific assessment of implant performance, concluding that the subjects received benefit from the implant with minimal risk.[47] From this, the cochlear prosthesis gained the

legitimacy needed to justify funded research efforts toward a multichannel device. Furthermore, while the world waited for the multichannel implant, the single-channel device was viable.

◆ Development of a Multichannel Device

With the Bilger study confirming the utility of a single-channel device, Dr. House moved forward with refinement of his implant. He and Jack Urban joined forces with the 3M Company. The House/3M single-channel device (**Fig. 1–4**) was implanted into several thousand patients by the early 1980s, and in 1984 the Food and Drug Administration (FDA) granted approval for the device. Other centers, however, concentrated their efforts on researching and developing a multichannel device. At the forefront of this competition were Merzenich, Michelson, Robert Schindler and colleagues at UCSF (**Fig. 1–5**), and Graham Clark at University of Melbourne in Australia.

Clark, a clinically trained otolaryngologist, began investigating the cochlear implant as a graduate student in the 1960s. He realized as early as his graduate thesis in 1969 that the single-channel device had limited utility,[48] and he sought to use a systematic scientific approach to developing a multielectrode device. The approach had several fronts: developing speech processing strategies, optimizing the electrode array, and developing a safe, reliable implantable receiver-stimulator. The efforts toward what would become the Cochlear Corporation's (Sydney, Australia) Nucleus multichannel implant was primarily an Australian venture,

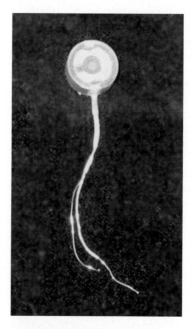

Figure 1–4 House/3M single-channel device, early version. Shown is the implanted receiver/stimulator and wire electrodes. (Courtesy of John Q. Adams Center for the History of Otolaryngology–Head and Neck Surgery, Alexandria, VA.)

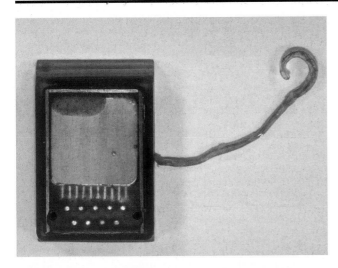

Figure 1–5   Early eight-channel electrode and epoxy-coated receiver designed by Robin Michelson and assembled by Mel Bartz. The intracochlear portion of the electrode array was formed from Silastic to fill scala tympani. (Courtesy of John Q. Adams Center for the History of Otolaryngology–Head and Neck Surgery, Alexandria, VA.)

stimuli must be different. Several studies in the late 1970s and early 1980s demonstrated that significant interference (known as "interaction") resulted from simultaneous stimulation of multiple electrodes.[54,55] It was found that electrode interaction could be minimized by stimulating the electrodes in a staggered, nonsimultaneous pattern.[54] Another discovery was that nonsimultaneous stimulation at pulse rates greater than 1 kHz was especially effective at improving an implant subject's speech understanding. A collaboration between UCSF and the Research Triangle Institute resulted in the implementation and testing of a speech processing scheme that utilized this concept. The concept was patented and became known as "continuous interleaved sampling" (CIS). The implementation of CIS provided a tremendous improvement in implant recipients' performance with speech recognition.[56]

Since that time there have been numerous noteworthy technological developments in both device design and coding. And the future promises even greater advances to further enhance performance in the implanted hearing impaired population.

as funding came from Australian national telethons, government-associated engineering firms, and partly through government grants.[49] Several of the important findings that Clark and his colleagues made were that inserting the electrode array in an anterograde direction through a single cochleostomy at the round window niche into scala tympani was less traumatic to the cochlear structures than either retrograde insertion or multiple cochleostomies[50,51] and dissolution of platinum electrodes with biphasic pulsatile stimuli was minimal, implying safe long-term stimulation.[52] Clark first implanted a human subject in 1978, and by 1981 he showed that subjects were able to understand some open-set speech with their implants and without the aid of lipreading.[53] The FDA approval for the Nucleus multichannel implant was granted for adult patients in 1985 and children as young as 2 years in 1990.

As several technical challenges were overcome in the 1980s, multichannel cochlear implants became a safe option for profoundly deaf adults and children. Patients with the implant were expected to have a quality of life improvement and some open-set speech recognition. Another development was required, however, to dramatically improve the speech recognition provided by the implant, and this was the development of high rate interleaved stimulation. Multiple electrode stimulation relies on the place principle of coding auditory stimuli along the cochlea. For separate electrodes to be effective in eliciting different frequency responses, the spatial extent of their

◆ Conclusion

The development of the cochlear implant began in 1957 with the first attempts to restore hearing with direct electrical stimulation of the auditory nerve. In the years that followed, the primary proponents of implants were a few otologists trying to help their patients with single-channel devices, despite considerable opposition from leaders in the field. If it were not for these pioneers, cochlear implants may well have been delayed by many years. Following the Bilger study, cochlear implant research gained mainstream support and efforts toward a marketable multichannel device were underway. Improvements are ongoing and offer a bright future to the hearing impaired population.

Acknowledgment

The author wishes to acknowledge the assistance of Tracy Sullivan at the John Q. Adams Center for the History of Otolaryngology–Head and Neck Surgery for her assistance with the figures. Gratitude is also extended to the following individuals for their interviews: Stephen Rebscher, Patricia Leake, Michael Merzenich, Robert Schindler, Harry Levitt, C. Robert Pettit, William House, F. Terry Hambrecht, Mark White, Merle Lawrence, and the late Robert Bilger.

References

1. Dudley H. Remaking speech. J Acoust Soc Am 1939;11:169–177

2. Wever EG, Bray CW. The nature of the acoustic response: the relation between sound frequency of impulses in the auditory nerve. J Exp Psychol 1930;13:373–387

3. Stevens SS. On hearing by electrical stimulation. J Acoust Soc Am 1937;8:191–195

4. Shah SB, Chung JH, Jackler RK. Lodestones, quackery, and science: electrical stimulation of the ear before cochlear implants. Am J Otol 1997;18:665–670

5. Djourno A, Strohl A. Modifications du courant de peau de grenouille pendant l'excitation électrique. CR Soc Biol (Paris) 1937; 125:625

6. Djourno A. Variation de l'excitabilite du sciatique de grenouille suivant l'écart des électrodes. CR Soc Biol (Paris) 1946;140:183

7. Djourno A. Sur la mésure instantanée de la fréquence du pouls. Paris Médical 1938;37:83

8. Djourno A, Masmonteil, Roucayrol JC. Une application de la haute fréquence a l'extraction de protheses métalliques. Soc Electrother Radiol 1948;29:637–638

9. Djourno A, Delay J, Verdeaux G. Un cas de narcolepsie avec étude électroencephalographique. Congres d'Electro-encephalographie de Langue francaise, Paris, 1949

10. Djourno A. La respiration électrophrenique. Presse Med 1952;60:1532–1533

11. Djourno A. Excitation électrique localisée à distance. C R Acad Sci 1953;236:2337–2338

12. Djourno A, Kayser D. La méthode des excitations induites a distance. J Radiol 1954;36:117–118

13. Djourno A, Kayser D, Guyon L. Sur la tolérance par le nerf d'appareils électriques d'excitation inclus à démeure. CR Soc Biol (Paris) 1955;149:1882–1883

14. Eyries C. Traitement de l'ozene par un nouveau précède de prothèse chirurgicale. Ann Otolaryngol 1946;13:581–586

15. Olivier G, Eyries C. Repères chirurgicaux et aspects du nerf facial extra petreux. Med Trop 1953;13:720–723

16. Eyries C. Expérience personelle. Cahiers d'Oto-Rhino-Laryngologie 1979;14:679–681

17. Djourno A. Interview with Phillip Seitz, January 12, 1994. Alexandria, VA: John Q. Adams Center Archives, 1994

18. Djourno A, Eyries C, Vallancien B. De l'excitation électrique du nerf cochleaire chez l'homme, par induction à distance, à l'aide d'un micro-bobinage inclus à demeure. CR Soc Biol (Paris) 1957;151:423–425

19. Eyries C. Interview with Phillip Seitz, January 10, 1994. Alexandria, VA: John Q. Adams Center Archives, 1994

20. Djourno A. Analyse oscillographique instantanée de la voix parlée. CR Soc Biol (Paris) 1959;153:197–198

21. Djourno A. A propos de prothèse sensorielle totale. Bull Acad Nat Méd 1977;161:282–283

22. Chouard CH. Entendre Sans Oreilles. Paris: Robert Laffont, 1973

23. Eisen MD. Djourno, Eyries, and the first implanted electrical neural stimulator to restore hearing. Otol Neurotol 2003;24:500–506

24. House WF. A personal perspective on cochlear implants. In: Schindler RA, Merzenich MM, eds. Cochlear Implants. New York: Raven Press, 1985:13–16

25. House WF. Cochlear Implants: My Perspective. Newport Beach, CA: AllHear, 1995

26. Doyle JB. Interview with Philip Seitz, August 22, 1993. Alexandria, VA: John Q. Adams Center Archives, 1993

27. House WF. Cochlear implants. Ann Otol Rhinol Laryngol 1976; 85(suppl 27):1–93

28. Doyle JB, Ballantyne EW, inventors. Artificial sense organ. U.S. patent 3,449,768. June 17, 1969

29. Anonymous. California electronics firm readies "artificial ear" implant. Space Age News 1961;3:1

30. Doyle JB, Doyle JH, Turnbull FM, Abbey J, House L. Electrical stimulation in eighth nerve deafness. Bull Los Angeles Neurol Soc 1963;28:148–150

31. Doyle JH, Doyle JB, Turnbull FM. Electrical stimulation of the eighth cranial nerve. Arch Otolaryngol 1964;80:388–391

32. Simmons FB, Mongeon CJ, Lewis WR. Electrical stimulation of acoustical nerve and inferior colliculus; results in man. Arch Otolaryngol 1964;79:559–567

33. Simmons FB, Epley JM, Lummis RC, et al. Auditory nerve: electrical stimulation in man. Science 1965;148:104–106

34. Simmons FB. Electrical stimulation of the auditory nerve in man. Arch Otolaryngol 1966;84:2–54

35. House WF, Urban J. Long term results of electrode implantation and electronic stimulation of the cochlea in man. Ann Otol Rhinol Laryngol 1973;82:504–517

36. Michelson RP. Interview with Phillip Seitz, November 7, 1995. Alexandria, VA: John Q. Adams Center Archives, 1995

37. Michelson RP. Interview with Philip Seitz, Nov. 7, 1995. San Francisco, California. Joh Q. Adams Center Archives, 1995

38. Michelson RP. Electrical stimulation of the human cochlea. Arch Otolaryngol 1971;93:317–323

39. Merzenich MM. Interview with Marc Eisen, March 26, 2004

40. Merzenich MM, Michelson RP, Pettit CR, Schindler RA, Reid M. Neural encoding of sound sensation evoked by electrical stimulation of the acoustic nerve. Ann Otol Rhinol Laryngol 1973;82:486–503

41. Hannaway C. Contributions of the National Institutes of Health to the Development of Cochlear Prostheses. Bethesda, MD: National Institutes of Health, 1996

42. Kerr A, Schuknecht HF. The spiral ganglion in profound deafness. Acta Otolaryngol 1968;65:586–598

43. Kiang NYS, Moxon EC. Physiological considerations in artificial stimulation of the inner ear. Ann Otol Rhinol Laryngol 1972;81:714–730

44. Lawrence M, Johnsson LG. The role of the organ of Corti in auditory nerve stimulation. Ann Otol Rhinol Laryngol 1973;82:464–472

45. Schuknecht HF. Lesions of organ of Corti. Trans Am Acad Ophthalmol Otolaryngol 1953;57:366–383

46. Merzenich MM, Sooy FA. Report on a workshop on cochlear implants. University of California at San Francisco, October 23–25, 1974

47. Bilger RC, Black FO. Auditory prostheses in perspective. Ann Otol Rhinol Laryngol Suppl. 1977; 86(3Pt. 2 Suppl. 38):3–10

48. Clark G. Middle ear and neural mechanisms in hearing and in the management of deafness. Doctor of Philosophy thesis. Sydney, Australia: University of Sydney, 1969

49. Clark G. Sounds from Silence. Adelaide: Allen & Unwin, 2000

50. Clark GM, Hallworth RJ, Zdanius K. A cochlear implant electrode. J Laryngol Otol 1975;89:787–792

51. Clark GM. An evaluation of per-scalar cochlear electrode implantation techniques: an histopathological study in cats. J Laryngol Otol 1977;91:I85–I99

52. Black FO, Wall C III, O'Leary DP, Bilger RC, Wolf RV. Galvanic disruption of vestibulospinal postural control by cochlear implant devices. J Otolaryngol 1978;7:519–527

53. Clark GM, Tong YC, Martin LF. A multiple-channel cochlear implant: an evaluation using open-set CID sentences. Laryngoscope 1981;91:628–634

54. Eddington DK, Dobelle WH, Brackmann DE, Mladejovsky MG, Parkin JL. Auditory prostheses research with multiple channel intracochlear stimulation in man. Ann Otol Rhinol Laryngol 1978;87:1–39

55. White M. Design Considerations of a Prosthesis for the Profoundly Deaf. Berkeley, CA: University of California, Berkeley, 1978

56. Wilson BS, Finley CC, Lawson DT, Wolford RD, Eddington DK, Rabinowitz WM. Better speech recognition with cochlear implants. Nature 1991;352:236–238

2

Genetic Predictors of Cochlear Implant Outcome

Andrew K. Patel and

Anil K. Lalwani

Congenital or acquired severe to profound loss sustained prior to the development of language is estimated to occur between 0.5 and 4.0 per 1000 births (Morton, 1991). The most common cause of childhood deafness is genetic, accounting for approximately one half to two thirds of all cases (Marazita et al, 1993). The remainder of cases of childhood deafness is due to nongenetic or environmental causes; however, it is likely that genetic factors contribute to many of these forms of congenital deafness.

Several hundred genes are thought to cause hereditary hearing loss and deafness (Gorlin et al, 1995). A large number of genetic hearing loss cases are single-gene mutations, and this proportion has continued to increases as public health improves, leading to a decrease in the incidence of hearing loss resulting from infection. Hereditary hearing loss is classified into syndromic and nonsyndromic forms. The syndromic forms, in which hearing loss is associated with a variety of other anomalies, account for 30% of genetic deafness; several hundred syndromes associated with hearing loss have been described (Gorlin et al, 1995). Among hereditary nonsyndromic deafness, autosomal recessive forms predominate (accounting for ~85% of cases), followed by autosomal dominant, X-linked, and mitochondrial forms (Petit, 1996; Van Camp, 2005). The last few years have seen major advances in the elucidation of the genetic causes of childhood-onset hearing impairment. Since 1992, nearly 120 loci for nonsyndromic deafness have been mapped to human chromosomes and 40 responsible genes have been identified—quite a remarkable feat given that only one deafness gene had been mapped in 1992 (Petit, 1996; Van Camp et al, 1997; Snoeckx et al, 2005).

◆ Modes of Inheritance in Nonsyndromic Deafness

Recessive Hearing Impairment

Recessive hearing impairment is typified by profound hearing loss at birth and accounts for nearly 85% of genetic hearing impairment. An autosomal recessive trait is characterized by having two unaffected parents who are heterozygous carriers for mutant forms of the gene in question but in whom the phenotypic expression of the mutant allele is masked by the normal allele (**Fig. 2–1**). These heterozygous parents (A/a) can each generate two types of gametes, one carrying the mutant copy of the gene (a) and the other having a normal copy of the gene (A). Of the four possible combinations of these two gamete types from each of the parents, only the offspring that inherits both mutant copies (a/a) will exhibit the trait. Of the three remaining possibilities, all will have a normal hearing phenotype but two of the three will be heterozygous carriers for the mutant form of the gene, similar to the carrier parents. Marriage among close relatives greatly increases the potential to produce a child affected by a recessive disorder.

Autosomal recessive deafness is extremely heterogeneous. Over 59 separate nonsyndromic recessive loci (noted as DFNBX, where X represents the order in which it was identified) have been reported, and already at least 21 of these genes have been identified. The most important of these is *GJB2* encoding for a gap junction protein connexin 26. Mutations in this gene, which facilitates transport of small solutes across cells, are responsible for half of childhood recessive deafness. Other recessive genes identified thus far

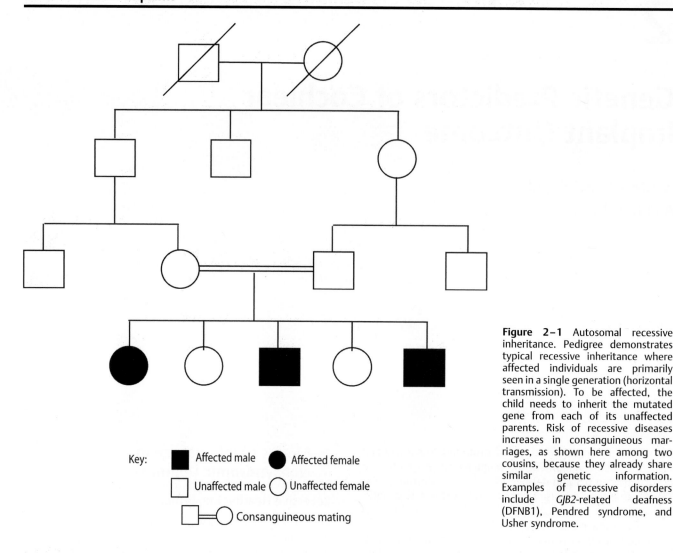

Key:

■ Affected male   ● Affected female

□ Unaffected male   ○ Unaffected female

□—=○ Consanguineous mating

Figure 2–1 Autosomal recessive inheritance. Pedigree demonstrates typical recessive inheritance where affected individuals are primarily seen in a single generation (horizontal transmission). To be affected, the child needs to inherit the mutated gene from each of its unaffected parents. Risk of recessive diseases increases in consanguineous marriages, as shown here among two cousins, because they already share similar genetic information. Examples of recessive disorders include *GJB2*-related deafness (DFNB1), Pendred syndrome, and Usher syndrome.

encode proteins involved in the structure or maintenance of the inner ear, particularly of hair cells, or in the maintenance ionic balances within the inner ear.

Autosomal Dominant Hearing Impairment

Autosomal dominant hearing impairment is characterized by delayed-onset, progressive hearing loss and accounts for 10 to 15% of genetic hearing impairment. For autosomal dominant disorders, the transmission of a rare allele of a gene by a single heterozygous parent is sufficient to generate an affected child (**Fig. 2–2A**). A heterozygous parent can produce two types of gametes. One gamete carries the mutant form of the gene of interest, and the other carries the normal form. Each of these gametes then has an equal chance of being utilized in the formation of a zygote. Thus the chance that an offspring of an autosomal dominant affected parent will be affected is 50%. Equal numbers of affected males and females are expected for an autosomal dominant trait and roughly half of the offspring of an affected individual will be affected.

Autosomal dominant traits often exhibit incomplete penetrance and variable expressivity. Variable expressivity refers to the differences in the observed effects of a given allele in related and unrelated individuals. Variable expression of different aspects of syndromes including hearing loss is common. The range of variation observed in dominant disorders is generally wider than in recessive disorders. Incomplete penetrance is an extreme form of variable expressivity and is characterized by the total absence of expression in persons known to carry the mutant allele (**Fig. 2–2B**). Variation in the age of onset for symptoms associated with a genetic disorder is common for traits that are not expressed at birth or prenatally. If the mutant phenotype is always expressed in individuals carrying the disease allele, then its penetrance is said to be complete, otherwise it is incomplete. Complete penetrance of the dominant allele results in the expression of the disease phenotype in all carriers of that allele without skipping generations.

Similar to autosomal recessive nonsyndromic hearing impairment, autosomal dominant nonsyndromic hearing impairment is genetically heterogeneous. To date, 54 chromosomal regions have been shown to contain a gene that is involved in an autosomal dominant type of nonsyndromic hearing impairment, the so-called DFNA loci. Twenty-one of the corresponding genes have been identified, including channel and gap junction proteins, unconventional

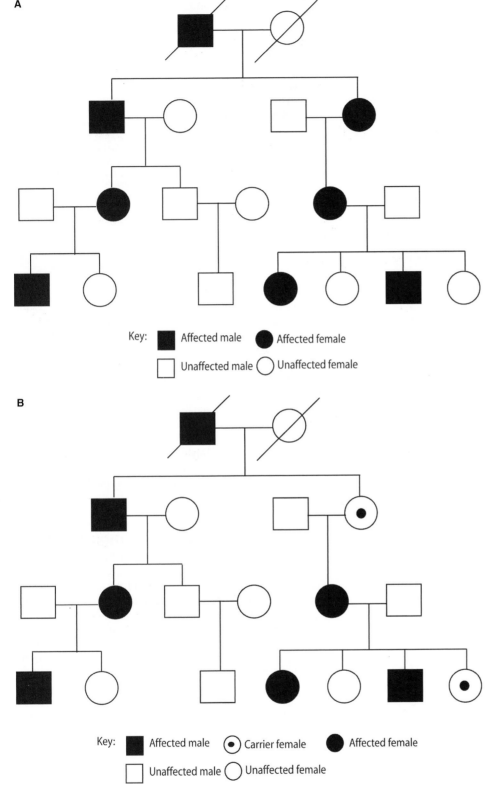

A

Key: ■ Affected male ● Affected female

□ Unaffected male ○ Unaffected female

B

Key: ■ Affected male ◉ Carrier female ● Affected female

□ Unaffected male ○ Unaffected female

Figure 2–2 Autosomal dominant inheritance. **(A)** Pedigree showing typical autosomal dominant inheritance pattern where affected individual are seen in multiple generations (vertical transmission). To be affected, an offspring needs to inherit only a single copy of the mutated gene from either parent. This pedigree demonstrates *complete penetrance* as every individual with the affected gene is affected. **(B)** In contrast, this pedigree demonstrates *incomplete penetrance* of a dominant trait: every individual who harbors the mutated gene does not have the associated disease. Examples of dominant diseases include Waardenburg syndrome, neurofibromatosis type 2, and Alport syndrome.

myosins, transcription factors, extracellular matrix proteins, and genes with an unknown function. These gene identifications are increasing knowledge of the molecular basis of hearing, and potentially may lead to new therapeutic measures for hearing impairment in the future.

X-linked Hearing Impairment

X-chromosomal inherited nonsyndromic hearing impairment accounts for about 2 to 3% of all hearing impairment and is therefore less common than autosomal hereditary

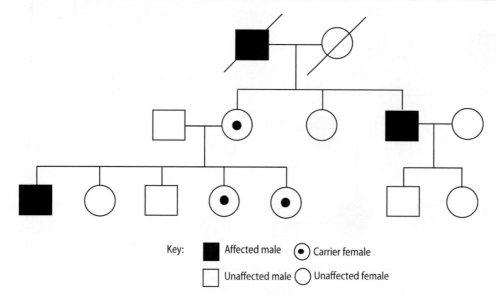

Figure 2–3 X-linked inheritance. Pedigree showing a typical X-linked inheritance with affected males and unaffected carrier females. Notice that fathers cannot pass along the X chromosome harboring the mutation to their sons as they contribute the Y chromosome; further, the daughters are only carriers as they inherit a normal X chromosome from their mother. In contrast, carrier mothers have affected and unaffected sons and carrier daughters. Examples of X-linked disorders include stapes gusher syndrome, Duchenne muscular dystrophy, and color blindness.

Key: ■ Affected male   ⊙ Carrier female
      □ Unaffected male ○ Unaffected female

hearing impairment (**Fig. 2–3**). The X-linked or DFN phenotype displays a high grade of clinical and genetic heterogeneity. In humans, females have 22 pairs of autosomes and a pair of X chromosomes (46, XX); males have 22 autosomes, one X chromosome, and one Y chromosome (46, XY). Accordingly, males always receive their Y chromosome from their father and their X chromosome from their mother, whereas females receive one of their X chromosomes from each of their two parents. Men are affected more often and, because of hemizygosity, affected males usually show a more severe, distinctive hearing impairment phenotype. Diseases that are rarely expressed clinically in heterozygous females are called X-linked recessive; if they commonly present in females, it is designated X-linked dominant. Currently, five nonsyndromic loci and one syndromic locus have been identified and two genes have been cloned. Stapes gusher syndrome is an X-linked disorder for which the responsible gene, *POU3F4*, has been identified. Patients often show a prelingual onset of hearing impairment.

Mitochondrial Mutations and Hearing Impairment

Not all genes are equally inherited from both parents. The extranuclear genome is inherited solely through the mother. Male mitochondria are not contributed to newly formed zygotes. This inheritance pattern gives rise to pedigrees in which all the children of an affected mother may be affected and none of the children of an affected father will be affected (**Fig. 2–4**). In practice, the expression of mitochondrially inherited disorders is often variable and may be incompletely penetrant.

The last decade has seen the identification of several mitochondrial DNA mutations associated with hearing loss. Because the only known function of the human mitochondrial chromosome is to participate in the production of chemical energy through oxidative phosphorylation, it was not unexpected that mitochondrial mutations

interfering with energy production could cause systemic neuromuscular disorders, which have as one of their features hearing impairment. Surprisingly, however, inherited mitochondrial mutations have also been found to be a cause of nonsyndromic hearing loss and to predispose to aminoglycoside-induced hearing loss, whereas acquired mitochondrial mutations have been proposed as one of the causes of presbycusis. Clinical expression of these mitochondrial mutations is dependent on environmental exposures and nuclear-encoded modifier genes. Emphasis on preventive or therapeutic strategies requires identification and avoidance of the environmental exposures, and the identification of the nuclear-encoded modifier genes.

◆ The Impact of Cochlear Implantation on Hereditary Hearing Impairment

Cochlear implantation has been used to restore the sense of audition to deaf children since the mid-1980s, when the first single-channel devices followed by multichannel devices were permanently implanted. Since that time, significant advances have been made in both device design and implantation techniques. These have allowed the technology to be more broadly and successfully applied. Candidacy guidelines based in part on consistent, reliable documentation of postoperative performance have evolved greatly since the mid-1980s. Patient selection has emerged as one of the most important determinants of successful outcome after pediatric cochlear implantation (Daya et al, 1999).

To determine suitability for cochlear implantation, fulfillment of several criteria is necessary. These include confirmation that there is a profound sensorineural hearing loss (SNHL), an absence of medical contraindications to implantation, and the presence of an implantable cochlea. Further evaluation of speech and language development, educational setting, home environment, developmental milestones, and other handicaps facilitates determining the degree and type of rehabilitation appropriate for the

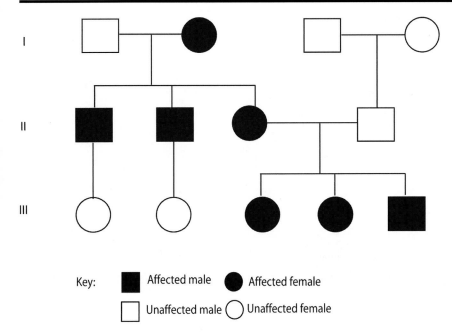

Key: ■ Affected male   ● Affected female
      □ Unaffected male ○ Unaffected female

Figure 2–4 Mitochondrial inheritance. Pedigree showing mitochondrial inheritance in a three-generation (I, II, III) family. As the mitochondrial DNA is only present in the egg and not the sperm, the mitochondrial disease can only be passed on by an affected mother. An example of mitochondrial disease includes hearing loss due to exaggerated sensitivity to aminoglycosides associated with A1555G mutation in 12S ribosomal RNA.

implant candidate. Finally, assessment of factors such as age at onset of deafness, duration of deafness, and speech perception performance may provide some indication of expected outcome. Assessment therefore requires a multidisciplinary approach. Many centers have developed a structured approach to evaluate potential candidates to select those who would benefit the most from implantation.

Cochlear implantation (CI) is an effective but controversial intervention that poses multiple challenges to both purchasers and providers of health care. Although offering a potentially life-transforming benefit for patients, the relative expense for the procedure and the subsequent rehabilitation may be high. Cochlear implant manufacturers seek to expand the market by promoting relaxations of cochlear implant candidate criteria. Although more than 90% of congenitally deaf children are born to hearing parents who wish to communicate with their children by speaking rather than signing, the question arises whether CI is sufficiently effective and cost-effective to justify elective surgery on a young child (Lane & Bahan, 1998); recent long-term follow-up in children implanted under the age 2 strongly suggests that CI is effective in rehabilitation of the deaf. Finally, CI is a low-volume intervention at most hospital centers, with variable outcomes whose overall effectiveness is difficult to judge from outcomes obtained in any individual hospital.

several prospective and retrospective case series, comparative case series, and matched-pair case series. The reported benefit in children has varied widely across individual users. Therefore, although one can inform the patient or the patient's parents that most do well with implants, it is not possible to predict the outcome for any given patient.

With the advances in our understanding of genetics of deafness, recent work has focused on the ability of genetic testing to predict CI outcome. Currently, genetic testing is available for many different types of syndromic and nonsyndromic deafness, though most are only available on a research basis. However, DNA-based testing can be performed to diagnose Pendred syndrome (*SLC26A4* gene), Usher syndrome type IIA (*USH2A* gene), branchio-oto-renal (BOR) syndrome (*EYA1* gene), Mohr-Tranebjaerg syndrome (deafness-dystonia-optic atrophy syndrome; *TIMM8A* gene), one mutation in *USH3A*, DFNB1 (*GJB2* gene), DFN3 (*POU3F4* gene), DFNB4 (*SLC26A4* gene), and DFNA6/14 (*WFS1* gene) (Van Camp, 2005). Diagnostic testing for mutations in the *GJB2* gene causing deafness (which encodes the connexin 26 protein) and in the *GJB6* gene (which encodes the connexin 30 protein) also plays a prominent role in diagnosis and genetic counseling due to the high proportion of nonsyndromic hearing loss caused by these mutations.

◆ Prediction of Successful Outcomes with Cochlear Implantation

It is strongly desirable to identify factors that predict cochlear implantation outcome. At this time, no single test can predict which patients will achieve success with CI. Evidence supporting the efficacy of cochlear implants in sensorineural deafness exists primarily in the form of data from

◆ Evaluation of Specific Causes of Hereditary Hearing Impairment and Cochlear Implant Outcome

GJB2-Related Deafness and Cochlear Implant Outcome

After a newborn screening test indicates hearing loss, the neonate is referred for evaluation by a multidisciplinary team experienced in the evaluation of neonatal deafness. Hearing loss is categorized by the portion of the hearing

Table 2–1 *GJB2*-Related Deafness and Cochlear Implant Outcome (Alphabetical by Author)

Disorder	No. of Patients	Study Type	Variable	Statistically Significant Findings	References
GJB2	22	Case control	Reading comprehension, nonverbal cognitive measure after CI	65% of *GJB2* versus 45% of non-*GJB2* read at age level	(Bauer et al, 2003)
GJB2	20	Retrospective case review	Speech performance (closed- or open-set recognition) after CI	No impact on speech performance at 12, 24, or 36 months	(Cullen et al, 2004)
GJB2	15	Case control	Language and speech perception	No significant difference	(Dahl et al, 2003)
GJB2	3	Cohort study	Speech performance after CI	Mean vocabulary and developmental quotient higher in *GJB2* patients	(Fukushima et al, 2002)
GJB2	13	Prospective cohort	Rehabilitative outcome	No difference in outcome from rest of CI population	(Lustig et al, 2004)
GJB2– 233delC	4	Retrospective analysis	Primary speech perception measured by Meaningful Auditory Integration Scale (MAIS)	MAIS score of speech perception higher in *GJB2* group	(Matsushiro et al, 2002)
GJB2	11	Observational cohort	Iowa Matrix and GASP sentence scores	GASP scores were higher (equal/better speech discrimination)	(Sinnathuray et al, 2004b)
GJB2	14	Observational retrospective cohort	Speech intelligibility rating and mainstream school setting	Speech intelligibility rating scores were higher, larger proportion in mainstream school	(Sinnathuray et al, 2004a)

CI, cochlear implantation; GASP, Glendonald Auditory Screening Procedure.

system affected (conductive, sensorineural, or mixed); whether it is primarily due to a genetic cause or environmental one (hereditary or acquired), and if genetic, whether or not it is a component of a genetic syndrome (syndromic or nonsyndromic). If genetic, 50% are due to DFNB1 mutations. DFNB1 related hearing loss has approximate prevalence in the general population of 14/100,000 (~1/7,000), with an estimated carrier frequency of 1 in 31 in the general population.

DFNB1-related hearing loss is characterized by congenital (present at birth), nonprogressive sensorineural hearing impairment. Usually, the hearing impairment is severe or severe-to-profound; however, it can range from mild to severe in different families and within a family. Except for the hearing impairment, affected individuals are healthy and enjoy a normal life span. Vestibular function is normal; affected infants and young children do not experience balance problems and learn to sit and walk at age-appropriate times.

DFNB1-related hearing loss is suspected in patients who have congenital, nonprogressive sensorineural hearing impairment that is mild-to-profound by auditory brainstem response (ABR) testing or pure tone audiometry, and no related systemic findings identified by medical history or physical examination. They may also have a family history consistent with autosomal recessive inheritance of hearing loss (for example, an affected sibling). However, the majority of people with autosomal recessive diseases represent the first known case in their family. The diagnosis of DFNB1-related hearing loss is confirmed if the patient has recognized disease-causing mutations in the gene *GJB2* (chromosome 13q11–12) that alters the connexin 26 (Cx26) protein. DNA-based testing of the *GJB2* gene detects ~95% of disease-causing mutations. The most common

mutation, 35delG, is found in over two thirds of persons with DFNB1.

About 30% of patients with DFNB1 have other identifiable disease-causing mutations in *GJB2*; more than two dozen other disease-causing mutations have been identified. Available methods of screening for Cx26 mutations have failed to identify disease-causing mutations in some families in whom the diagnosis of DFNB1 has been established by linkage studies; thus, failure to detect a Cx26 mutation does not exclude the diagnosis of DFNB1.

The GJB2 test has prognostic value. Children with profound deafness due to Cx26 mutations have an excellent outcome with cochlear implants (**Table 2–1**). The isolated insult to the cochlea created by *GJB2* allele variants allows for preservation of central cognitive function. Better reading performance is seen in children with GJB2-related deafness compared with children with other nonsyndromic deafness (Bauer et al, 2003). Given that children with *GJB2*-related deafness do not have other handicaps, improved outcome in this group may reflect the exclusion of children with multiple handicaps in whom the outcome is more heterogeneous. Regardless, excellent outcome in children with *GJB2*-related deafness is an important piece of information for parents to know as they make decisions regarding rehabilitative intervention in their child.

Syndromic Autosomal Recessive–Related Deafness and Cochlear Implant Outcome

The experience with cochlear implantation in a variety of recessive hearing disorders is summarized in **Table 2–2** and is discussed here. Usher syndrome is an autosomal recessive disorder manifested by hearing impairment, retinitis pigmentosa (RP), and variable vestibular deficit,

Table 2–2 Autosomal Recessive Syndromes (in Decreasing Frequency)

Syndrome	Frequency	Hearing Loss	Associated Findings	Gene(s) Involved/ Genetic Testing	Cochlear Implants Attempted?
Usher	Most common autosomal recessive syndrome (3.5/ 100,000 births, 10% of congenital deafness)	Sensorineural; degeneration of cochlear sensory epithelium	Retinitis pigmentosa	Research only	Yes (Loundon et al, 2003)
Pendred	Second most common (up to 10% of recessive hereditary hearing loss)	Bilateral, more prominent in higher frequencies; abnormal bony labyrinth	Euthyroid goiter at puberty; vestibular symptoms	*PDS* gene *SLC26A4* (chrom locus 7q22-q31)/clinical	Yes (Vescan et al, 2002)
Jervell and Lange-Nielsen	Third most common (1% of recessive hereditary hearing loss, 1:100000)	Congenital bilateral severe hearing loss with organ of Corti/spiral ganglion atrophy and PAS+ deposits in the membranous labyrinth	Syncopal episodes and sudden death (prolonged QTc)	High-risk families	Yes (Chorbachi et al, 2002; Green et al, 2000)
Refsum disease	Rare	Sensorineural with degeneration of organ of Corti and stria vascularis	Retinitis pigmentosa; faulty phytanic acid metabolism, polyneuropathy	Clinical	None reported

PAS, periodic acid–Schiff.

and affects 50% of the deaf-blind patients in the United States. Recent progress in the characterization of the genetics of Usher syndrome has shown that this disorder is phenotypically and genetically complex (Kimberling & Moller, 1995). Furthermore, successful cochlear implantation for patients with Usher syndrome has been reported (Han et al, 2004; Loundon et al, 2003).

Pendred syndrome is the second most common type of autosomal recessive deafness. *PDS* mutation screening (research testing) is available. This test is performed by SSCP, or single-stranded conformational polymorphism, is a technique for detecting point mutations in genes by amplifying a region of genomic DNA (using asymmetric PCR) and running the resulting product on a high quality gel. Single base substitutions can alter the secondary structure of the fragment in the gel, producing a visible shift in its mobility of the 21 exons, with sequencing as indicated. Four mutations account for greater than 60% of all *PDS* mutations. To date, sensitivity and specificity rates are not known. *PDS* mutation screening is appropriate in persons with inner ear defects, especially Mondini malformations or dilated vestibular aqueducts. All patients who have *PDS* screening also have *GJB2* screening. Vescan et al (2000) have reported cochlear implantation in two patients with Pendred syndrome and enlarged vestibular aqueduct syndrome. Implantation in patients with Pendred syndrome or isolated large vestibular aqueduct syndrome is uniformly associated with excellent outcome.

Jervell and Lange-Nielsen (1957) originally reported four siblings with profound congenital SNHL, syncopal attacks, sudden death, and a prolonged corrected QT interval (QTc) shown on electrocardiography. The deafness is usually profound; vestibular dysfunction has not been documented (Cusimano et al, 1991). Cardiogenic syncope is common and sudden death occurs in 70% of untreated cases due to

ventricular arrhythmias (torsades de pointes), which are usually precipitated by a sudden increase in autonomic activity (Cusimano et al, 1991). Secondary focal seizures may also occur. The syndrome is autosomal recessive (Sanchez Cascos et al, 1990). The underlying pathophysiology is due to an abnormality in the function of the potassium channel complex (Gordon, 1994). Cardiac investigation should part of the diagnostic workup of all patients with congenital or early-onset hearing loss. Furthermore, two separate case reports describe successful cochlear implantation in patients with Jervell and Lange-Nielsen syndrome (Chorbachi et al, 2002; Green et al, 2000).

Autosomal Dominant–Related Deafness and Cochlear Implantation Outcomes

The experience with cochlear implantation in a variety of dominant hearing disorders is summarized in **Table 2–3** and is discussed here. Auditory-pigmentary syndromes are caused by physical absence of melanocytes from the skin, hair (white forelock), eyes (heterochromia iridis), or the stria vascularis of the cochlea (Reed et al, 1967). Dominantly inherited examples with patchy depigmentation are the most common example of autosomal dominant syndromic hearing loss and are usually labeled Waardenburg syndrome (WS), of which there are four types based on the presence of other abnormalities (Read & Newton, 1997; Waardenburg, 1951). All these forms show marked variability even within families, and at present it is not possible to predict the severity, even when a mutation is detected (Lalwani et al, 1996). Deafness has been more commonly reported in WSII than WSI (Read & Newton, 1997). Testing is currently available for WSI and WSIII from the *PAX3* gene; some cases of WSII (20%) are caused by mutations

Table 2–3   Autosomal Dominant Inheritance (in Decreasing Frequency)

Syndrome	Frequency	Hearing Loss	Associated Findings	Gene(s) Involved	Cochlear Implants Attempted?
Waardenburg	Most common autosomal dominant inheritance (1 per 42,000: 1–2% of congenital deafness)	Sensorineural	Pigmentary abnormalities; ±limb abnormalities; Hirschsprung's (defective neural crest migration and development)	PAX3, MITF, EDNRB, EDN3, SOX10	Yes (Sugii et al, 2000)
Branchio-oto-renal	Second most common (1 per 45,000; 1–2% of congenital deafness)	Conductive, sensorineural, or mixed	Branchial cleft cysts or fistulae, malformations of the external ear including preauricular pits, and renal anomalies	EYA1 gene in 30%	Yes (MacArdle et al, 2002)
Neurofibromatosis type 1 (NF1)	More common (1 in 3000)	Bilateral, profound, sensorineural	Multiple endocrine neoplasia (MEN) 2B; adult development of cutaneous and subcutaneous neurofibromas, café-au-lait spots, elephantoid overgrowth of skin and other cutaneous lesions, such as hemangiomas, giant hairy nevi, and depigmented macules	NF1	Yes (Poissant et al, 2003)
Stickler	Many undiagnosed (1 in 10,000)	Sensorineural	Cleft palate, and spondyloepiphyseal dysplasia resulting in osteoarthritis (truncated type II collagen protein)	STL1, STL2, and STL3.	None reported
Osteogenesis imperfecta	Rare (1 in 20,000)	Initially conductive, but may develop sensorineural or mixed	Bowing of long bones, fractures, limb shortening, and decreased skull echogenicity; easy bruising; repeated fracture after mild trauma that heals readily; deafness (50% by age 40 in type I)	Hearing loss most often associated with mutation in type I collagen A1 gene	Yes (Huang et al, 1998; Mens & Mulder, 2002; Migirov et al, 2003; Szilvassy et al, 1998)
Neurofibromatosis type 2 (NF2)	Rare (1 in 30,000)	Secondary to bilateral vestibular schwannomas	Invariably, bilateral acoustic neuromas; flat dysplastic tumors or subcutaneous spherical nodules of the peripheral nerves on the limbs, and trunk at risk for a variety of other tumors including meningiomas, astrocytomas, ependymomas, and meningio-angiomatosis	NF2	Yes (Belal, 2001; Hoffman et al, 1992; Hulka et al, 1995; Shin et al, 1998)

STL, Stickler syndrome.

in the *MITF* gene; and WSIV has been associated with mutations in endothelin-3 (*EDN3*) or the endothelin-B receptor (*EDNRB*) genes, and *SOX10* (Lalwani et al, 1995; Tassabehji et al, 1993, 1994, 1995). A congenital SNHL is associated in an estimated 25% of cases of WSI. Cochlear implantation has been performed in patients with Waardenburg syndrome, with good outcome to date (Sugii et al, 2000).

Branchio-oto-renal (BOR) syndrome was first described by Melnick et al (1975). In *Drosophila*, the *eyes-absent* phenotype is characterized by a reduction or absence of the adult compound eye, and loss of *eya* function in the eye primordium causes an increase in programmed cell death, suggesting the gene product plays a role in cell death or apoptosis. *EYA1* mutations have been found in about 15 to 20% of patients with BOR syndrome. If persons have the BOR syndrome phenotype, *EYA1* mutation screening is available. The 16 exons are screened by SSCP, with direct sequencing as indicated. A common mutation has not been reported, and sensitivity and specificity rates are not known. Absence of a mutation in *EYA1* in a person with the BOR syndrome phenotype does not exclude the diagnosis of BOR syndrome (current available screening methods, including direct nucleotide sequencing, fail to identify mutations in more than 70% of families with a clinical BOR syndrome). Characteristic BOR temporal bone findings include cochlear hypoplasia (four-fifths of normal size with only two turns), dilation of the vestibular aqueduct, bulbous internal auditory canals, deep posterior fossae, and acutely angled promontories, with 70 to 93% of individuals demonstrating hearing loss (Chen et al, 1995). Ostri et al (1991) reported that computed tomography studies of the temporal bone in patients with BOR demonstrated inner ear malformations of hypoplastic cochleae with reduced vertical diameters, and absent or hypoplastic semicircular canals and normal endolymphatic ducts. The single report of cochlear implantation in a patient with branchio-oto-facial syndrome notes that although benefits in detection, recognition, and identification of environmental sounds and gains in receptive spoken language skills were achieved, intelligible speech did not result, and that rehabilitation was prolonged to twice the duration required for children without special needs (MacArdle et al, 2002).

Neurofibromatosis type 1 (NF1) was first described by Frederick von Recklinghausen, who proposed that the characteristic dermal tumors observed in NF1 arose from the fibrous tissue surrounding peripheral nerves, leading to the term *neurofibroma*. In addition to neurofibromas, individuals affected with NF1 may exhibit a multitude of other clinical manifestations that affect different organ systems, with neurologic, dermatologic, ophthalmologic, and orthopedic impairments being most common. Loss of neurofibromin in cells lacking NF1 generates high levels of the guanosine triphosphatase (GTPase) activating protein RAS, resulting in dysregulated cell growth and tumor formation (Sherman et al, 2000). Most patients with neurofibromatosis (NF) and hearing loss suffer from NF2, and hearing loss in NF1 is often conductive in nature (related to the presence of neurofibromas in the external auditory canal or middle ear), though SNHL has also been reported (Lustig & Jackler, 1996; McKennan, 1991; Pensak et al, 1989; Shamboul & Grundfast, 1999). The pathophysiology of SNHL in NF1, however, has yet to be defined. However, based on a successful cochlear implantation and rehabilitation, Poissant et al (2003) concluded that standard cochlear implantation should be considered a viable option and the first line of therapy for the treatment of bilateral, severe to profound SNHL in patients with NF1 and normal VIIIth nerve radiographic findings (Poissant et al, 2003). However, the authors note that disparities in potential NF1 lesions resulting in severe to profound SNHL are significant, because the presence of a retrocochlear lesion would suggest that CI would potentially be a less than ideal treatment option.

Osteogenesis imperfecta (OI) designates a heterogeneous group of heritable disorders of connective tissue that in addition to bone may affect tendons, ligaments, fascia, skin, sclerae, blood vessels, teeth, and hearing, with four major subtypes. In 201 patients examined in one study, 39% had a conductive or mixed hearing loss, whereas SNHL or anacusis was seen in 11%, and 50% of patients affected with either form by age 50 (Paterson et al, 2001; Pedersen, 1984). In most cases the onset of hearing impairment was noted in the second or third decade and progressing with increasing age, especially after the age of 60. Tympanometry and acoustic reflex measurements suggest that the cause of conductive or mixed hearing loss is stapedial fixation or occasionally ossicular discontinuity due to aplasia or fracture of the stapedial crura. Reports of CI in two adults with OI, as well as in a child with OI and otospongiosis, noted that it was successful (though the electrode array of a third patient with OI was improperly placed in the internal auditory meatus); however, CI in these patients was noted to be extremely rare (Huang et al, 1998; Mens & Mulder, 2002; Migirov et al, 2003; Szilvassy et al, 1998).

Neurofibromatosis type 2 (NF2) is characterized by bilateral acoustic neuromas. Additionally, other tumors of the central and peripheral nervous systems such as schwannomas, meningiomas, ependymomas, as well as ocular abnormalities, can be found (Evans et al, 1992). NF2 is caused by mutations in a gene coding for the tumor suppressor merlin or schwannomin, and tumor formation follows the two-hit model (Trofatter et al, 1993). Cochlear implantation in patients with NF2 has been reported at the time of or after acoustic tumor removal (Belal, 2001; Hoffman et al, 1992; Hulka et al, 1995). These descriptions noted the requirement of both cochlear nerve survival (confirmed by a positive preoperative promontory test) and cochlear patency [confirmed by preoperative high-resolution computed tomography (CT) or magnetic resonance imaging (MRI)] (Shin et al, 1998). In addition, it was noted that CI was best performed at the time of acoustic tumor removal in translabyrinthine surgery, or 1 to 3 months after middle fossa surgery, before cochlear ossification completes (Belal, 2001). Belal (2001) noted that brainstem implantation must be chosen for cases of cochlear neuroma (due to mandatory cochlear nerve sacrifice) or for extension of the acoustic neuroma to the cochlea.

Mitochondrial Mutation–Related Deafness and Cochlear Implant Outcome

The first molecular defect for nonsyndromic hearing loss was identified in 1993, and was a mitochondrial mutation (Jaber et al, 1992; Prezant et al, 1992). Since then, several inherited mitochondrial DNA (mtDNA) mutations have been implicated in hearing loss, and acquired mtDNA mutations have been proposed as one of the causes of the hearing loss associated with aging—presbyacusis (Hutchin & Cortopassi, 2000). Such mtDNA mutations may not be readily detected in all tissues equally, as reported by Mancuso et al (2004) in describing a patient with nonsyndromic hearing loss caused by very low levels of the mtDNA A3243G mutation, which was detectable by restriction fragment length polymorphism analysis in muscle and urine but not in serum. Furthermore, the prevalence of mitochondrial mutations in groups of patients with aminoglycoside-induced hearing loss and subsequent cochlear implantation may be as high as 10% (Usami et al, 2000). The major clinical relevance of mitochondrial mutations to hearing loss remains the prevention of aminoglycoside-induced hearing loss (Fischel-Ghodsian, 1998). These mutations derive their clinical importance from their status both among the few currently preventable forms of genetic hearing loss, and in countries where aminoglycoside antibiotics are used commonly, as a major cause of hearing loss (Fischel-Ghodsian, 1999, 2003; Hu et al, 1991).

Successful CI in a patient with a previously undescribed mitochondrial DNA defect was reported in a patient who no longer received benefit from conventional hearing aids (Counter et al, 2001) (**Table 2–4**). In addition, Cullington (1999) also reported successful CI in a patient with mitochondrial cytopathy causing progressive deafness, and stated that is likely that other patients with this unusual disorder will present for cochlear implant assessment. Furthermore, Tono et al (1998) note that the excellent clinical outcome after CI in a patient with an A1555G mitochondrial mutation suggests that hearing loss associated with this mutation is primarily caused by insult to the cochlear tissue containing rich mitochondria such as hair cells, stria vascularis, or both, while sparing the cochlear nerve and its central connections. Cochlear implantation, therefore, can be offered to patients with profound mitochondrial SNHL.

Mitochondrial Encephalopathy, Lactic Acidosis, and Stroke-Like Episodes (MELAS)-Related Deafness and Cochlear Implant Outcome

The MELAS syndrome, first described in 1984, is one of a group of mitochondrial cytopathies that is associated with point genetic mutations (Pavlakis et al, 1984). Characteristic brain abnormalities include basal ganglia calcifications in addition to focal lesions of cerebellar and cerebral atrophy, resulting from cellular rather than vascular dysfunction (Sue et al, 1998). Although it does not feature in the acronym, hearing loss is a common finding in MELAS. Large kindreds and patient series have been reported, demonstrating that over 50% of patients have moderate or severe SNHL: 21 of 28 Australian patients with MELAS in a series were deaf, as were eight of 14 British patients in a series (Morgan-Hughes et al, 1995; Sue et al, 1998). Three constraints control the phenotypic expression of the mutation: the percentage of mutant mitochondrial DNA in the target tissue (though this percentage carries at most a loose correlation with clinical lesions), the degree of exposure to oxidative stress of different organs or cell populations, and unidentified collaborating somatic mutations that selectively enhance aspects of the syndrome.

The cochlea is an organ extremely vulnerable to oxidative stress. The outer hair cells have a tenuous, indirect metabolic support from Deiter cells, and the stria vascularis is both metabolically very active and nonmitotic, hence further subject to mutation accumulation. Recently detailed audiological findings have been reported in 18 patients with MELAS, and the authors argued that the hearing loss in their patients was entirely due to cochlear lesions (Sue et al, 1998). Excellent speech discrimination scores

Table 2–4   Mitochondrial Mutation-Related Deafness and Cochlear Implant Outcome

Disorder	No. of Patients	Study Type	Variable	Outcome	References
Mitochondrial mutations causing hearing loss	12	Literature review	CI outcomes	The data were not amenable to formal meta-analysis or valid data summarization, other than descriptive statistics; however, the authors present an overview of those patients successfully rehabilitated by cochlear implantation	(Sinnathuray et al, 2003)
Mitochondrial DNA defect	1	Case study	Auditory rehabilitation	Successful, with marked sentence recognition improvement and environmental sound recognition	(Counter et al, 2001)
Mitochondrial cytopathy	1	Case study	Auditory rehabilitation	Very successful with greatly improved quality of life	(Counter et al, 2001; Cullington, 1999)
A1555G (12S rRNA) mitochondrial mutation	1	Case study	Auditory rehabilitation	Excellent auditory performance; 78% monosyllable recognition using native language word lists for speech audiometry	(Tono et al, 1998)

Table 2–5 MELAS-Related Deafness and Cochlear Implant Outcome (Alphabetical by Author)

Disorder	No. of Patients	Study Type	Variable	Outcome	References
MELAS or maternally inherited diabetes mellitus with deafness (MIDD)–A3243G	2	Case report	Cochlear implantation and rehabilitation	Successful implantation with BKB scores in top 5% of patient series	(Hill et al, 2001; Sinnathuray et al, 2002)
MELAS	1	Case report	Cochlear implantation and rehabilitation	Open-set speech recognition and communication using the auditory/oral mode	(Rosenthal et al, 1999)
MELAS–A3243G	1	Case report	Cochlear implantation and rehabilitation	Restoration of good functional hearing	(Sue et al, 1998)
MELAS	1	Case report	Cochlear implantation and rehabilitation	Successful implantation, able to use the telephone, very satisfied with improvement in communication	(Yasumura et al, 2003)

BKB, Bamford-Kowal-Bench; MELAS, mitochondrial encephalopathy, lactic acidosis, and stroke-like episodes.

were found in six of 12 patients with mild to moderate deafness, and after excluding severe and profoundly deaf patients with a complete absence of responses, there were normal and symmetric brainstem evoked responses in 18 of 20 latencies recorded from 10 patients. Promontory stimulation testing in two patients was normal, and CT and MRI were reported as showing no lesions that could contribute to hearing loss. In addition, central auditory lesions have been reported as a cause of hearing loss in MELAS.

To date, five case reports describing CI in patients with MELAS and hearing loss have demonstrated successful implantation outcomes in these patients, including open-set speech recognition in some patients (**Table 2–5**).

Auditory Neuropathy–Related Deafness and Cochlear Implant Outcome

Normal outer hair cell (OHC) function and dyssynchronous neural responses characterize auditory neuropathy/auditory dyssynchrony (AN/AD). A combination of measures of OHC function and neural synchrony are necessary to correctly identify these patients. Otoacoustic emissions (OAEs) and cochlear microphonics (CM) reflect OHC function, and the results on these tests, in the absence of middle-ear problems, are normal.

The variation of characteristics between patients in combination with the fact that several possible underlying mechanisms can result in normal OHC function and poor neural synchrony suggest that AN/AD is not a single entity with a single underlying etiology (Starr et al, 2000). Due to the possibility that some of the mechanisms and etiologies may not be specifically neural in nature, the term *auditory dyssynchrony* has been suggested to provide a more comprehensive view of auditory neuropathy that logically connects to current viable management options (Berlin et al, 2001).

Localization of the site of injury in AN/AD has been hypothesized to include the inner hair cells (IHC), the synaptic juncture between the IHC and auditory nerve, or the auditory nerve itself (Deltenre et al, 1997b). Each of these sites of injury could result in normal OAEs and a

dyssynchronous ABR. Several sources of information support the possible involvement of IHC, including animal models and recent human histological data (Amatuzzi et al, 2001; Steel & Bussoli, 1999). Some patients with AN/AD have demyelinating conditions such as hereditary motor sensory neuropathy, Charcot-Marie-Tooth disease, or other neural conditions.

Although numerous patients have risk factors related to hearing loss in their history, a significant number of patients have no identifiable risk factors. Factors observed in infants include hyperbilirubinemia, exchange transfusion, premature birth, and perinatal asphyxia (Deltenre et al, 1997a; Rance et al., 1999; Simmons & Beauchaine, 2000). Heredity is another possible underlying factor, as several families have been identified with multiple (two or more) members with AN/AD.

Cochlear implants are a viable management option for patients with AN/AD. Though some patients may have absent or malfunctioning IHC with intact neural function, in those patients with impaired neural elements the electrical stimulation from a cochlear implant may improve synchrony. AN/AD children with cochlear implants demonstrate synchronous neural responses and performance on behavioral tests comparable to non-AN/AD children with cochlear implants (Shallop et al, 2001; Trautwein et al, 2000). Unfortunately, there is currently no way to specifically determine the involvement of either cochlear (IHC) or neural sites in individual patients. Despite this obstacle, the data gathered to date suggest that the outcome of CI in these patients is not significantly different from that in other pediatric cochlear implant patients, and physiologic data suggest that the implant was able to overcome the desynchronization hypothesized to underlie auditory neuropathy (Buss et al, 2002) (**Table 2–6**).

◆ Conclusion

The promise of utilizing genetic testing to predict cochlear implantation outcome is near. Early experience with CI in patients with *GJB2*-related deafness, autosomal recessive

Table 2–6 Auditory Neuropathy–Related Deafness and Cochlear Implant Outcome

Disorder	No. of Patients	Study Type	Variable	Outcome	References
Auditory neuropathy (AN/AD)	?	?	?	CI is effective in the 93% of patients with AN who have hearing impairment	Berlin et al, 2002 *Seminars in Hearing*
Auditory neuropathy	4	Case control	Evoked auditory brainstem responses and reflex measures, obtained contra-lateral to the implant	CI outcome similar to that of other pediatric CI patients	(Buss et al, 2002)
Auditory neuropathy	4 (of 18 with AN)	Retrospective case review	Performance results after CI	All showed improvement in auditory and verbal development, but this improvement was variable	(Madden et al, 2002)
Auditory neuropathy	4	Retrospective review	Brainstem auditory evoked responses (BAERs), audiological performance	Patients with CI demon-strated implant-evoked BAER and improved audiological performance	(Mason et al, 2003)
Auditory neuropathy	1	Case control (single-subject, repeated measures design)	Closed-set and open-set word recognition abilities	Slightly lower vowel recognition, significantly lower consonant and open-set word recognition	(Miyamoto et al, 1999)
Auditory neuropathy	13 (10 children and 3 adults)	Case control	Program threshold and comfort current levels; program strategy, communi-cation mode, edu-cational placement, sound field thresholds, speech perception measures, neural response telemetry (NRT) measures, electrical stapedius reflex measures	CI patients with and without AN have very similar variable outcomes	(Peterson et al, 2003) (publi-cation of first five pediatric cases in Shallop reference)
Auditory neuropathy	5	Retrospective case series	Electrode impedance, electrical auditory brainstem responses (EABRs), otoacoustic emissions and NRT	Significant improvements in sound detection, speech perception, communication skills and NRT results	(Shallop et al, 2001)
Auditory neuropathy	1	Case control	Speech perception	Significant improvement in speech perception was found post-CI	(Trautwein et al, 2000)

AN, auditory neuropathy.

and dominant deafness, mitochondrial hearing loss, and auditory neuropathy suggest that, in the setting of normal anatomy of the inner ear and an intact central auditory pathway, the outcome in uniformly excellent. Genetic testing may assist in identifying those implant candidates, such as children with multiple handicaps, requiring additional intervention and more aggressive ancillary therapies to optimize outcome.

References

Amatuzzi MG, Northrop C, Liberman MC, et al. (2001). Selective inner hair cell loss in premature infants and cochlea pathological patterns from neonatal intensive care unit autopsies. Arch Otolaryngol Head Neck Surg 127:629–636

Bauer PW, Geers AE, Brenner C, Moog JS, Smith RJ. (2003). The effect of GJB2 allele variants on performance after cochlear implantation. Laryngoscope 113:2135–2140

Belal A. (2001). Is cochlear implantation possible after acoustic tumor removal? Otol Neurotol 22:497–500

Berlin C, Hood L, Rose K. (2001). On renaming auditory neuropathy as auditory dys-synchrony. Audiology Today 13:15–17

Berlin et al (2002). Auditory neuropathy/dyssynchrony: its many forms and outcomes. Seminars in Hearing 23:209–214

Buss E, Labadie RF, Brown CJ, Gross AJ, Grose JH, Pillsbury HC. (2002). Outcome of cochlear implantation in pediatric auditory neuropathy. Otol Neurotol 23:328–332

Chen A, Francis M, Ni L, et al. (1995). Phenotypic manifestations of branchio-oto-renal syndrome. Am J Med Genet 58:365–370

Chorbachi R, Graham JM, Ford J, Raine CH. (2002). Cochlear implantation in Jervell and Lange-Nielsen syndrome. Int J Pediatr Otorhinolaryngol 66:213–221

Counter PR, Hilton MP, Webster D, et al. (2001). Cochlear implantation of a patient with a previously undescribed mitochondrial DNA defect. J Laryngol Otol 115:730–732

Cullen RD, Buchman CA, Brown CJ, et al. (2004). Cochlear implantation for children with GJB2-related deafness. Laryngoscope 114:1415–1419

Cullington HE. (1999). Cochlear implantation of a deaf blind patient with mitochondrial cytopathy. J Laryngol Otol 113:353–354

Cusimano F, Martines E, Rizzo C. (1991). The Jervell and Lange-Nielsen syndrome. Int J Pediatr Otorhinolaryngol 22:49–58

Dahl HH, Wake M, Sarant J, Poulakis Z, Siemering K, Blamey P. (2003). Language and speech perception outcomes in hearing-impaired children with and without connexin 26 mutations. Audiol Neurootol 8:263–268

Daya H, Figueirido JC, Gordon KA, Twitchell K, Gysin C, Papsin BC. (1999). The role of a graded profile analysis in determining candidacy and outcome for cochlear implantation in children. Int J Pediatr Otorhinolaryngol 49:135–142

Deltenre P, Mansbach AL, Bozet C, Clercx A, Hecox KE. (1997a). Auditory neuropathy: a report on three cases with early onsets and major neonatal illnesses. Electroencephalogr Clin Neurophysiol 104:17–22

Deltenre P, Mansbach AL, Bozet C, Clercx A, Hecox KE. (1997b). Temporal distortion products (kernel slices) evoked by maximum-length-sequences in auditory neuropathy: evidence for a cochlear pre-synaptic origin. Electroencephalogr Clin Neurophysiol 104:10–16

Evans DG, Huson SM, Donnai D, et al. (1992). A genetic study of type 2 neurofibromatosis in the United Kingdom. II. Guidelines for genetic counselling. J Med Genet 29:847–852

Fischel-Ghodsian N. (1998). Mitochondrial mutations and hearing loss: paradigm for mitochondrial genetics. Am J Hum Genet 62:15–19

Fischel-Ghodsian N. (1999). Mitochondrial deafness mutations reviewed. Hum Mutat 13:261–270

Fischel-Ghodsian N. (2003). Mitochondrial deafness. Ear Hear 24:303–313

Fukushima K, Sugata K, Kasai N, et al. (2002). Better speech performance in cochlear implant patients with GJB2-related deafness. Int J Pediatr Otorhinolaryngol 62:151–157

Gordon N. (1994). The long Q-T syndromes. Brain Dev 16:153–155

Gorlin RJ, Toriello HV, Cohen MM, eds. (1995). Hereditary Hearing Loss and Its Syndromes. New York: Oxford University Press

Green JD, Schuh MJ, Maddern BR, Haymond J, Helffrich RA. (2000). Cochlear implantation in Jervell and Lange-Nielsen syndrome. Ann Otol Rhinol Laryngol Suppl 185:27–28

Han DY, Wu WM, Xi X, Huang DL, Yang WY. (2004). Cochlear implant in patients with congenital malformation of inner ear. Zhonghua Er Bi Yan Hou Ke Za Zhi 39:85–88

Hill D, Wintersgill S, Stott L, Cadge B, Graham J. (2001). Cochlear implantation in a profoundly deaf patient with MELAS syndrome. J Neurol Neurosurg Psychiatry 71:281

Hoffman RA, Kohan D, Cohen NL. (1992). Cochlear implants in the management of bilateral acoustic neuromas. Am J Otol 13:525–528

Hu DN, Qui WQ, Wu BT, et al. (1991). Genetic aspects of antibiotic induced deafness: mitochondrial inheritance. J Med Genet 28:79–83

Huang TS, Yen PT, Liu SY. (1998). Cochlear implantation in a patient with osteogenesis imperfecta and otospongiosis. Am J Otolaryngol 19:209–212

Hulka GF, Bernard EJ, Pillsbury HC. (1995). Cochlear implantation in a patient after removal of an acoustic neuroma. The implications of magnetic resonance imaging with gadolinium on patient management. Arch Otolaryngol Head Neck Surg 121:465–468

Hutchin TP, Cortopassi GA. (2000). Mitochondrial defects and hearing loss. Cell Mol Life Sci 57:1927–1937

Jaber L, Shohat M, Bu X, et al. (1992). Sensorineural deafness inherited as a tissue specific mitochondrial disorder. J Med Genet 29:86–90

Jervell A, Lange-Nielsen F. (1957). Congenital deaf-mutism, functional heart disease with prolongation of the Q-T interval and sudden death. Am Heart J 54:59–68

Kimberling WJ, Moller C. (1995). Clinical and molecular genetics of Usher syndrome. J Am Acad Audiol 6:63–72

Lalwani AK, Brister JR, Fex J, et al. (1995). Further elucidation of the genomic structure of PAX3, and identification of two different point mutations within the PAX3 homeobox that cause Waardenburg syndrome type 1 in two families. Am J Hum Genet 56:75–83

Lalwani AK, Mhatre AN, San Agustin TB, Wilcox ER. (1996). Genotype-phenotype correlations in type 1 Waardenburg syndrome. Laryngoscope 106:895–902

Lane H, Bahan B. (1998). Ethics of cochlear implantation in young children: a review and reply from a deaf-world perspective. Otolaryngol Head Neck Surg 119:297–313

Loundon N, Marlin S, Busquet D, et al. (2003). Usher syndrome and cochlear implantation. Otol Neurotol 24:216–221

Lustig LR, Jackler RK. (1996). Neurofibromatosis type I involving the external auditory canal. Otolaryngol Head Neck Surg 114:299–307

Lustig LR, Lin D, Venick H, et al. (2004). GJB2 gene mutations in cochlear implant recipients: prevalence and impact on outcome. Arch Otolaryngol Head Neck Surg 130:541–546

MacArdle BM, Bailey C, Phelps, PD, Bradley J, Brown T, Wheeler A. (2002). Cochlear implants in children with craniofacial syndromes: assessment and outcomes. Int J Audiol 41:347–356

Madden C, Hilbert L, Rutter M, Greinwald J, Choo D. (2002). Pediatric cochlear implantation in auditory neuropathy. Otol Neurotol 23:163–168

Mancuso M, Filosto M, Forli F, et al. (2004). A non-syndromic hearing loss caused by very low levels of the mtDNA A3243G mutation. Acta Neurol Scand 110:72–74

Marazita ML, et al. (1993). Genetic epidemiological studies of early-onset deafness in the U.S. school-age population. Am J Med Genet 46(5):486–491

Mason JC, De Michele A, Stevens C, Ruth RA, Hashisaki GT. (2003). Cochlear implantation in patients with auditory neuropathy of varied etiologies. Laryngoscope 113:45–49

Matsushiro N, Doi K, Fuse Y, et al. (2002). Successful cochlear implantation in prelingual profound deafness resulting from the common 233delC mutation of the GJB2 gene in the Japanese. Laryngoscope 112:255–261

McKennan KX. (1991). Neurofibromatosis type I–a rare case resulting in conductive hearing loss. Otolaryngol Head Neck Surg 104:868–872

Melnick M, Bixler D, Silk K, Yune H, Nance WE. (1975). Autosomal dominant branchiootorenal dysplasia. Birth Defects Orig Artic Ser 11:121–128

Mens LH, Mulder JJ. (2002). Averaged electrode voltages in users of the Clarion cochlear implant device. Ann Otol Rhinol Laryngol 111:370–375

Migirov L, Henkin Y, Hildesheimer M, Kronenberg J. (2003). Cochlear implantation in a child with osteogenesis imperfecta. Int J Pediatr Otorhinolaryngol 67:677–680

Miyamoto RT, Kirk KI, Renshaw J, Hussain D. (1999). Cochlear implantation in auditory neuropathy. Laryngoscope 109(2 pt 1):181–185

Morgan-Hughes JA, Sweeney MG, Cooper JM, et al. (1995). Mitochondrial DNA (mtDNA) diseases: correlation of genotype to phenotype. Biochim Biophys Acta 1271:135–140

Morton NE. (1991). Genetic epidemiology of hearing impairment. Ann N Y Acad Sci 630:16–31

Ostri B, Johnsen T, Bergmann I. (1991). Temporal bone findings in a family with branchio-oto-renal syndrome (BOR). Clin Otolaryngol 16:163–167

Paterson CR, Monk EA, McAllion SJ. (2001). How common is hearing impairment in osteogenesis imperfecta? J Laryngol Otol 115:280–282

Pavlakis SG, Phillips PC, DiMauro S, De Vivo DC, Rowland LP. (1984). Mitochondrial myopathy, encephalopathy, lactic acidosis, and strokelike episodes: a distinctive clinical syndrome. Ann Neurol 16:481–488

Pedersen U. (1984). Hearing loss in patients with osteogenesis imperfecta. A clinical and audiological study of 201 patients. Scand Audiol 13:67–74

Pensak ML, Keith RW, Dignan PS, Stowens DW, Towbin RB, Katbamna B. (1989). Neuroaudiologic abnormalities in patients with type 1 neurofibromatosis. Laryngoscope 99(7 pt 1):702–706

Peterson A, Shallop J, Driscoll C, et al. (2003). Outcomes of cochlear implantation in children with auditory neuropathy. J Am Acad Audiol 14:188–201

Petit C. (1996). Genes responsible for human hereditary deafness: symphony of a thousand. Nat Genet 14:385–391

Poissant SF, Megerian CA, Hume D. (2003). Cochlear implantation in a patient with neurofibromatosis type 1 and profound hearing loss: evidence to support a cochlear site of lesion. Otol Neurotol 24:751–756

Prezant RT, Shohat M, Jaber L, Pressman S, Fischel-Ghodsian N. (1992). Biochemical characterization of a pedigree with mitochondrially inherited deafness. Am J Med Genet 44:465–472

Rance G, Beer DE, Cone-Wesson B, et al. (1999). Clinical findings for a group of infants and young children with auditory neuropathy. Ear Hear 20:238–252

Read AP, Newton VE. (1997). Waardenburg syndrome. J Med Genet 34:656–665

Reed WB, Stone VM, Boder E, Ziprkowski L. (1967). Pigmentary disorders in association with congenital deafness. Arch Dermatol 95:176–186

Rosenthal EL, Kileny PR, Boerst A, Telian SA. (1999). Successful cochlear implantation in a patient with MELAS syndrome. Am J Otol 20: 187–190 discussion 190–181

Sanchez Cascos A, Sanchez Pernaute R, Cifuentes S. (1990). A child affected by the Romano-Ward syndrome born of a mother with the Jervell and Lange-Nielsen syndrome. Rev Esp Cardiol 43:406–407

Shallop JK, Peterson A, Facer GW, Fabry LB, Driscoll CL. (2001). Cochlear implants in five cases of auditory neuropathy: postoperative findings and progress. Laryngoscope 111(4 pt 1):555–562

Shamboul K, Grundfast K. (1999). Hearing loss in neurofibromatosis type 1: report of two cases. East Afr Med J 76:117–119

Sherman LS, Atit R, Rosenbaum T, Cox AD, Ratner N. (2000). Single cell Ras-GTP analysis reveals altered Ras activity in a subpopulation of neurofibroma Schwann cells but not fibroblasts. J Biol Chem 275: 30740–30745

Shin YJ, Fraysse B, Sterkers O, Bouccara D, Rey A, Lazorthes Y. (1998). Hearing restoration in posterior fossa tumors. Am J Otol 19:649–653

Simmons JL, Beauchaine KL. (2000). Auditory neuropathy: case study with hyperbilirubinemia. J Am Acad Audiol 11:337–347

Sinnathuray AR, Raut V, Awa A, Magee A, Toner JG. (2003). A review of cochlear implantation in mitochondrial sensorineural hearing loss. Otol Neurotol 24:418–426

Sinnathuray AR, Raut V, Toner JG, Magee A. (2002). Cochlear implantation in a profoundly deaf patient with MELAS syndrome. J Neurol Neurosurg Psychiatry 73:97; author reply 97–98

Sinnathuray AR, Toner JG, Clarke-Lyttle J, Geddis A, Patterson CC, Hughesm AE. (2004a). Connexin 26 (GJB2) gene-related deafness and speech intelligibility after cochlear implantation. Otol Neurotol 25: 935–942

Sinnathuray AR, Toner JG, Geddis A, Clarke-Lyttle J, Patterson CC, Hughes AE. (2004b). Auditory perception and speech discrimination after cochlear implantation in patients with connexin 26 (GJB2) gene-related deafness. Otol Neurotol 25:930–934

Snoeckx RL, et al. (2005). GJB2 mutations and degree of hearing loss: a multicenter study. Am J Hum Genet 77(6):945–957

Starr A, Sininger YS, Pratt H. (2000). The varieties of auditory neuropathy. J Basic Clin Physiol Pharmacol 11:215–230

Steel KP, Bussoli TJ. (1999). Deafness genes: expressions of surprise. Trends Genet 15:207–211

Sue CM, Lipsett LJ, Crimmins DS, et al. (1998). Cochlear origin of hearing loss in MELAS syndrome. Ann Neurol 43:350–359

Sugii A, Iwaki T, Doi K, et al. (2000). Cochlear implant in a young child with Waardenburg syndrome. Adv Otorhinolaryngol 57:215–219

Szilvassy J, Jori J, Czigner J, Toth F, Szilvassy Z, Kiss JG. (1998). Cochlear implantation in osteogenesis imperfecta. Acta Otorhinolaryngol Belg 52:253–256

Tassabehji M, Newton VE, Liu XZ, et al. (1995). The mutational spectrum in Waardenburg syndrome. Hum Mol Genet 4:2131–2137

Tassabehji M, Newton VE, Read AP. (1994). Waardenburg syndrome type 2 caused by mutations in the human microphthalmia (MITF) gene. Nat Genet 8:251–255

Tassabehji M, Read AP, Newton VE, et al. (1993). Mutations in the PAX3 gene causing Waardenburg syndrome type 1 and type 2. Nat Genet 3:26–30

Tono T, Ushisako Y, Kiyomizu K, et al. (1998). Cochlear implantation in a patient with profound hearing loss with the A1555G mitochondrial mutation. Am J Otol 19:754–757

Trautwein PG, Sininger YS, Nelson R. (2000). Cochlear implantation of auditory neuropathy. J Am Acad Audiol 11:309–315

Trofatter JA, MacCollin MM, Rutter JL, et al. (1993). A novel moesin-, ezrin-, radixin-like gene is a candidate for the neurofibromatosis 2 tumor suppressor. Cell 72:791–800

Usami S, Abe S, Akita J, et al. (2000). Prevalence of mitochondrial gene mutations among hearing impaired patients. J Med Genet 37:38–40

Van Camp GSR. (2005). Hereditary Hearing Loss Homepage. http://dnalab-www.uia.ac.be/dnalab/hhh/

Van Camp J, Coucke PJ, Kunst H, et al. (1997). Linkage analysis of progressive hearing loss in five extended families maps the DFNA2 gene to a 1.25-Mb region on chromosome 1p. Genomics 41:70–74

Vescan A, Parnes LS, Cucci RA, Smith RJ, MacNeill C. (2002). Cochlear implantation and Pendred's syndrome mutation in monozygotic twins with large vestibular aqueduct syndrome. J Otolaryngol 31:54–57

Waardenburg PJ. (1951). A new syndrome combining developmental anomalies of the eyelids, eyebrows and nose root with pigmentary defects of the iris and head hair and with congenital deafness. Am J Hum Genet 3:195–253

Yasumura S, Aso S, Fujisaka M, Watanabe Y. (2003). Cochlear implantation in a patient with mitochondrial encephalopathy, lactic acidosis and stroke-like episodes syndrome. Acta Otolaryngol 123:55–58

3

Consequences of Deafness and Electrical Stimulation on the Peripheral and Central Auditory System

Robert K. Shepherd,

Noah E. Meltzer,

James B. Fallon, and

David K. Ryugo

Cochlear implants provide important auditory cues necessary for auditory awareness and speech perception in severe to profoundly deaf subjects. Over the past three decades more than 80,000 adults and children worldwide have received these devices. Clinical experience has shown, however, a large variability in outcome among implant users. Factors predicting a successful clinical outcome reflect the importance of auditory experience—either before an acquired hearing loss or with use of a cochlear implant. Moreover, deaf children, with little or no prior auditory experience, can obtain significant benefit from a cochlear implant provided that their device is fitted at a young age. This clinical experience suggests that such a response can be at least partially attributed to plasticity within the auditory system.

This chapter reviews the response of the auditory system to both deafness and its reactivation through a cochlear implant, and includes experimental data from animal models as well as human material where applicable. Understanding the complexities of this response will help provide a substrate for understanding the clinical variability evident among cochlear implant users.

◆ The Cochlea

Cochlear Pathophysiology Following Deafness

Spiral ganglion neurons (SGNs), whose cell bodies are located within Rosenthal's canal (**Fig. 3–1**), are the target neurons for cochlear implants. These devices electrically depolarize local populations of SGNs, initiating the generation of action potentials via an electrode array typically located in the scala tympani (a description of the initiation of an action potential via an electrical stimulus is provided elsewhere[1]). It is important to emphasize that once the action potential has been initiated, the implant plays no further role in its propagation along the ascending auditory pathway; saltatory conduction along the central process of the SGN and its passage across synapses within the cochlear nucleus (CN) or higher auditory centers are performed via normal physiologic processes.

Survival of these neurons is dependent on the integrity of the organ of Corti; SGNs are subject to atrophic and degenerative changes that occur secondary to a sensorineural hearing loss (SNHL). Although the minimum number of SGNs required to achieve acceptable clinical performance with a cochlear implant is unclear, the greater number of viable SGNs available for stimulation is likely to result in improved clinical performance.[2,3] Here we discuss the pathophysiologic changes that occur to the cochlea following SNHL and describe techniques that may lead to SGN preservation.

Cochlear Pathology

Hair cells of the organ of Corti are sensitive to many forms of pathologic damage including acoustic trauma, ototoxic drugs, congenital abnormalities, and aging. Unlike avian hair cells, mammalian hair cells cannot spontaneously regenerate; loss of hair cells results in a permanent SNHL. Several atrophic and pathologic changes occur to SGNs following the loss of the sensory epithelium and the support cells of the organ of Corti. First, there is a rapid

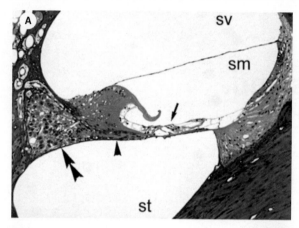

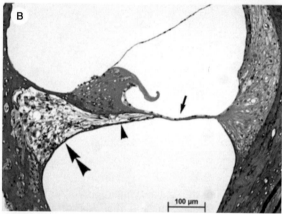

Figure 3–1 Photomicrographs of the upper basal turn from **(A)** normal hearing and **(B)** 10-week deafened rat cochleae. The normal organ of Corti evident in the control animal contrasts with the complete degeneration of both hair cells and their supporting structure in the deafened cochlea (arrow). Other deafness-induced degenerative changes evident here include a loss of peripheral processes that would normally innervate the organ of Corti (arrowhead), and loss of the spiral ganglion neuron (SGN) soma within Rosenthal's canal (double arrowhead). sv, scala vestibuli; sm, scala media; st, scala tympani.

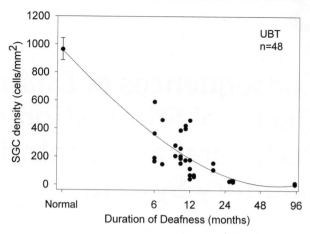

Figure 3–2 Graph illustrating the rate of loss of SGNs in the upper basal turn (UBT) of the cat cochlea as a function of duration of deafness. Although there is a relatively wide individual variability in the data, there is a clear reduction in SGN survival with increased durations of deafness. Similar degenerative patterns are observed in other mammals albeit at different rates. Although rodents such as guinea pigs exhibit a more rapid loss of SGNs compared with the cat, it is important to emphasize that ganglion cell loss is significantly slower in humans. These data are based on counts from 48 cat cochleae including 16 normal hearing controls. Error bar = +/−1 SEM.

and extensive loss of the unmyelinated peripheral processes within the organ of Corti.[4] This process is followed by a more gradual degeneration of the myelinated portion of the peripheral processes within the osseous spiral lamina and of the cell bodies within Rosenthal's canal[5–7] (**Fig. 3–1**). The degenerative process also results in demyelination of residual SGN soma and possibly part of their central processes.[5,7,8] Finally, the perikaryon of residual SGNs undergoes considerable shrinkage,[9–11] a response that is repeated throughout the central auditory pathway following an SNHL (see below), although the functional effects of this atrophy are unknown.

The secondary degeneration of SGNs following loss of the organ of Corti is an ongoing process, eventually resulting in very small numbers of surviving neurons[6,7] (**Fig. 3–2**). As we will describe below, these pathologic changes affect the physiologic response of SGNs to an electrical stimulus. The ongoing degeneration of SGNs has been widely reported across mammalian species following various etiologies that

target the organ of Corti: mouse,[12] rat,[13,14] chinchilla,[15] guinea pig,[16] and cat.[6,7,17–21] It is important to emphasize that the rate of SGN degeneration exhibits considerable variation across species—a theme we shall return to when discussing SGN loss in humans.

In the majority of forms of SNHL, SGN degeneration is secondary to the loss of hair cells and support cells of the organ of Corti.[22–24] These changes appear due, at least in part, to the withdrawal of neurotrophic factors normally expressed by the hair cells[25–28] and nerve growth factors released by support cells.[29] This pathway of SGN loss is common to many forms of SNHL described clinically, and would be expected to result in a gradual but ongoing secondary degeneration of SGNs as reported above. Importantly, etiologies that directly target SGNs, including viral and bacterial labyrinthitis, mechanical trauma, and disruption to cochlear vasculature, are likely to result in a more rapid and extensive loss of auditory neurons.

Reports of degeneration patterns of SGNs in human cochleae following a profound SNHL are generally consistent with the experimental studies already summarized. Degeneration of peripheral processes is more extensive than that of the SGN soma or central processes, and the extent of the pathology typically varies with distance along the cochlear partition in a manner that reflects the extent of damage to the organ of Corti, being most extensive in the basal turn with less extensive pathology apicalward.[3,22,23,30–33]

Analysis of SGN survival from profoundly deaf adult temporal bones reveals a moderate to severe loss of auditory neurons. Otte and colleagues[32] studied 62 profoundly deaf ears and demonstrated that 45% of cochleae had a SGN population in excess of 10,000, that is, approximately one third of normal ($28,418 \pm 3,675$[3]). Nadol and colleagues[3] studied 66 profoundly deaf ears and showed that the mean SGN population was approximately half that of normal ears, although the standard deviation, as in all studies of this sort, was large ($14,061 \pm 8,063$). Total SGN loss tended to be greater in older compared with younger subjects and, consistent with animal studies, greater loss was observed with longer durations of deafness. However, the single most significant determinant of SGN loss in humans was etiology,[3,31] with loss most extensive in patients with postnatal viral labyrinthitis, congenital or genetic deafness, or bacterial meningitis, that is, pathologies that directly target SGNs or patients having long durations of deafness. Patients deafened with aminoglycoside antibiotics or sudden idiopathic deafness typically exhibited the smallest levels of SGN pathology.

Although many of the findings observed in adult temporal bones have also been reported in temporal bones from profoundly deaf children, two important differences were noted: (1) the SGN population in children did not show evidence of ongoing loss with duration of deafness within the age range of 0 to 9 years; and (2) there was a more even distribution of SGNs throughout the cochleae.[34] These results provide encouraging findings for pediatric cochlear implantation, and emphasize the relatively slow rate of SGN degeneration evident in humans compared with experimental animals. This situation may reflect, at least in part, the lack of a long-term decrease in clinical performance with device use.[35]

Physiologic Response of the Spiral Ganglion Neuron to Deafness

Despite the extensive pathologic changes that occur to SGNs following an SNHL, these neurons remain capable of initiating and propagating action potentials elicited via an electrical stimulus, even in cochleae deafened for many years, with surviving neural populations of <5% of normal.[6] In general, the basic response properties of SGNs in deafened cochleae remain similar to those observed in normal cochleae; that is, the cells show an increase in the probability of firing and a decrease in both response latency and the jitter in the timing of the response with increasing stimulus current. There are, however, more subtle changes seen in neural response properties in cochleae subjected to long periods of deafness; these pathology-induced changes have the potential to degrade the perceptual quality of cochlear implants. First, loss of peripheral process and ongoing loss of SGNs results in an increase in threshold.[14,36-38] This change likely has an adverse effect on power consumption and results in a reduction in spatial selectivity of the electrode array.[39] Second, demyelination results in an increase in membrane capacitance,[40,41] reducing the efficiency of a neuron in initiating and propagating action potentials in response to electrical stimuli. In the auditory system, there is evidence of reduced temporal resolution in myelin-deficient or deafened cochleae,[42] as well as a significant increase in the refractory properties of auditory nerve fibers[14] and evidence of conduction block.[17]

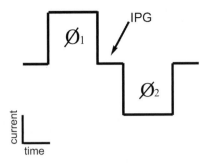

Figure 3–3 Schematic diagram illustrating the charge balanced biphasic current pulses typically used in cochlear implants. Charge in the second phase ($\varnothing_2$) is equal in magnitude but opposite in polarity to the charge in the first phase ($\varnothing_1$). The duration of each phase typically varies between ~10 and 50 μs/phase for monopolar stimulation and 50 and 200 μs/phase for the less efficient bipolar stimulation. IPG, interphase gap.

Effects of Electrical Stimulation

Safety Issues

Nondamaging electrical stimulation consists of short-duration (<200 μs/phase) charge-balanced biphasic current pulses (**Fig. 3–3**) delivered using platinum electrodes and operating at charge densities of <60 μC/cm^{-2} geom per phase.[43-49] These stimulus guidelines ensure that the charge injection process is achieved using reversible electrochemical reactions localized to the electrode–tissue interface, minimizing the chance of releasing potentially harmful electrochemical products into the tissue environment.[50-52] Contemporary cochlear implants operating in a monopolar electrode configuration would typically produce charge densities of an order of magnitude below these levels.

Although theoretically, charge-balanced biphasic current pulses should not result in the production of potentially damaging direct current, in practice it is not possible to generate perfectly balanced stimuli. Neural damage and new bone formation is observed following chronic stimulation with direct current levels greater than 0.4 μA.[53,54] Protection against direct current, and the local pH changes that occur as a result of charge imbalance, can be achieved by either shorting electrodes between current pulses or by placing a capacitor in series with each electrode.[55,56] One or a combination of these techniques is used to ensure complete charge recovery in contemporary cochlear implant systems.

Trophic Effects of Electrical Stimulation on Spiral Ganglion Neuron Survival

In deafness, there is a lack of both driven neural activity and significant reductions in the levels of spontaneous activity,[17,20,21,37] such that SGNs rarely undergo depolarization. However, neural activity is known to play an important role in SGN survival; depolarization is sufficient to maintain neuronal survival in vitro without the addition of neurotrophic factors.[57] Membrane depolarization appears to promote SGN survival by elevating intracellular calcium levels and cascading several intracellular signaling pathways.[57] Finally, the trophic support of SGNs via depolarization in vitro appears to be additive with the actions of some neurotrophins.[58]

Several in vivo studies have described significant increases in SGN survival—to levels of up to 70% greater than nonstimulated control cochleae—in ototoxically deafened animals following chronic electrical stimulation of the auditory nerve.[59-67] However, it is important to emphasize that this is not a universal finding; work from other laboratories has reported no such trophic influence.[43,45,68,69] Given the subtle methodological differences across studies, this variation in results is not surprising. Indeed, it is expected that these differences will ultimately provide further insight into the mechanisms underlying stimulus-induced trophic support of SGNs.

There is agreement, however, that chronic electrical stimulation in deafened ears results in subtle morphologic changes to SGNs. For example, there is a small but significant increase in the soma area of SGNs in deafened, chronically stimulated cochleae compared with deafened controls.[43,67] This increase in soma area presumably reflects an increase in biosynthetic activity within the SGN soma following reactivation via an electrical stimulus.

Neurotrophin Support of the Spiral Ganglion

Several growth factor families have been shown to play important roles in the development, maintenance, and protection against injury of SGNs.[70] Both presynaptic hair cells and postsynaptic neurons within the CN are necessary for SGN survival, reflecting complementary neurotrophic support from both sources. These neurotrophins include both brain-derived neurotrophic factor (BDNF) and neurotrophin-3 (NT-3)[25,26,71], with receptors for both of these neurotrophins expressed on SGNs.[25,26] Moreover, survival of SGNs in the absence of hair cells has been promoted by exogenous BDNF or NT-3 in vivo.[13,16,72-74]

This research has recently been extended to demonstrate enhanced SGN survival in deafened cochleae treated with both exogenous neurotrophins and electrical stimulation[63,69] (**Fig. 3–4**). Importantly, this work has also shown a functional advantage, in the form of significantly reduced electrically evoked auditory brainstem response thresholds in ears treated with neurotrophins,[69,75] that may be associated with a neurotrophin-mediated growth of SGN peripheral processes toward the scala tympani.[74,76] Reductions in electrical thresholds would reduce the power consumption of a cochlear implant, thereby providing several engineering advantages including the possibility of smaller, more numerous electrode contacts.

Although these results are promising, from a clinical perspective further research is necessary before neurotrophins can be combined with cochlear implants. First, the long-term safety and efficacy of neurotrophin delivery to the cochlea must be examined, as there is evidence that the removal of exogenous BDNF leads to an accelerated loss of SGNs,[77] implying that the neurotrophin must be supplied continuously. The perilymph of scala tympani is connected to the cerebrospinal fluid via the cochlear aqueduct; therefore, safety studies must be directed at both the level of the cochlea and the central nervous system (CNS). Second, an appropriate strategy for longterm delivery of neurotrophins must be established. The use of pumps should be discouraged because of the risks of introducing infection into the inner ear. Alternative delivery methods using viral vectors or cell-based therapies hold promise in this area.[63] Finally, while neurotrophin therapy has been shown to protect SGNs following an insult to the organ of Corti, it is not clear whether neurotrophins would be effective in etiologies that directly target SGNs.

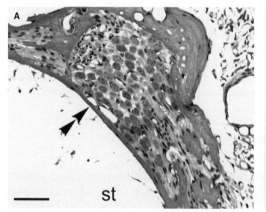 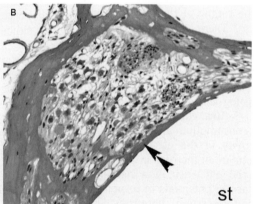

Figure 3–4 Photomicrographs of Rosenthal's canal (double arrowhead) and the SGNs of the upper basal turn from deafened guinea pig cochleae **(A)** treated with the neurotrophin brain-derived neurotrophic factor (BDNF) and electrically stimulated via a cochlear implant and **(B)** the contralateral deafened untreated control. The near-normal SGN population in the BDNF-treated cochlea contrasts with the ~50% SGN loss after 4 weeks of deafening in the deafened control cochlea. st, scala tympani. Scale bar = 50 μm.

◆ The Cochlear Nucleus

Deafness and the Cochlear Nucleus

The role of acoustically generated activity on the structural and functional development of the central auditory system is a subject of intense research. Auditory deprivation in the developing animal produces severe abnormalities in the central pathway, whereas older animals are less affected.[78-84] Postmortem studies of those rare human cases where the profound hearing loss of the individual is documented has revealed up to 50% somatic shrinkage in the CN, with acknowledgment that many variables contribute to the nonuniform results.[85-88] Clinical observations related to congenital deafness suggest that the best candidates for cochlear implants are very young children, and that with increasing age the outcomes become less optimal.[89-91] The implication is that sensory stimulation, whether natural or prosthetic, is necessary during early life to ensure the normal development of the central auditory system.

In the auditory system, there is a period during which the normal development of speech and hearing is adversely affected by sound deprivation, and thereafter it cannot be remedied even if sound is fully restored. The nature of this epoch, called the "critical period," is conceptually similar across species but undoubtedly varies in timing and magnitude of effect. Intervention strategies in the case of pediatric patients with a profound SNHL have concentrated on cochlear implants, and there is a growing tendency to implant deaf children at earlier and earlier ages. It seems necessary, however, to acquire better knowledge of those factors affecting the structure and function of the auditory system when electrical stimulation is used.

In an effort to understand the influence of acoustic stimulation on the developing brain, there have been experimental manipulations on the end organs to deprive the system of input. Deafening has been produced by surgical or pharmacologic manipulations of the auditory periphery as well as by congenital or hereditary defects. Each form of deafness is accompanied by its own potential complication. One must be vigilant for indirect surgical trauma, nonspecific drug effects, and downstream genetic influences.

Models of Deafness and the Cochlear Nucleus

The least invasive manipulation on the auditory system is produced by the introduction of conductive hearing loss. This method basically involves the "plugging" of the ear canal with a malleable substance or removing one of the ossicles. Results from ear plugging have been inconsistent, probably because of the high rates of spontaneous discharges in auditory nerve fibers, which are not affected by this manipulation.[92] Even with extreme plugging strategies, the effects are relatively small and show signs of recovery.[93-95]

Surgical ablation of the cochleae in neonatal animals produces a profound SNHL and results in ∼50% ipsilateral volume loss, 30 to 40% cell body shrinkage, and >50% neural death in the CN.[81,96,97] Importantly, the loss of central neurons following cochlear ablation is restricted to a critical period that appears to end at the onset of hearing.[98,99] Although deafferentation during cochlear development results in widespread neural loss in the CN, similar cochlear damage after the onset of hearing results in atrophic changes but not neural loss. Given that most forms of SNHL occur following the onset of hearing,[100-102] these results imply that the major transneuronal effects of deafness are atrophic, with relatively small amounts of neural loss.

An alternative form of deafening is provided by the administration of ototoxic drugs. These drugs (e.g., amikacin, neomycin, kanamycin, ethacrynic acid) are known to cause a loss of hair cell receptors and deafness[7,103-105] as described above. Following ganglion cell loss, there is a reduction in CN volume and distinct cell shrinkage in cats, gerbils, and guinea pigs,[6,106-108] with the effect on the ventral CN much greater compared with that on the dorsal CN. This form of deafening represents the model of choice for current investigations of this topic.

The congenitally deaf white cat (DWC) represents a third alternative for these kinds of studies.[19,20,82,109-114] DWCs have long been of interest because an autosomal dominant gene links coat color, eye pigment, and deafness.[115-119] This well-documented syndrome is probably a variably penetrant and variably expressive syndrome affecting several characteristics including cochlear pathology[120] that was first described in congenitally deaf patients.[121,122] The pathology in the DWC ranges from moderate hair cell loss to complete collapse of the organ of Corti with corresponding degrees of hearing loss.[19,20,110,123-125] For those animals with a profound SNHL, deafness is manifest by the collapse of Reissner's membrane onto the undifferentiated organ of Corti, thinning of the stria vascularis, and malformation of the tectorial membrane. A variable degree of SGN degeneration proceeds over time,[118,124] and distinct atrophic features are evident in the CN including a 50% reduction in nuclear volume and a differential shrinkage of separate cell types.[20,109,126,127] Furthermore, a hypertrophy of synapses is seen on some but not other CN neurons.[82] Spherical and globular bushy cells represent two major cell classes in the ventral CN. Spherical bushy cells receive large axosomatic endings called endbulbs of Held, whereas globular bushy cells received smaller endbulbs. Congenital deafness results in a reduction in endbulb branching, reduction of presynaptic vesicles, flattening and hypertrophy of postsynaptic densities, and loss of intermembranous channels. Synapses on spherical bushy cells are severely affected by a SNHL, whereas those on globular bushy cells are less so. In contrast, synapses on multipolar cells exhibit only slight structural abnormalities[82,113,128] (**Fig. 3–5**).

The structural abnormalities in CN neurons in response to a SNHL seem a natural consequence of abnormal inputs from the auditory nerve. Congenital and ototoxic deafness significantly reduces the levels of spontaneous activity in auditory nerve fibers of the cat.[17,20] Variations in spontaneous activity in auditory nerve fibers have an effect on spherical bushy cells even in normal hearing cats.[129] Deafness-induced changes are expressed as increased thresholds to activation,[14] smaller action potentials, smaller after-hyperpolarizations, and shorter membrane time constants.[130]

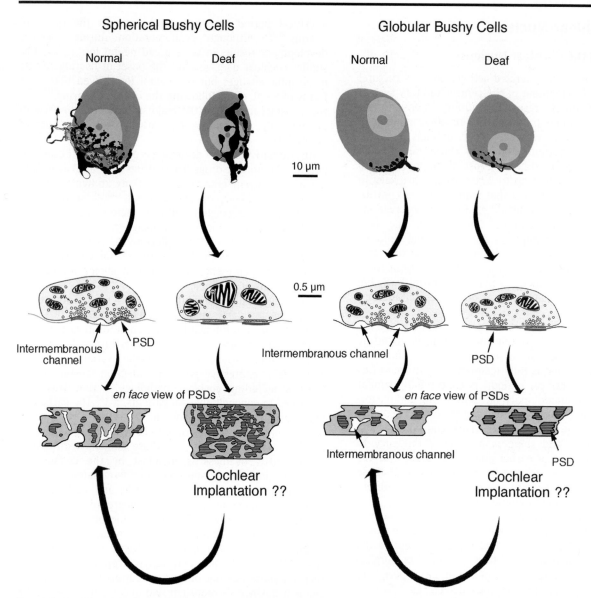

Figure 3–5 Schematic diagram summarizing the effects of deafness on bushy cells of the cochlear nucleus (CN). Congenital deafness results in shrinkage of the bushy cell body, a reduction in endbulb branching, reduction of presynaptic vesicles, flattening and hypertrophy of postsynaptic densities, and loss of intermembranous channels. Although globular bushy cells show similar deafness-induced changes, they are not as extensive as those observed in the spherical bushy cell. The question is whether neural activity induced by cochlear implantation can reverse or reduce these abnormalities. PSD, postsynaptic density. (Adapted from Redd EE, Pongstaporn T, Ryugo DK. The effects of congenital deafness on auditory nerve synapses and globular bushy cells in cats. Hear Res 2000;147:160–174.) *Note*: Recent observations demonstrated that cochlear implantation in young kittens prevented the formation of abnormal auditory nerve synapses (Ryugo et al, Science 310:1490–1492, 2005).

Effects of Electrical Stimulation

The question naturally arises as to whether electrical stimulation of the auditory nerve can effectively prevent, ameliorate, or reverse the deleterious effects of deafness. Inherent to the interpretation of implantation and stimulation results is a consideration that either or both manipulations can contribute to changes additional to those caused by SNHL, and the nature of these changes is not necessarily predictable. Nevertheless, given the notion of a "critical period" in auditory system development, deafened animals are being used to develop experimental models. Furthermore, children, especially prelingually deaf children, are postulated

to receive additional benefit from early electrical stimulation via cochlear implants. The rationale is that the preservation of neurons and synapses represents the substrate for improved development of language skills.

The results of electrical stimulation of the auditory nerve on CN structure have not been uniform. In deafened guinea pigs, chronic electrical stimulation of one cochlea resulted in an increase in the size of octopus cells in the ipsilateral CN compared with those on the contralateral side.[131] If specific cell types were not considered, analysis of all neurons suggested that there was no effect of electrical stimulation. Likewise, there was no statistically significant difference in nuclear volume between the ipsilateral and contralateral sides. In a similar study using unilateral electrical stimulation of ototoxically deafened cats, the size of spherical bushy cells was reduced 20% by deafening, but stimulation did not produce any difference between the ipsilateral and contralateral sides.[132] In related studies, these same comparisons revealed a small (6%) but statistically significant increase in somatic cross-sectional area between ipsilateral and contralateral spherical bushy cells.[106,133] There were also mixed results regarding difference in volumes of the cochlear nuclei and somatic sizes of various cell types in the stimulated and non-stimulated sides. Finally, no work has yet examined the effects of chronic electrical stimulation of the auditory nerve on ultrastructural changes to endbulb synapses on spherical or globular bushy cells in the anteroventral CN (**Fig. 3–5**).

The conclusion from these observations is that electrical stimulation of the cochlea in deaf animals exerts, at best, a small increase in cell body size for CN neurons. There are, however, several considerations that temper this interpretation. First, it isn't always clear that the cells sampled were those that were stimulated. Because the stimulating electrodes are placed in the basal (high frequency) end of the cochlea, the sampling must also occur in the high-frequency regions of the nuclei. In several studies the sampling was from spherical busy cells in the rostral pole of the anteroventral CN, and this region is known to be responsive primarily to low frequencies.[134] Second, using the contralateral CN as a control may not be appropriate with evidence of strong commissural connections between cochlear nuclei.[135–139] Stimulation of the ipsilateral CN by auditory nerve fibers undoubtedly produces activity in the contralateral CN via the commissural projections, thereby negating the idea that there is a simple dichotomy produced by the manipulation.

What emerges from these studies is the conclusion that congenital deafness, regardless of its cause, results in transneuronal changes that are expressed at the level of the CN. We shall now examine deafness-induced effects at higher centers of the auditory system. Ascending projections out of the CN exhibit abnormal pathways[97,140–142] that impact on the structure of the target brainstem nuclei, including the superior olivary nuclei[109,111,143] and inferior colliculus.[144–147] These wide-ranging abnormalities are implicated as part of the explanation of why cochlear implants do not always produce beneficial outcomes.

◆ Higher Auditory Centers

The variable synaptic abnormalities within the CN in response to an SNHL, summarized in **Fig. 3–5**, may contribute to differential transmission delays along the central pathways, leading to corrupted temporal processing of auditory information initiated by cochlear implants. Changes within the CN could obviously have widespread effects because this structure serves as the gateway to the central auditory system. As one ascends the auditory pathway, it seems that transneuronal changes can occur at all levels.

Deafness and the Superior Olivary Complex

The deleterious effects of deafness evident within the CN, are also seen in more central structures. In the DWC, microscopic analysis of the lateral and medial superior olive and the medial nucleus of the trapezoid body demonstrated that neural soma and nuclei areas were 33 to 50% smaller in deaf compared with hearing cats.[109] The size of cerebellar Purkinje cells was not affected by an SNHL. There was also a 35% decrease in the number of synapses per unit somatic length in these nuclei in DWCs.[111] Analysis of the medial superior olive from deaf humans suggests a 20 to 30% reduction in neural soma area for the denervated structure.[88]

Deafness and the Inferior Colliculus

In the midbrain, the central nucleus of the inferior colliculus (ICC) represents a key structure in the central auditory pathway. It is tonotopically organized and receives strong excitatory input from the contralateral ear, although most ICC neurons are binaurally influenced. Inputs to the ICC arise bilaterally from the superior olivary complex via the lateral lemniscus (decussating fibers represent the major pathway) and contralaterally from the dorsal and ventral cochlear nuclei.[148,149]

Following a SNHL, significant structural abnormalities are observed in unilaterally deaf young animals when compared with both normal hearing and bilaterally deafened animals. Such studies revealed an increase in the afferent projection from the normal CN to the ipsilateral ICC.[140,141,150] In contrast, bilaterally deaf animals show symmetry of the ascending projection that is similar to that in normal hearing animals.[112,151] It would appear that these changes are driven by asymmetrical input to the central auditory system as a result of unilateral deafness. It is worth noting that the great majority of cochlear implant subjects also receive a strongly asymmetrical input via a single cochlear implant.

No difference was found between hearing and unilaterally deaf animals when studying ICC ultrastructure after 1 year of chemically induced deafness, although in bilaterally deaf cats, there was a reduction in the number of synapses compared with partial hearing or normal hearing cats.[144] A small but statistically significant reduction in neuronal soma area may be present in bilaterally but not unilaterally deaf cats.[146]

Anatomic Changes Due to Electrical Stimulation

In patients who had some exposure to electrical stimulation via a cochlear implant, the range of neuronal soma size in the ICC was found to be as much as 30% smaller than normal.[88] Small study size, sampling bias, and laterality of stimulation may have obscured trophic effects if they were present, because all cell area averages were smaller than normal hearing controls. Cell soma area was smaller in cases of cochlear pathology than in cases of auditory nerve sectioning. This finding was postulated to be due to a dystrophic effect on neurons from a diseased cochlea, rather than the loss of trophic activity. This inference may have implications for models of deafness based on cochlear abnormalities.

Alternatively, neuronal soma size may not be a relevant (or is at best a crude) parameter in evaluating CNS changes due to deafness and electrical stimulation.

Metabolic Changes Due to Electrical Stimulation

Metabolic markers such as 2-deoxyglucose (2-DG) have been used to study the extent of neural activation in the ICC in response to electrical stimulation of the auditory nerve. Brown et al[152] compared the effects of electrical versus auditory stimulation on 2-DG uptake in cats. Using acute, unilaterally deafened animals, the 2-DG uptake that was evoked from the deafened, electrically stimulated cochlea resembled that seen in the acoustically stimulated contralateral ICC. The location and extent of 2-DG uptake was dependent on the electrode configuration, electrode location, and stimulus intensity, although any increase in 2-DG uptake may also reflect an additive component arising from the ipsilateral auditory stimulation. In a different set of experiments, bilaterally deafened guinea pigs did not exhibit significantly reduced 2-DG activity in the ICC, and remained responsive to acute electrical stimulation after 15 months of deafness.[153] Schwartz et al[154] similarly observed normal 2-DG uptake in electrically stimulated deaf guinea pigs. The 2-DG labeling equaled but did not surpass levels observed in acoustically stimulated normal hearing controls. This effect was seen at increasing levels of stimulation, and with chronic stimulation. Collectively these studies suggest that in the unstimulated state, basic pathways for auditory information to the ICC in deafened animals remain largely functionally and structurally intact, indicating a powerful role for genetic programming of auditory connections.

Physiologic Changes Due to Electrical Stimulation

Frequency Representation in the Inferior Colliculus

Single cell activity evoked by electrical stimulation of the auditory nerve in neonatally deafened cats has revealed that major physiologic features of the ICC are preserved over wide durations of deafness.[145] The spatial tuning of the ICC studied in these acutely stimulated cats revealed that long-term deafness reduced the distance between basal and apical electrode neural representation in the ICC compared with that seen in cats with more auditory experience.

Experiments using neonatally deafened, chronically electrically stimulated cats have also been performed. Snyder et al[155] observed an increase in the ICC neural representation of the electrically stimulated sectors of auditory nerve. Correlating ICC recording depth with neural activity demonstrated a significant increase in neural representation of that sector of auditory nerve subject to chronic stimulation. Moreover, chronic electrical stimulation of the auditory nerve can induce a similar degree of plastic expansion in the ICC of adult-deafened implanted cats.[156] More recently, ICC recordings using multielectrode arrays have been implemented.[157] When applied chronically, this technique promises to provide a longitudinal view of neural activity across the ICC in response to cochlear implantation.

Alternating stimulation of separate areas of the auditory nerve may preserve, or perhaps even sharpen, ICC representation of those stimulated sectors of auditory nerve.[158] These studies indicate that even in prolonged early-onset deafness, basic cochleotopic and neural representation of electrical stimuli may be elicited in the ICC. This developmental feature, however, is clearly modifiable by sensory experience. Neural plasticity of the ICC seems to expand the neural representation of chronically stimulated sectors of auditory nerve, even when those sectors receive stimulation long after the onset of deafness.

Temporal Response Properties

The ability of neurons in the ICC to synchronize their spike discharges to an auditory stimulus is referred to as temporal response properties. These properties allow for the encoding of sound features for speech recognition and word discrimination. Properties such as latency, jitter, and spike rate have been studied. Data are collected by presenting different electrical stimuli to deaf implanted animals, and modifying the duration of deafness, the duration of electrical stimulation, or the stimulus characteristics. Evidence suggests that early-onset deafness followed by chronic electrical stimulation of the auditory nerve may enhance the capacity of the ICC to encode high pulse frequencies, beyond those seen in normal hearing animals.[159] In addition, there is a maximum electrical pulse rate that may be encoded by the ICC, findings that have implications for stimulus parameters in the application of cochlear implants.[145,159] Neurons in the ICC also appear to have higher temporal resolution when stimulated using amplitude-modulated electrical pulses compared with unmodulated stimuli.[160] Most ICC neurons are able to encode frequency-modulated stimuli up to 40 Hz. The carrier pulse rate eliciting response of neurons in the ICC was 104 pulses per second in unmodulated stimuli. By amplitude-modulating the stimuli, carrier pulse rate could exceed 600 pulses per second. Distortion of the neural response was observed as the ratio of modulation to carrier rate approached one fourth to one sixth. This observation may be significant, because cochlear implants can exceed these parameters. Following chronic stimulation at high rates, the ICC seems able to increase its average maximum following-frequency.[161] High stimulation rates do not appear to impact the peak maximum following-frequency.

Increased latency and jitter of single unit responses were seen in long-term deaf, acutely stimulated cats.[145] Elevated stimulus levels ameliorated these changes. Significantly, chronically stimulating deaf cats at high rates reduced the median latency below that seen in normal-hearing cats.[161] Overall, the ICC appears to retain the basic neural properties exhibited by normal-hearing animals. Chronic electrical stimulation may increase the temporal resolving capacity of the ICC, but the significance of this observation remains unknown.

◆ The Auditory Cortex

In 1942 Woolsey and Walzl[162] reported the first cortical responses to electrical stimulation of the auditory nerve in normal-hearing cats. Subsequently, the primary auditory cortex (AI) in the normal-hearing animal was shown to be cochleotopically organized, and individual neurons within layer III/IV have well-characterized input-output functions for electrical stimulation and decreasing response latencies (to a minimum around 8 milliseconds) with increasing stimulus strength.[163–166]

The changes in the auditory cortex after a SNHL are dependent on many factors, including the severity of the SNHL, whether the SNHL is unilateral or bilateral, and the developmental stage at the time of the SNHL. A further complication in the interpretation of changes in the auditory cortex in response to a SNHL, is that many "downstream" changes occur as a result of the SNHL (see previous sections), which effect the input, and the organization of that input, into the auditory cortex. At least some of the changes that occur in the auditory cortex as a result of a SNHL are plastic, and the return of input to the auditory cortex, via electrical stimulation of the auditory nerve, results in the reorganization of the auditory cortex. It is the plastic nature of the auditory cortex that is likely to be an underlying factor in the continued improvement in performance of cochlear implant patients with device use.[167]

Morphological Changes Following Deafness

In contrast to the lower auditory centers, there is a scarcity of data on the morphologic changes that occur in the auditory cortex as a result of a long-term SNHL.[168] Nonetheless, reports of research in rabbits that were unilaterally deafened as neonates indicate that there is no change in neuron soma area, number of dendritic branches, or total basal dendritic length.[169] However, there is an apparent reduction in the number of spines along basal dendrites of lamina III/IV pyramidal neurons of the auditory cortex,[170] and a reorganization of "spine-free" but not "spiny" dendrites, with an increase in "nonspiny" dendrite length mostly in a tangential direction.[171] In combination, these results indicate a loss of synapses within the auditory cortex after a prolonged deprivation of auditory input during development.

Although there have been reports that after pure tone stimulation the location of c-FOS–positive neurons within the auditory cortex (c-FOS is a protein associated with learning[172]) matched the expected tonotopic organization,[173] there have been no reports of the effects of SNHL on either its localization or expression.

Physiologic Changes Following Deafness

The motto "use it or lose it" is often apt for cortical centers, and so reports of the activation of the auditory cortex by other modalities after an early SNHL are not surprising.[174–176] However, as is the case for the ICC, there is evidence of the development of a "rudimentary cochleotopic representation" within AI, even when completely deprived of input.[168,177] Other "higher-order" cortical auditory centers, including the secondary auditory cortex, on the

other hand, appear to be more susceptible to "infiltration" from other modalities and exhibit more plasticity than AI in the cat.[178,179]

Field potentials and single- and multiunit recordings from layers III/IV of the auditory cortex in the DWC have shown that not only is a rudimentary cochleotopic representation present, but basic response properties, including growth functions and latencies, were similar to those in normal-hearing cats.[177] Corroborating results have been reported for short-term neonatally deafened cats,[180] although the cochleotopic organization was less robust, particularly in the dorsal part of AI, and became further degraded throughout the entire AI with extended periods of deafness.

Clearly, the AI does not develop entirely normally in the absence of sensory input; in fact there are different changes in the development of different layers within AI. Although the DWC develops a rudimentary cochleotopic representation in layers III/IV, there is a decrease in current sinks (and, therefore, presumably synaptic currents) at long (>30 milliseconds) latencies in layers II, III, and IV.[181] The decrease in current sinks is even more evident in the deeper (infragranular) layers IV, V, and VI, and in these deeper layers the decrease is evident at all latencies. The infragranular layers are considered to be the output layers of AI, and therefore, in the DWC "efferent projections of the primary auditory cortex to sub-cortical structures and possibly also to higher-order cortical areas are probably substantially diminished."[182]

The effects of a restricted unilateral SNHL in adult animals, resulting from a cochlea lesion, and subsequent exposure to at least some auditory input, rather than a complete bilateral SNHL, are apparent in the reorganization of the contralateral AI. Under such conditions, the normal cochleotopic organization of the contralateral AI is distorted, and acoustic frequencies that correspond to regions of cochlea near the lesion-edge become grossly overrepresented.[183–186] A unilateral SNHL not only affects the contralateral AI, but also results in the ipsilateral AI becoming more sensitive.[185,187–189] Such reorganization could be due to "rapid disinhibition or true plastic reorganization with morphological changes,"[182] and a contribution from the reorganization of interhemispheric corticocortical projections cannot be excluded.

Many of the studies of SNHL-induced changes in the auditory cortex utilize congenitally or neonatally deafened animal models, which allow access to the early critical period in development. However, changes in the response of neurons within the auditory cortex to a SNHL are not limited to this critical period, but can occur later in development.[189] There is a growing body of work supporting the plasticity of the adult auditory cortex, including AI.[190–192]

Response to Chronic Electrical Stimulation

Chronic, behaviorally relevant, intracochlear electrical stimulation results in plastic changes in the deaf auditory cortex. Compared with unstimulated deaf controls, cats subjected to chronic electrical stimulation exhibit an increase in long-latency (>150 milliseconds) field potentials, larger current source densities (particularly in layers II and III) and more sustained single- and multiunit activity.[193] There is also an expansion in the area of cortex activated by the electrical stimulation of the auditory nerve.[193] The resulting response properties of AI in chronically stimulated deaf cats are similar to those reported in normal-hearing animals. The long-latency responses are thought to be mediated by corticothalamic loops, and are proposed to be essential for short-term memory and processing in higher-order auditory centers.[182] Therefore, behaviorally relevant, chronic intracochlear electrical stimulation appears to allow the auditory cortex to achieve an experience-dependent maturation, albeit not precisely as it would have occurred in the absence of a SNHL.

Clinical Changes Following Deafness

Many of the reports of changes in the auditory cortex in deaf patients, as in the animal studies of the cortex, have been focused on the "use it or lose it" scenario.[194] Therefore, it comes as no surprise that it has been reported that in prelingual deaf patients "the brain region usually reserved for hearing may be activated by other sensory modalities."[195] However, the auditory deprivation–induced "takeover" of auditory areas appears to be limited to secondary auditory areas (supratemporal gyrus/perisylvian region), which are normally used for auditory processing and language.[195–197]

Consistent with results reported from the animal models, the connections to AI appear to be more robustly organized than those to the secondary auditory areas, as there is no evidence of cross-modal activation of AI using either positron emission tomography (PET)[198] or functional magnetic resonance imaging (fMRI).[199] Auditory evoked potentials recorded from both cochlear implant and normal hearing subjects also suggest near-normal maturation of middle (IV and deep III) cortical layers. However, there appears to be altered maturation or input to the superficial (II, upper III) layers,[200] particularly in the absence of auditory input during the early critical period.[201,202] Therefore, as in the animal models, it appears that the auditory cortex, and in particular AI, remains in an immature state in prelingual deaf patients.[203]

Ipsilateral-contralateral differences in the responses of the auditory cortex in unilaterally deaf subjects are smaller than in normal-hearing subjects [magnetoencephalogram (MEG)[204–207] and fMRI[208]]. The ipsilateral-contralateral changes can also occur in adult subjects as a result of a late-onset unilateral hearing loss,[209] again highlighting the plasticity of the auditory system in the adult brain. Some changes may manifest within weeks of the hearing loss,[210] but changes continue to occur over a prolonged time course of 2 years or more,[209] suggesting there may be both an unmasking of ordinarily silent inputs and morphologic changes. Interestingly, changes in the response of the ipsilateral auditory cortex may also be dependent on which side the unilateral deafness occurred,[211] indicating that these changes may be at least partially a result of changes peripheral to the auditory cortex. These results emphasize the difficulties in determining if functional changes in the response of the auditory cortex are the result of changes within the cortex itself, or a result of downstream changes.

Despite many years of auditory deprivation, during which very low levels of activity are evident in AI, its activation can be seen using a variety of imaging techniques after the return of auditory input via a cochlear implant.[212–215] In fact, after long-term cochlear implant use, auditory evoked potentials recorded from prelingual deaf patients, implanted in early childhood, appear nearly normal, suggesting an activation-induced maturation of the auditory cortex.[216] There are also plastic changes within the "higher-order" auditory centers, with the amount of activity in these centers in prelingual deaf patients with a cochlear implant decreasing with experience in using the implant.[217] There also is less activity seen in the higher-order auditory centers in prelingual deaf cochlear implant patients than in postlingual deaf cochlear implant patients.[218] Finally, long-term cochlear implant use also appears to enhance "top-down" feedback modulation of processing within lower auditory centers.[194]

A final interesting observation is that there is a positive correlation between speech perception and low resting activity in AI prior to cochlear implantation for the prelingual deaf.[217] This relationship suggests that although AI and other higher-order auditory centers are capable of plastic change, as evident in the continued improvement in auditory performance with increasing experience using a cochlear implant,[167] the best clinical outcomes for cochlear implant patients may in fact occur with the most immature auditory cortex, or the "cleanest sheet."

◆ Conclusions

Auditory experience plays a key role in laying down the fine organizational structure of the auditory pathway onto a framework generated by genetic cues. A lack of auditory experience during development results in a more rudimentary pathway; however, this reduced level of organization appears sufficient to provide both the temporal and spatial cues necessary for speech perception using a cochlear implant. Importantly, the ability of this pathway to undergo plastic reorganization following cochlear implantation is now recognized as a major factor underlying the clinical success of these devices. This chapter reviewed the degenerative and atrophic changes that occur within the auditory pathway following a SNHL and the trophic and functional reorganization that occurs following reafferentation via a cochlear implant.

Acknowledgments

This work was funded by the National Institutes of Health–National Institute on Deafness and Other Communication Disorders (NIDCD) (DC00232 and DC00027 and NO1-DC-3–1005), the Wagstaff Fellowship from the Royal Victorian Eye and Ear Hospital, and the Bionic Ear Institute. Sarah McGuiness, Rodney Millard, Stephanie Epp, and Anne Coco made important contributions to this work, and Dexter Irvine provided critical comment on an earlier version of this chapter, for which we are most grateful.

References

1. Grill WM. Electrical stimulation of the peripheral nervous system: biophysics and excitation properties. In: Horch KW, Dhillon GS, eds. Neuroprosthetics: Theory and Practice, vol 2. Singapore: World Scientific Publishing, 2004:319–341

2. Gantz BJ, Woodworth GG, Knutson JF, Abbas PJ, Tyler RS. Multivariate predictors of audiological success with multichannel cochlear implants. Ann Otol Rhinol Laryngol 1993;102:909–916

3. Nadol JB Jr, Young YS, Glynn RJ. Survival of spiral ganglion cells in profound sensorineural hearing loss: implications for cochlear implantation. Ann Otol Rhinol Laryngol 1989;98:411–416

4. Terayama Y, Kaneko Y, Kawamoto K, Sakai N. Ultrastructural changes of the nerve elements following disruption of the organ of Corti. I. Nerve elements in the organ of Corti. Acta Otolaryngol 1977;83:291–302

5. Spoendlin H. Factors inducing retrograde degeneration of the cochlear nerve. Ann Otol Rhinol Laryngol Suppl 1984;112:76–82

6. Hardie NA, Shepherd RK. Sensorineural hearing loss during development: morphological and physiological response of the cochlea and auditory brainstem. Hear Res 1999;128:147–165

7. Leake PA, Hradek GT. Cochlear pathology of long term neomycin induced deafness in cats. Hear Res 1988;33:11–33

8. Shepherd RK, Hardie NA. Deafness induced changes in the auditory pathway: implications for cochlear implants. Audiol Neurootol 2001;6:305–318

9. Spoendlin H, Schrott A. Analysis of the human auditory nerve. Hear Res 1989;43:25–38

10. Elverland HH, Mair IW. Hereditary deafness in the cat. An electron microscopic study of the spiral ganglion. Acta Otolaryngol 1980;90:360–369

11. Nadol JB Jr. Degeneration of cochlear neurons as seen in the spiral ganglion of man. Hear Res 1990;49:141–154

12. Steel KP, Bock GR. Electrically-evoked responses in animals with progressive spiral ganglion degeneration. Hear Res 1984;15:59–67

13. McGuinness SL, Shepherd RK. Exogenous BDNF rescues rat spiral ganglion neurons in vivo. Otol Neurotol 2005;26:1064–1072

14. Shepherd RK, Roberts LA, Paolini AG. Long-term sensorineural hearing loss induces functional changes in the rat auditory nerve. Eur J Neurosci 2004;20:3131–3140

15. Takeno S, Wake M, Mount RJ, Harrison RV. Degeneration of spiral ganglion cells in the chinchilla after inner hair cell loss induced by carboplatin. Audiol Neurootol 1998;3:281–290

16. Gillespie LN, Clark GM, Marzella PL. Delayed neurotrophin treatment supports auditory neuron survival in deaf guinea pigs. Neuroreport 2004;15:1121–1125

17. Shepherd RK, Javel E. Electrical stimulation of the auditory nerve. I. Correlation of physiological responses with cochlear status. Hear Res 1997;108:112–144

18. Heid S, Hartmann R, Klinke R. A model for prelingual deafness, the congenitally deaf white cat–population statistics and degenerative changes. Hear Res 1998;115:101–112

19. Mair IW. Hereditary deafness in the white cat. Acta Otolaryngol Suppl 1973;314:1–48

20. Ryugo DK, Rosenbaum BT, Kim PJ, Niparko JK, Saada AA. Single unit recordings in the auditory nerve of congenitally deaf white cats: morphological correlates in the cochlea and cochlear nucleus. J Comp Neurol 1998;397:532–548

21. Liberman MC, Kiang NY. Acoustic trauma in cats. Cochlear pathology and auditory-nerve activity. Acta Otolaryngol Suppl 1978;358:1–63

22. Johnsson LG. Sequence of degeneration of Corti's organ and its first-order neurons. Ann Otol Rhinol Laryngol 1974;83:294–303

23. Suzuka Y, Schuknecht HF. Retrograde cochlear neuronal degeneration in human subjects. Acta Otolaryngol Suppl 1988;450:1–20

24. Imamura S, Adams JC. Distribution of gentamicin in the guinea pig inner ear after local or systemic application. J Assoc Res Otolaryngol 2003;4:176–195

25. Ylikoski J, Pirvola U, Moshnyakov M, Palgi J, Arumae U, Saarma M. Expression patterns of neurotrophin and their receptor mRNAs in the rat inner ear. Hear Res 1993;65:69–78

26. Schecterson LC, Bothwell M. Neurotrophin and neurotrophin receptor mRNA expression in developing inner ear. Hear Res 1994;73:92–100

27. Fritzsch B, Barbacid M, Silos-Santiago I. Nerve dependency of developing and mature sensory receptor cells. Ann N Y Acad Sci 1998;855:14–27

28. Ernfors P, Van De Water T, Loring J, Jaenisch R. Complementary roles of BDNF and NT-3 in vestibular and auditory development. Neuron 1995;14:1153–1164

29. Stankovic K, Rio C, Xia A, et al. Survival of adult spiral ganglion neurons requires erbB receptor signaling in the inner ear. J Neurosci 2004;24:8651–8661

30. Hinojosa R, Marion M. Histopathology of profound sensorineural deafness. Ann N Y Acad Sci 1983;405:459–484

31. Nadol JB Jr. Patterns of neural degeneration in the human cochlea and auditory nerve: implications for cochlear implantation. Otolaryngol Head Neck Surg 1997;117(3 pt 1):220–228

32. Otte J, Schuknecht HF, Kerr AG. Ganglion cell populations in normal and pathological human cochleae. Implications for cochlear implantation. Laryngoscope 1978;88(8 pt 1):1231–1246

33. Felix H, Pollak A, Gleeson M, Johnsson LG. Degeneration pattern of human first-order cochlear neurons. Adv Otorhinolaryngol 2002;59:116–123

34. Miura M, Sando I, Hirsch BE, Orita Y. Analysis of spiral ganglion cell populations in children with normal and pathological ears. Ann Otol Rhinol Laryngol 2002;111(12 pt 1):1059–1065

35. Waltzman SB, Cohen NL, Green J, Roland JT Jr. Long-term effects of cochlear implants in children. Otolaryngol Head Neck Surg 2002;126:505–511

36. Javel E, Shepherd RK. Electrical stimulation of the auditory nerve. III. Response initiation sites and temporal fine structure. Hear Res 2000;140:45–76

37. Hartmann R, Topp G, Klinke R. Discharge patterns of cat primary auditory fibers with electrical stimulation of the cochlea. Hear Res 1984;13:47–62

38. van den Honert C, Stypulkowski PH. Physiological properties of the electrically stimulated auditory nerve. II. Single fiber recordings. Hear Res 1984;14:225–243

39. Frijns JH, de Snoo SL, ten Kate JH. Spatial selectivity in a rotationally symmetric model of the electrically stimulated cochlea. Hear Res 1996;95:33–48

40. Tasaki I. New measurements of the capacity and the resistance of the myelin sheath and the nodal membrane of the isolated frog nerve fiber. Am J Physiol 1955;181:639–650

41. Koles ZJ, Rasminsky M. A computer simulation of conduction in demyelinated nerve fibres. J Physiol 1972;227:351–364

42. Zhou R, Abbas PJ, Assouline JG. Electrically evoked auditory brainstem response in peripherally myelin-deficient mice. Hear Res 1995;88:98–106

43. Araki S, Kawano A, Seldon L, Shepherd RK, Funasaka S, Clark GM. Effects of chronic electrical stimulation on spiral ganglion neuron survival and size in deafened kittens. Laryngoscope 1998;108:687–695

44. Xu J, Shepherd RK, Millard RE, Clark GM. Chronic electrical stimulation of the auditory nerve at high stimulus rates: a physiological and histopathological study. Hear Res 1997;105:1–29

45. Shepherd RK, Matsushima J, Martin RL, Clark GM. Cochlear pathology following chronic electrical stimulation of the auditory nerve: II. Deafened kittens. Hear Res 1994;81:150–166

46. Ni D, Shepherd RK, Seldon HL, Xu S-A, Clark GM, Millard RE. Cochlear pathology following chronic electrical stimulation of the auditory nerve. I: normal hearing kittens. Hear Res 1992;62:63–81

47. Shepherd RK, Clark GM, Black RC. Chronic electrical stimulation of the auditory nerve in cats. Physiological and histopathological results. Acta Otolaryngol Suppl 1983;399:19–31

48. Leake-Jones PA, Rebscher SJ. Cochlear pathology with chronically implanted scala tympani electrodes. Ann N Y Acad Sci 1983;405:203–223

49. Walsh SM, Leake-Jones PA. Chronic electrical stimulation of auditory nerve in cat: physiological and histological results. Hear Res 1982;7:281–304

50. Brummer SB, Turner MJ. Electrochemical considerations for safe electrical stimulation of the nervous system with platinum electrodes. IEEE Trans Biomed Eng 1977;24:59–63

51. Robblee LS, McHardy J, Agnew WF, Bullara LA. Electrical stimulation with Pt electrodes. VII. Dissolution of Pt electrodes during electrical

stimulation of the cat cerebral cortex. J Neurosci Methods 1983;9:301–308

52. Rose TL, Robblee LS. Electrical stimulation with Pt electrodes. VIII. Electrochemically safe charge injection limits with 0.2 ms pulses. IEEE Trans Biomed Eng 1990;37:1118–1120

53. Shepherd RK, Linahan N, Xu J, Clark GM, Araki S. Chronic electrical stimulation of the auditory nerve using non-charge-balanced stimuli. Acta Otolaryngol 1999;119:674–684

54. Shepherd RK, Matsushima J, Millard RE, Clark GM. Cochlear pathology following chronic electrical stimulation using non-charge balanced stimuli. Acta Otolaryngol 1991;111:848–860

55. Huang CQ, Carter PM, Shepherd RK. Stimulus induced pH changes in cochlear implants: an in vitro and in vivo study. Ann Biomed Eng 2001;29:791–802

56. Huang CQ, Shepherd RK, Carter PM, Seligman PM, Tabor B. Electrical stimulation of the auditory nerve: direct current measurement in vivo. IEEE Trans Biomed Eng 1999;46:461–470

57. Hegarty JL, Kay AR, Green SH. Trophic support of cultured spiral ganglion neurons by depolarization exceeds and is additive with that by neurotrophins or cAMP and requires elevation of [Ca2+]i within a set range. J Neurosci 1997;17:1959–1970

58. Hansen MR, Zha XM, Bok J, Green SH. Multiple distinct signal pathways, including an autocrine neurotrophic mechanism, contribute to the survival-promoting effect of depolarization on spiral ganglion neurons in vitro. J Neurosci 2001;21:2256–2267

59. Lousteau RJ. Increased spiral ganglion cell survival in electrically stimulated, deafened guinea pig cochleae. Laryngoscope 1987;97:836–842

60. Hartshorn DO, Miller JM, Altschuler RA. Protective effect of electrical stimulation in the deafened guinea pig cochlea. Otolaryngol Head Neck Surg 1991;104:311–319

61. Miller CA, Faulkner MJ, Pfingst BE. Functional responses from guinea pigs with cochlear implants. II. Changes in electrophysiological and psychophysical measures over time. Hear Res 1995;92:100–111

62. Mitchell A, Miller JM, Finger PA, Heller JW, Raphael Y, Altschuler RA. Effects of chronic high-rate electrical stimulation on the cochlea and eighth nerve in the deafened guinea pig. Hear Res 1997;105:30–43

63. Kanzaki S, Stover T, Kawamoto K, et al. Glial cell line-derived neurotrophic factor and chronic electrical stimulation prevent VIII cranial nerve degeneration following denervation. J Comp Neurol 2002;454:350–360

64. Leake PA, Hradek GT, Rebscher SJ, Snyder RL. Chronic intracochlear electrical stimulation induces selective survival of spiral ganglion neurons in neonatally deafened cats. Hear Res 1991;54:251–271

65. Leake PA, Snyder RL, Hradek GT, Rebscher SJ. Chronic intracochlear electrical stimulation in neonatally deafened cats: effects of intensity and stimulating electrode location. Hear Res 1992;64:99–117

66. Leake PA, Snyder RL, Hradek GT, Rebscher SJ. Consequences of chronic extracochlear electrical stimulation in neonatally deafened cats. Hear Res 1995;82:65–80

67. Leake PA, Hradek GT, Snyder RL. Chronic electrical stimulation by a cochlear implant promotes survival of spiral ganglion neurons after neonatal deafness. J Comp Neurol 1999;412:543–562

68. Li L, Parkins CW, Webster DB. Does electrical stimulation of deaf cochleae prevent spiral ganglion degeneration? Hear Res 1999;133:27–39

69. Shepherd R, Coco A, Epp S, Crook JM. Chronic depolarization enhances the trophic effects of BDNF in rescuing auditory neurons following a sensorineural hearing loss. J Comp Neurol 2005;486:145–158

70. Fritzsch B, Pirvola U, Ylikoski J. Making and breaking the innervation of the ear: neurotrophic support during ear development and its clinical implications. Cell Tissue Res 1999;295:369–382

71. Lefebvre PP, Weber T, Rigo J-M, Staecker H, Moonen G, Van De Water TR. Peripheral and central target-derived trophic factor(s) effects on auditory neurons. Hear Res 1992;58:185–192

72. Ernfors P, Duan ML, ElShamy WM, Canlon B. Protection of auditory neurons from aminoglycoside toxicity by neurotrophin-3. Nat Med 1996;2:463–467

73. Miller JM, Chi DH, O'Keeffe LJ, Kruszka P, Raphael Y, Altschuler RA. Neurotrophins can enhance spiral ganglion cell survival after inner hair cell loss. Int J Dev Neurosci 1997;15:631–643

74. Staecker H, Kopke R, Malgrange B, Lefebvre P, Van de Water TR. NT-3 and/or BDNF therapy prevents loss of auditory neurons following loss of hair cells. Neuroreport 1996;7:889–894

75. Shinohara T, Bredberg G, Ulfendahl M, et al. Neurotrophic factor intervention restores auditory function in deafened animals. Proc Natl Acad Sci U S A 2002;99:1657–1660

76. Wise AK, Richardson R, Hardman J, Clark G, O'Leary S. Resprouting and survival of guinea pig cochlear neurons in response to the administration of the neurotrophins brain-derived neurotrophic factor and neurotrophin-3. J Comp Neurol 2005;487:147–165

77. Gillespie LN, Clark GM, Bartlett PF, Marzella PL. BDNF-induced survival of auditory neurons in vivo: Cessation of treatment leads to an accelerated loss of survival effects. J Neurosci Res 2003;71:785–790

78. Powell TPS, Erulkar SD. Transneuronal cell degeneration in the auditory relay nuclei of the cat. J Anat 1962;96:249–268

79. Webster DB. A critical period during postnatal auditory development of mice. Int J Pediatr Otorhinolaryngol 1983;6:107–118

80. Webster DB. Conductive hearing loss affects the growth of the cochlear nuclei over an extended period of time. Hear Res 1988;32:185–192

81. Hashisaki GT, Rubel EW. Effects of unilateral cochlea removal on anteroventral cochlear nucleus neurons in developing gerbils. J Comp Neurol 1989;283:5–73

82. Ryugo DK, Pongstaporn T, Huchton DM, Niparko JK. Ultrastructural analysis of primary endings in deaf white cats: morphologic alterations in endbulbs of Held. J Comp Neurol 1997;385:230–244

83. Sininger YS, Doyle KJ, Moore JK. The case for early identification of hearing loss in children. Auditory system development, experimental auditory deprivation, and development of speech perception and hearing. Pediatr Clin North Am 1999;46:1–14

84. Marianowski R, Liao WH, Van Den Abbeele T, et al. Expression of NMDA, AMPA and GABA(A) receptor subunit mRNAs in the rat auditory brainstem. I. Influence of early auditory deprivation. Hear Res 2000;150:1–11

85. Clark GM, Shepherd RK, Franz BK, et al. The histopathology of the human temporal bone and auditory central nervous system following cochlear implantation in a patient. Correlation with psychophysics and speech perception results. Acta Otolaryngol Suppl 1988;448:1–65

86. Seldon HL, Clark GM. Human cochlear nucleus: comparison of Nissl-stained neurons from deaf and hearing patients. Brain Res 1991;551:185–194

87. Moore JK, Niparko JK, Miller MR, Linthicum FH. Effect of profound hearing loss on a central auditory nucleus. Am J Otol 1994;15:588–595

88. Moore JK, Niparko JK, Perazzo LM, Miller MR, Linthicum FH. Effect of adult-onset deafness on the human central auditory system. Ann Otol Rhinol Laryngol 1997;106:385–390

89. Waltzman SB, Cohen NL, Shapiro WH. Effects of chronic electrical stimulation on patients using a cochlear prosthesis. Otolaryngol Head Neck Surg 1991;105:797–801

90. Niparko JK, Kirk KI, Mellon NK, Robbins AM, Tucci DL, Wilson BS. Cochlear Implants: Principles and Practices. Philadelphia: Lippincott Williams & Wilkins, 2000

91. Sarant JZ, Blamey PJ, Dowell RC, Clark GM, Gibson WP. Variation in speech perception scores among children with cochlear implants. Ear Hear 2001;22:18–28

92. Tucci DL, Rubel EW. Afferent influences on brain stem auditory nuclei of the chicken: effects of conductive and sensorineural hearing loss on n. magnocellularis. J Comp Neurol 1985;238:371–381

93. Hood LJ, Webster DB. Reversible conductive hearing loss in mice. Ann Otol Rhinol Laryngol 1988;97(3 pt 1):281–285

94. Doyle WJ, Webster DB. Neonatal conductive hearing loss does not compromise brainstem auditory function and structure in rhesus monkeys. Hear Res 1991;54:145–151

95. Moore DR, Hine JE, Jiang ZD, Matsuda H, Parsons CH, King AJ. Conductive hearing loss produces a reversible binaural hearing impairment. J Neurosci 1999;19:8704–8711

96. Trune DR. Influence of neonatal cochlear removal on the development of mouse cochlear nucleus: I. Number, size, and density of its neuronal. J Comp Neurol 1982;209:409–424

97. Moore DR, Kowalchuk NE. Auditory brainstem of the ferret: effects of unilateral cochlear lesions on cochlear nucleus volume and projections to the inferior colliculus. J Comp Neurol 1988;272:503–515

98. Tierney TS, Russell FA, Moore DR. Susceptibility of developing cochlear nucleus neurons to deafferentation-induced death abruptly ends just before the onset of hearing. J Comp Neurol 1997;378:295–306

99. Mostafapour SP, Cochran SL, Del Puerto NM, Rubel EW. Patterns of cell death in mouse anteroventral cochlear nucleus neurons after unilateral cochlea removal. J Comp Neurol 2000;426:561–571

100. Marot M, Uziel A, Romand R. Ototoxicity of kanamycin in developing rats: relationship with the onset of the auditory function. Hear Res 1980;2:111–113

101. Shepherd RK, Martin RL. Onset of ototoxicity in the cat is related to onset of auditory function. Hear Res 1995;92:131–142

102. O'Leary SJ, Moore DR. Development of cochlear sensitivity to aminoglycoside antibiotics. Ann Otol Rhinol Laryngol 1998;107:220–226

103. Hawkins JE Jr. Comparative otopathology: aging, noise, and ototoxic drugs. Adv Otorhinolaryngol 1973;20:125–141

104. Russell NJ, Fox KE, Brummett RE. Ototoxic effects of the interaction between kanamycin and ethacrynic acid. Cochlear ultrastructure correlated with cochlear potentials and kanamycin levels. Acta Otolaryngol 1979;88:369–381

105. Fleckeisen CE, Harrison RV, Mount RJ. Effects of total cochlear haircell loss on integrity of cochlear nucleus. A quantitative study. Acta Otolaryngol Suppl 1991;489:23–31

106. Lustig LR, Leake PA, Snyder RL, Rebscher SJ. Changes in the cat cochlear nucleus following neonatal deafening and chronic intracochlear electrical stimulation. Hear Res 1994;74:29–37

107. Lesperance MM, Helfert RH, Altschuler RA. Deafness induced cell size changes in rostal AVCN of the guinea pig. Hear Res 1995;86:77–81

108. Russell FA, Moore DR. Effects of unilateral cochlear removal on dendrites in the gerbil medial superior olivary nucleus. Eur J Neurosci 1999;11:1379–1390

109. West CD, Harrison JM. Transneuronal cell atrophy in the congenitally deaf white cat. J Comp Neurol 1973;151:377–398

110. Bosher SK, Hallpike CS. Observations on the histological features, development and pathogenesis of the inner ear degeneration of the deaf white cat. Proc R Soc Lond B Biol Sci 1965;162:147–170

111. Schwartz IR, Higa JF. Correlated studies of the ear and brainstem in the deaf white cat: changes in the spiral ganglion and the medial superior olivary nucleus. Acta Otolaryngol 1982;93:9–18

112. Heid S, Jähn-Siebert TK, Klinke R, Hartmann R, Langner G. Afferent projection patterns in the auditory brainstem in normal and congenitally deaf white cats. Hear Res 1997;110:191–199

113. Redd EE, Pongstaporn T, Ryugo DK. The effects of congenital deafness on auditory nerve synapses and globular bushy cells in cats. Hear Res 2000;147:160–174

114. Brown KS, Bergsma DR, Barrow MV. Animal models of pigment and hearing abnormalities in man. Birth Defects Orig Artic Ser 1971;7:102–109

115. Rawitz B. Gehörorgan und gehirn eines weissen Hundes mit blauen Augen. Morphol Arbeit 1896;6:545–554

116. Bamber RC. Correlation between white coat colour, blue eyes and deafness in cats. J Genet 1933;27:407–413

117. Wolff D. Three generations of deaf white cats. J Hered 1942;33:39–43

118. Wilson TG, Kane F. Congenital deafness in white cats. Acta Otolaryngol 1959;50:269–275 discussion 275–267

119. Bergsma DR, Brown KS. White fur, blue eyes, and deafness in the domestic cat. J Hered 1971;62:171–185

120. Ryugo DK, Cahill HB, Rose LS, Rosenbaum BT, Schroeder ME, Wright AL. Separate forms of pathology in the cochlea of congenitally deaf white cats. Hear Res 2003;181:73–84

121. Scheibe A. A case of deaf-mutism with auditory atrophy and anomalies of development in the membranous labyrinth of both ears. Arch Otolaryngol 1892;21:12–22

122. Scheibe A. Bildungsanomalien im hautigen labyrinth bei taubstummheit. Z Ohrenheilk 1895;27:95–99

123. Pujol R, Rebillard M, Rebillard G. Primary neural disorders in the deaf white cat cochlea. Acta Otolaryngol 1977;83:59–64

124. Rebillard M, Rebillard G, Pujol R. Variability of the hereditary deafness in the white cat. I. Physiology. Hear Res 1981;5:179–187

125. Rebillard M, Pujol R, Rebillard G. Variability of the hereditary deafness in the white cat. II. Histology. Hear Res 1981;5:189–200

126. Larsen SA, Kirchhoff TM. Anatomical evidence of synaptic plasticity in the cochlear nuclei of white-deaf cats. Exp Neurol 1992;115:151–157

127. Saada AA, Niparko JK, Ryugo DK. Morphological changes in the cochlear nucleus of congenitally deaf white cats. Brain Res 1996;736:315–328

128. Redd EE, Cahill HB, Pongstaporn T, Ryugo DK. The effects of congenital deafness on auditory nerve synapses: type I and type II multipolar cells in the anteroventral cochlear nucleus of cats. J Assoc Res Otolaryngol 2002;3:403–417

129. Ryugo DK, Sento S. Auditory nerve terminals and cochlear nucleus neurons: endbulb of Held and spherical bushy cells. In: Ainsworth WA, ed. Advances in Speech, Hearing and Language Processing. London: Jai Press, 1996:19–40

130. Francis HW, Manis PB. Effects of deafferentation on the electrophysiology of ventral cochlear nucleus neurons. Hear Res 2000;149:91–105

131. Chouard CH, Meyer B, Josset P, Buche JF. The effect of the acoustic nerve chronic electric stimulation upon the guinea pig cochlear nucleus development. Acta Otolaryngol 1983;95:639–645

132. Hultcrantz M, Snyder R, Rebscher S, Leake P. Effects of neonatal deafening and chronic intracochlear electrical stimulation on the cochlear nucleus in cats. Hear Res 1991;54:272–280

133. Matsushima J-I, Shepherd RK, Seldon HL, Xu S-A, Clark GM. Electrical stimulation of the auditory nerve in deaf kittens: effects on cochlear nucleus morphology. Hear Res 1991;56:133–142

134. Bourk TR, Mielcarz JP, Norris BE. Tonotopic organization of the anteroventral cochlear nucleus of the cat. Hear Res 1981;4:215–241

135. Cant NB, Gaston KC. Pathways connecting the right and left cochlear nuclei. J Comp Neurol 1982;212:313–326

136. Wenthold RJ. Evidence for a glycinergic pathway connecting the two cochlear nuclei: an immunocytochemical and retrograde transport study. Brain Res 1987;415:183–187

137. Shore SE, Godfrey DA, Helfert RH, Altschuler RA, Bledsoe SC Jr. Connections between the cochlear nuclei in guinea pig. Hear Res 1992;62:16–26

138. Schofield BR, Cant NB. Projections from the ventral cochlear nucleus to the inferior colliculus and the contralateral cochlear nucleus in guinea pigs. Hear Res 1996;102:1–14

139. Schofield BR, Cant NB. Origins and targets of commissural connections between the cochlear nuclei in guinea pigs. J Comp Neurol 1996;375:128–146

140. Moore DR, Kitzes LM. Projections from the cochlear nucleus to the inferior colliculus in normal and neonatally cochlea-ablated gerbils. J Comp Neurol 1985;240:180–195

141. Nordeen KW, Killackey HP, Kitzes LM. Ascending projections to the inferior colliculus following unilateral cochlear ablation in the neonatal gerbil, *Meriones unguiculatus*. J Comp Neurol 1983;214:144–153

142. Russell FA, Moore DR. Afferent reorganisation within the superior olivary complex of the gerbil: development and induction by neonatal, unilateral cochlear removal. J Comp Neurol 1995;352:607–625

143. Jean-Baptiste M, Morest DK. Transneuronal changes of synaptic endings and nuclear chromatin in the trapezoid body following cochlear ablations in cats. J Comp Neurol 1975;162:111–134. http://www3.interscience.wiley.com/cgi-bin/abstract/109685039/ABSTRACT

144. Hardie NA, Martsi-McClintock A, Aitkin L, Shepherd RK. Neonatal sensorineural hearing loss affects synaptic density in the auditory midbrain. Neuroreport 1998;9:2019–2022

145. Shepherd RK, Baxi JH, Hardie NA. Response of inferior colliculus neurons to electrical stimulation of the auditory nerve in neonatally deafened cats. J Neurophysiol 1999;82:1363–1380

146. Nishiyama N, Hardie NA, Shepherd RK. Neonatal sensorineural hearing loss affects neurone size in cat auditory midbrain. Hear Res 2000;140:18–22

147. Vale C, Sanes DH. The effect of bilateral deafness on excitatory and inhibitory synaptic strength in the inferior colliculus. Eur J Neurosci 2002;16:2394–2404

148. Jahn AF, Santos-Sacchi J, eds. Physiology of the Ear. New York: Raven Press, 1988

149. Ehret G. The auditory midbrain, a "shunting-yard" of acoustical information processing. In: Ehret G, Romand R, eds. The Central Auditory System. Oxford: Oxford University Press, 1997:259–316

150. McAlpine D, Martin RL, Mossop JE, Moore DR. Response properties of neurons in the inferior colliculus of the monaurally deafened ferret to acoustic stimulation of the intact ear. J Neurophysiol 1997;78:767–779

151. Moore DR. Auditory brainstem of the ferret: bilateral cochlear lesions in infancy do not affect the number of neurons projecting from the cochlear nucleus to the inferior colliculus. Brain Res Dev Brain Res 1990;54:125–130

152. Brown M, Shepherd RK, Webster WR, Martin RL, Clark GM. Cochleo-topic selectivity of a multichannel scala tympani electrode array using the 2-deoxyglucose technique. Hear Res 1992;59: 224–240

153. el-Kashlan HK, Noorily AD, Niparko JK, Miller JM. Metabolic activity of the central auditory structures following prolonged deafferenta-tion. Laryngoscope 1993;103(4 pt 1):399–405

154. Schwartz DR, Schacht J, Miller JM, Frey K, Altschuler RA. Chronic elec-trical stimulation reverses deafness-related depression of electrically evoked 2-deoxyglucose activity in the guinea pig inferior colliculus. Hear Res 1993;70:243–249

155. Snyder RL, Rebscher SJ, Cao K, Leake PA, Kelly K. Chronic intracochlear electrical stimulation in the neonatally deafened cat. I: Expansion of central representation. Hear Res 1990;50:7–34

156. Moore CM, Vollmer M, Leake PA, Snyder RL, Rebscher SJ. The effects of chronic intracochlear electrical stimulation on inferior colliculus spatial representation in adult deafened cats. Hear Res 2002;164: 82–96

157. Snyder RL, Bierer JA, Middlebrooks JC. Topographic spread of inferior colliculus activation in response to acoustic and intracochlear electric stimulation. J Assoc Res Otolaryngol 2004;5:305–322

158. Leake PA, Snyder RL, Rebscher SJ, Moore CM, Vollmer M. Plasticity in central representations in the inferior colliculus induced by chronic single- vs. two-channel electrical stimulation by a cochlear implant after neonatal deafness. Hear Res 2000;147:221–241

159. Snyder R, Leake P, Rebscher S, Beitel R. Temporal resolution of neurons in cat inferior colliculus to intracochlear electrical stimulation: effects of neonatal deafening and chronic stimulation. J Neurophysiol 1995;73:449–467

160. Snyder RL, Vollmer M, Moore CM, Rebscher SJ, Leake PA, Beitel RE. Responses of inferior colliculus neurons to amplitude-modulated intracochlear electrical pulses in deaf cats. J Neurophysiol 2000;84:166–183

161. Vollmer M, Snyder RL, Leake PA, Beitel RE, Moore CM, Rebscher SJ. Temporal properties of chronic cochlear electrical stimulation determine temporal resolution of neurons in cat inferior colliculus. J Neurophysiol 1999;82:2883–2902

162. Woolsey CN, Walzl EM. Topical projection of nerve fibers from local regions of the cochlea to the cerebral cortex. Bull Johns Hopkins Hosp 1942;71:315–344

163. Popelar J, Hartmann R, Syka J, Klinke R. Middle latency responses to acoustical and electrical stimulation of the cochlea in cats. Hear Res 1995;92:63–77

164. Raggio MW, Schreiner CE. Neuronal responses in cat primary audi-tory cortex to electrical cochlear stimulation. I. Intensity dependence of firing rate and response latency. J Neurophysiol 1994;72: 2334–2359

165. Schreiner CE, Raggio MW. Neuronal responses in cat primary auditory cortex to electrical cochlear stimulation. II. Repetition rate coding. J Neurophysiol 1996;75:1283–1300

166. Raggio MW, Schreiner CE. Neuronal responses in cat primary auditory cortex to electrical cochlear stimulation: IV. Activation pattern for sinusoidal stimulation. J Neurophysiol 2003;89: 3190–3204

167. Blamey P, Arndt P, Bergeron F, et al. Factors affecting auditory per-formance of postlinguistically deaf adults using cochlear implants. Audiol Neurootol 1996;1:293–306

168. Shepherd RK, Hartmann R, Heid S, Hardie N, Klinke R. The central auditory system and auditory deprivation: experience with cochlear implants in the congenitally deaf. Acta Otolaryngol Suppl 1997;532: 28–33

169. McMullen NT, Goldberger B, Glaser EM. Postnatal development of lamina III/IV nonpyramidal neurons in rabbit auditory cortex: quan-titative and spatial analyses of Golgi-impregnated material. J Comp Neurol 1988;278:139–155

170. McMullen NT, Glaser EM. Auditory cortical responses to neonatal deafening: pyramidal neuron spine loss without changes in growth or orientation. Exp Brain Res 1988;72:195–200

171. McMullen NT, Goldberger B, Suter CM, Glaser EM. Neonatal deafening alters nonpyramidal dendrite orientation in auditory cortex: a com-puter microscope study in the rabbit. J Comp Neurol 1988;267: 92–106

172. Kandiel A, Chen S, Hillman DE. c-fos gene expression parallels auditory adaptation in the adult rat. Brain Res 1999;839:292–297

173. Zuschratter W, Gass P, Herdegen T, Scheich H. Comparison of frequency-specific c-Fos expression and fluoro-2-deoxyglucose uptake in auditory cortex of gerbils (Meriones unguiculatus). Eur J Neurosci 1995;7:1614–1626

174. Rebillard G, Rebillard M, Pujol R. Factors affecting the recording of visual-evoked potentials from the deaf cat primary auditory cortex (AI). Brain Res 1980;188:252–254

175. Rebillard G, Carlier E, Rebillard M, Pujol R. Enhancement of visual responses on the primary auditory cortex of the cat after an early destruction of cochlear receptors. Brain Res 1977;129:162–164

176. Ahn SH, Oh SH, Lee JS, et al. Changes of 2-deoxyglucose uptake in the rat auditory pathway after bilateral ablation of the cochlea. Hear Res 2004;196:33–38

177. Hartmann R, Shepherd RK, Heid S, Klinke R. Response of the primary auditory cortex to electrical stimulation of the auditory nerve in the congenitally deaf white cat. Hear Res 1997;112:115–133

178. Diamond DM, Weinberger NM. Physiological plasticity of single neurons in auditory cortex of the cat during acquisition of the pupil-lary conditioned response: II. Secondary field (AII). Behav Neurosci 1984;98:189–210

179. Weinberger NM, Hopkins W, Diamond DM. Physiological plasticity of single neurons in auditory cortex of the cat during acquisition of the pupillary conditioned response: I. Primary field (AI). Behav Neurosci 1984;98:171–188

180. Raggio MW, Schreiner CE. Neuronal responses in cat primary audi-tory cortex to electrical cochlear stimulation. III. Activation patterns in short- and long-term deafness. J Neurophysiol 1999;82:3506–3526

181. Kral A, Hartmann R, Tillein J, Heid S, Klinke R. Congenital auditory deprivation reduces synaptic activity within the auditory cortex in a layer-specific manner. Cereb Cortex 2000;10:714–726

182. Kral A, Hartmann R, Tillein J, Heid S, Klinke R. Delayed maturation and sensitive periods in the auditory cortex. Audiol Neurootol 2001;6:346–362

183. Robertson D, Irvine DR. Plasticity of frequency organization in audi-tory cortex of guinea pigs with partial unilateral deafness. J Comp Neurol 1989;282:456–471

184. Rajan R, Irvine DR, Wise LZ, Heil P. Effect of unilateral partial cochlear lesions in adult cats on the representation of lesioned and unlesioned cochleas in primary auditory cortex. J Comp Neurol 1993;338:17–49

185. Reale RA, Brugge JF, Chan JC. Maps of auditory cortex in cats reared after unilateral cochlear ablation in the neonatal period. Brain Res 1987;431:281–290

186. Reser DH, Fishman YI, Arezzo JC, Steinschneider M. Binaural inter-actions in primary auditory cortex of the awake macaque. Cereb Cortex 2000;10:574–584

187. Kitzes LM. Some physiological consequences of neonatal cochlear destruction in the inferior colliculus of the gerbil, Meriones unguicu-latus. Brain Res 1984;306:171–178

188. Kitzes LM, Hollrigel GS. Response properties of units in the posterior auditory field deprived of input from the ipsilateral primary auditory cortex. Hear Res 1996;100:120–130

189. Popelar J, Erre JP, Aran JM, Cazals Y. Plastic changes in ipsi-contralateral differences of auditory cortex and inferior colliculus evoked potentials after injury to one ear in the adult guinea pig. Hear Res 1994;72:125–134

190. Bao S, Chang EF, Davis JD, Gobeske KT, Merzenich MM. Progressive degradation and subsequent refinement of acoustic representations in the adult auditory cortex. J Neurosci 2003;23:10765–10775

191. Polley DB, Heiser MA, Blake DT, Schreiner CE, Merzenich MM. Associ-ative learning shapes the neural code for stimulus magnitude in primary auditory cortex. Proc Natl Acad Sci U S A 2004;101:16351–16356

192. Beitel RE, Schreiner CE, Cheung SW, Wang X, Merzenich MM. Reward-dependent plasticity in the primary auditory cortex of adult monkeys trained to discriminate temporally modulated signals. Proc Natl Acad Sci U S A 2003;100:11070–11075

193. Klinke R, Kral A, Heid S, Tillein J, Hartmann R. Recruitment of the auditory cortex in congenitally deaf cats by long-term cochlear elec-trostimulation. Science 1999;285:1729–1733

194. Giraud AL, Truy E, Frackowiak R. Imaging plasticity in cochlear implant patients. Audiol Neurootol 2001;6:381–393

195. Nishimura H, Hashikawa K, Doi K, et al. Sign language 'heard' in the auditory cortex. Nature 1999;397:116

196. Sadato N, Okada T, Honda M, et al. Cross-modal integration and plastic changes revealed by lip movement, random-dot motion and sign languages in the hearing and deaf. Cereb Cortex 2005;15:1113–1122

197. Petitto LA, Zatorre RJ, Gauna K, Nikelski EJ, Dostie D, Evans AC. Speech-like cerebral activity in profoundly deaf people processing

signed languages: implications for the neural basis of human language. Proc Natl Acad Sci U S A 2000;97:13961–13966

198.   Nishimura H, Doi K, Iwaki T, et al. Neural plasticity detected in short- and long-term cochlear implant users using PET. Neuroreport 2000;11:811–815

199.   Hickok G, Bellugi U, Klima ES. The basis of the neural organization for language: evidence from sign language aphasia. Rev Neurosci 1997;8:205–222

200.   Ponton CW, Eggermont JJ. Of kittens and kids: altered cortical maturation following profound deafness and cochlear implant use. Audiol Neurootol 2001;6:363–380

201.   Eggermont JJ, Ponton CW. Auditory-evoked potential studies of cortical maturation in normal hearing and implanted children: correlations with changes in structure and speech perception. Acta Otolaryngol 2003;123:249–252

202.   Sharma A, Dorman MF, Spahr AJ. A sensitive period for the development of the central auditory system in children with cochlear implants: implications for age of implantation. Ear Hear 2002;23:532–539

203.   Ponton CW, Don M, Eggermont JJ, Waring MD, Kwong B, Masuda A. Auditory system plasticity in children after long periods of complete deafness. Neuroreport 1996;8:61–65

204.   Vasama JP, Makela JP, Parkkonen L, Hari R. Auditory cortical responses in humans with congenital unilateral conductive hearing loss. Hear Res 1994;78:91–97

205.   Vasama JP, Makela JP. Auditory pathway plasticity in adult humans after unilateral idiopathic sudden sensorineural hearing loss. Hear Res 1995;87:132–140

206.   Vasama JP, Makela JP, Pyykko I, Hari R. Abrupt unilateral deafness modifies function of human auditory pathways. Neuroreport 1995;6:961–964

207.   Vasama JP, Makela JP. Auditory cortical responses in humans with profound unilateral sensorineural hearing loss from early childhood. Hear Res 1997;104:183–190

208.   Scheffler K, Bilecen D, Schmid N, Tschopp K, Seelig J. Auditory cortical responses in hearing subjects and unilateral deaf patients as detected by functional magnetic resonance imaging. Cereb Cortex 1998;8:156–163

209.   Ponton CW, Vasama JP, Tremblay K, Khosla D, Kwong B, Don M. Plasticity in the adult human central auditory system: evidence from late-onset profound unilateral deafness. Hear Res 2001;154:32–44

210.   Suzuki M, Kouzaki H, Nishida Y, Shiino A, Ito R, Kitano H. Cortical representation of hearing restoration in patients with sudden deafness. Neuroreport 2002;13:1829–1832

211.   Khosla D, Ponton CW, Eggermont JJ, Kwong B, Don M, Vasama JP. Differential ear effects of profound unilateral deafness on the adult human central auditory system. J Assoc Res Otolaryngol 2003;4:235–249

212.   Berthezene Y, Truy E, Morgon A, et al. Auditory cortex activation in deaf subjects during cochlear electrical stimulation. Evaluation by functional magnetic resonance imaging. Invest Radiol 1997;32:297–301

213.   Herzog H, Lamprecht A, Kuhn A, Roden W, Vosteen KH, Feinendegen LE. Cortical activation in profoundly deaf patients during cochlear implant stimulation demonstrated by H2(15)O PET. J Comput Assist Tomogr 1991;15:369–375

214.   Ito J, Sakakibara J, Iwasaki Y, Yonekura Y. Positron emission tomography of auditory sensation in deaf patients and patients with cochlear implants. Ann Otol Rhinol Laryngol 1993;102:797–801

215.   Ito J. Auditory cortex activities in severely hearing-impaired and cochlear implant patients. Positron emission tomographic study. Adv Otorhinolaryngol 1993;48:29–34

216.   Eggermont JJ, Ponton CW, Don M, Waring MD, Kwong B. Maturational delays in cortical evoked potentials in cochlear implant users. Acta Otolaryngol 1997;117:161–163

217.   Lee DS, Lee JS, Oh SH, et al. Cross-modal plasticity and cochlear implants. Nature 2001;409:149–150

218.   Naito Y, Hirano S, Honjo I, et al. Sound-induced activation of auditory cortices in cochlear implant users with post- and prelingual deafness demonstrated by positron emission tomography. Acta Otolaryngol 1997;117:490–496

4

Sound Processors in Cochlear Implants

Ward R. Drennan and
Jay T. Rubinstein

The sound processor provides the functional core of the cochlear implant, converting acoustic signals into electric signals. Sound processors have undergone extensive development over the past 40 years. Incremental improvements in hearing were achieved following each advancement. Sound processors evolved from single channel to multiple channels, from speech feature extractors to sound encoders, from simultaneous excitations to interleaved excitation, and from slow rates of presentation to high rates. From initial inception in the 1960s and early 1970s, the cochlear implant has changed from a device that provided merely a sensation of sound, improving acoustic awareness of the deaf, to a device that brings reliable speech understanding to the majority of users. Current research and development efforts continue to show improved hearing with new sound processing strategies.

Development of the cochlear implant has faced numerous challenges. First, hardware had to be developed that could safely deliver electrical signals into the inner ear. Second, processors had to be developed that could successfully transmit acoustic information to the auditory nerve. Third, the conditioners of the auditory systems in implant candidates are widely variable, so devices and processors had to be optimized to suit individuals. Outcomes were widely variable, yet, most users, particularly postlingually deafened adults and early-implanted deaf children, have enjoyed great benefit from their prostheses. This chapter reviews the historical development of sound processors and the current processing strategies, and highlights some promising new strategies.

◆ Single-Channel Implants

Early implants used a single channel. These implants provided some sensation of sound, but had extremely poor fidelity. The earliest single channel implant was the House/3M (St. Paul, MN) implant, developed by William F. House and his colleagues in Los Angeles, California. This single-channel implant succeeded in transmitting acoustic information electrically to the auditory nerve, but word recognition was not dramatically improved as there was minimal frequency-specific information delivered. A 16-kHz carrier provided a temporal envelope code that indicated when the sound was on or off. This could provide some periodicity information below 300 Hz,[1] but the device did not perform any compression, causing substantial peak clipping. Duration and some voicing cues in speech were discernible. Although a few "star" listeners could understand speech, this device primarily provided acoustic awareness and served as an aid to lipreading.

In the early 1980s, the Vienna/3M single-channel implant became available. This device incorporated loudness control and compression.[2,3] Compression minimized peak clipping and provided improved encoding for the temporal envelope. Nevertheless, minimal frequency information was available, so although outcomes improved,[4,5] performance was still marginal.

◆ Representing Frequency Spatially

It has long been known that the inner ear functions, in part, as a frequency analyzer, transforming acoustic frequency to specific place along the basilar membrane.[6] Although it was originally thought that an implant could not realistically achieve the fine frequency representation of 1000 inner hair cells, achieving some frequency representation was certainly possible. A linear array of electrode contacts was created and used to deliver multiple channels of current to different places along the basilar membrane dependent on the frequency of the input.

In the late 1970s and early 1980s, researchers in Australia introduced multichannel processors that extracted speech features from the acoustic input. For example, vowels are identified by the frequency of their spectral peaks (formants). This information could be delivered along with the fundamental frequency of the speaker (F0). (See *The Handbook of Speech Perception*[7] for broad reviews of speech perception issues.) The F0/F2 processor[8,9] identified an F0 and the second formant frequency (F2). F0, extracted with zero-crossings, determined the rate of electrical pulses delivered to a specific place corresponding to F2, re-creating the frequency encoding properties of the inner ear. The processing was implemented using a 22-channel cochlear implant. Such processing provided an improvement in performance over single-channel devices,[10] but the scheme still provided only a fraction of the information present in the speech stimulus.

Developments in the early 1980s led to the F0/F1/F2 processing strategy, which became available in 1985.[11] This processing scheme added first formant (F1) information. Central Institute for the Deaf (CID) sentence recognition more than doubled (from 16 to 35%) with the addition of the F1 component.[12] Northwestern University (NU)-6 word recognition increased more than threefold (from 8 to 28%). The processing strategy did not incorporate higher-frequency consonant information, which could improve speech understanding further.

A new strategy called MultiPEAK (MPEAK) was introduced in the late 1980s. This approach used the F0/F1/F2 encoder and added high-frequency information in which consonants were encoded. Three high-frequency bands (2000–2800 Hz, 2800–4000 Hz, and >4000 Hz) were encoded using an envelope detector. This information was passed to the more basal electrodes using electric pulses. Performance again improved markedly with the additional information. Consonant identification improved from 17 to 28%.[13] Sentence recognition also improved.[14,15]

These processors were intended to extract appropriate speech cues from the acoustic stimulus. If there was competing noise of any kind, particularly competing speech, the processors would often make errors in selection of the fundamental and formant frequencies. Later processors developed in Australia were also intended to encode speech, but they were not intended to extract specific speech cues.

◆ Compressed Analog and Continuous Interleaved Sampling

Concurrent with development of the Australian speech processors, a compressed analog (CA) strategy was developed in the United States.[16,17] The processor was multichannel, using continuous and simultaneous current flow at each electrode. Originally, using the Ineraid (Richards, Salt Lake City, UT) device, the incoming acoustic wave was compressed, filtered into four channels, and passed via electrical current to the appropriate electrode. The approach incorporated compression using an automatic gain control (AGC) that compressed the wide acoustic dynamic range

into the much more narrow electric dynamic range. Dorman et al[18] reported a broad range of abilities ranging from 0 to 100% word recognition within CID sentences. Average performance was 45% correct, far exceeding performance with single-channel implants.

The Ineraid device is no longer available; however, CA processing is currently implemented in the form of the simultaneous analog strategy[19] (SAS) with the Clarion (Advanced Bionics; Valencia, CA) device. SAS provided advancement over CA with a postfilter AGC, which limited spectral distortions caused by fast-acting compression implemented prior to filtering. SAS also used discrete current steps that change in intervals of 75 microseconds. The Clarion II can implement the SAS strategy with up to 16 channels. The CA and SAS approaches preserved the temporal waveform electrically including zero-crossings and temporal fine structure; however, users typically could perceive such fine structure only up to ~300 Hz.[1,20] Further, the simultaneous analog approach caused extensive channel interaction due to the summation of electric fields.[21] This limited spectral resolution and the effectiveness of simultaneous analog approaches.

Wilson et al[22] introduced continuous interleaved sampling (CIS), which addressed the problem of excessive channel interaction. CIS used rapid, nonsimultaneous sweeps of pulses across the electrode array to represent the time-varying acoustic spectrum. The incoming acoustic wave was filtered into multiple frequency channels corresponding to the number of electrodes. Then, the envelope of the wave was extracted using rectification and low-pass filtering. Finally, the amplitude envelopes were multiplied by non-simultaneous biphasic pulse trains. **Fig. 4–1**[23] shows a schematic of the process. Extraction of frequency-specific amplitude modulations successfully transmitted spectral information but eliminated periodicity and temporal fine-structure at frequencies above the maximum frequency of the low-pass filter. The Hilbert transform, used in the modern Med-El (Innsbruck, Austria) devices, can also accomplish the same goal. The Hilbert transform converts the original acoustic wave into two outputs: an envelope and temporal fine structure. The envelope provides a smooth envelope extraction, without jaggedness. The extracted envelope is multiplied by a series of biphasic pulses that are passed to the appropriate electrodes in the implant after compression of the input into the dynamic range of the user. Empirical studies[22] showed that speech can be understood well using the CIS approach. CIS often provided superior performance to SAS. All three implant companies offer CIS.

Several studies have compared SAS with interleaved strategies. The majority of people trying both strategies prefer CIS.[24–26] CIS has often shown superior outcomes[22]; however, Battmer et al[27] have shown that some SAS users can achieve excellent speech understanding. Osberger and Fisher[26] showed no significant difference in performance after 6 months of experience but noted a faster learning rate among SAS users. Preferences fro CIS or SAS can depend upon the specific hardware used. For example, the Clarion "HiFocus" electrode array is designed to sit closer to the center of the cochlea. In a group of 56 Clarion HiFocus users, Zwolan et al[28] reported that a majority

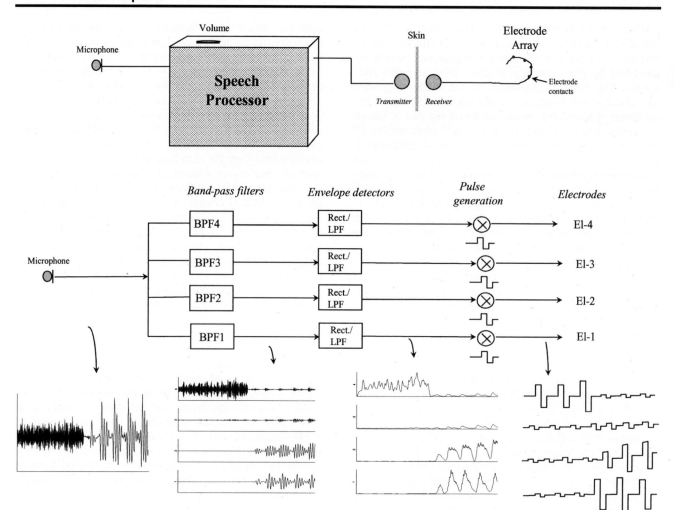

Figure 4–1 *Top*: Schematic of the cochlear implant. Middle: A more detailed schematic of the sound processor for continuous interleaved sampling (CIS). The input is filtered into four band-pass channels (only four channels are shown for simplicity). The band-pass outputs are rectified and low-pass filtered, creating a temporal envelope for each frequency band. The temporal envelopes are multiplied by nonsimultaneous biphasic pulse trains, which are delivered by electrical current through the cochlea via the electrode array. *Bottom*: The acoustic wave is transformed to a series of biphasic electrical pulses. (From Loizou P. Mimicking the human ear: an overview of signal-processing strategies for converting sound into electrical signals in cochlear implants. IEEE Signal Processing Magazine 1998;98:101–130, with permission.)

preferred SAS. In another group of similar size that did not use HiFocus, the majority preferred CIS, as in the other studies. Zwolan et al speculated that the HiFocus array limited channel interaction, allowing better performance with SAS. There has not yet been a demonstration of broad clinical superiority for either strategy, but most implantees use some form of interleaved processing.

◆ Spectral Peak Processors

Building on the CIS concept, an "*n*-of-*m*" approach, in which *m* is the maximum number of electrodes available in the implant and *n* is the total number of channels, was developed.[29] The Cochlear Corporation (Sydney, Australia) and Med-El (Innsbruck, Austria) devices currently use this approach. "*n*-of-*m*" worked much like CIS except that a

subset of electrodes with the maximum filter output was selected for presentation. The Australian group developed the spectral maxima sound processor (SMSP).[30] Sound was processed into 16 band-pass filters. Pulses were only delivered to the six channels having the maximum output. The current levels in filters with lower outputs were set to zero. Hence, *n* (6) of *m* (16) electrodes were activated on each sweep. The SMSP further reduced channel interaction. McKay et al[31] showed that the processor provided markedly better speech recognition than speech-feature-extraction approaches (MPEAK).

The SMSP processor was developed into the spectral peak strategy (SPEAK), which is currently available with the Cochlear Corporation implants. In SPEAK, as with SMSP, a subset of electrodes was selected to present on each sweep, based on the filters with the largest outputs, i.e. the spectral peaks. The total numbers of maxima were selected from 20 channels. The number of peaks selected was variable, using up to 10 channels. Channels below a certain noise threshold would not be selected even if they were among the strongest 10. The approach conserved power and further limited channel interaction. SPEAK showed superior performance to MPEAK independent of evolving and more liberal candidature characteristics.[32]

The SPEAK processor operated at a slow pulse rate [250 pulses per second per channel (pps/ch)]. Higher pulse rates would be expected to improve the temporal encoding of the processed sounds. The Advanced Combination Encoder[33] (ACE) was then implemented in the Nucleus (Cochlear Corporation, Englewood, CO) cochlear implants. ACE operated much like SPEAK, only using faster pulse rates. Evaluations of the ACE strategy have usually shown superior performance to SPEAK.[34,35] Such improvements were shown independent of changing candidature.[32] Most users preferred the ACE processing. The processing scheme that yielded the best speech perception performance usually corresponded with the preferred strategy. Kiefer et al[34] noted that, given the fact that most users prefer ACE, it would be appropriate to use that in the initial fitting; however, they caution that variability among different users was great. Vandali et al,[36] for example, noted wide variability in open-set speech recognition performance among five subjects with speech presented in multitalker noise. Loizou et al[37] also reported between-listener variability dependent on pulse rates and pulse durations. Thus, for implant users, one pulse rate does not fit all. Individual optimization of pulse rate and pulse duration parameters can lead to significantly improved performance.

Other processing schemes have been implanted that combine simultaneous and successive pulsatile stimulation. The paired pulsatile sampler (PPS) enabled the presentation of two pulses simultaneously such that two simultaneous sweeps could occur. The separation of the active electrodes is kept wide as to still maintain minimal channel interactions. The quadruple pulsatile sampler is similar to the PPS, but four electrodes are stimulated simultaneously. A "hybrid" can provide SAS stimulation to the apical electrodes and CIS presentation to the basal electrodes. SAS can provide temporal fine-structure information. The auditory system can only encode such information at low frequencies, so the hybrid approach can be used to provide fine temporal information in the low frequencies while still minimizing channel interaction in the high-frequency region. Loizou et al[38] compared these strategies. The results did not show many differences among strategies, but the participants did not have much experience with each strategy. Some trends were observed, however. Combination strategies can improve speech understanding over interleaved strategies or SAS alone. Further study will be required to document the extent to which these strategies might help over the long term.

◆ Further Improvements in Sound Processing

Ideally, an implant would perfectly re-create the neural excitation patterns of a normal-hearing person with acoustic stimulation. The implant achieves varying degrees of success depending on the type of information to be transferred.[39] A cochlear implant has many limitations. First, the dynamic range in implants is highly limited, leading to complex issues regarding the manner of compression required. Second, the spectral-resolving power of implants is poor. Finally, the ability of implants to deliver temporal fine structure is highly limited.

Small dynamic ranges in cochlear implant users require extensive compression. To decrease the amount of compression, and to minimize background noise, the softest sounds are often eliminated. Processed quiet sounds can also be masked easily by louder sounds. James et al[40] introduced adaptive dynamic range optimization (ADRO), which attempts to make all outputs comfortably loud. In doing so, ADRO increased the quieter speech sounds and improved intelligibility. With no background noise, ADRO improved open-set sentence recognition at low-to-moderate speech levels by 16 to 20%. Such increases in low-level pulses might reduce suprathreshold refractory effects, which can mask quiet sounds.[41] Using another approach, Geurts and Wouters[42] introduced "enhanced envelope" CIS (EECIS), which was intended to introduce rapid cochlear adaptation effects to electrical processing. EECIS could also increase lower level speech sounds (e.g., consonants). Word recognition ability was 7% better with EECIS than with CIS. The transient emphasis spectral maxima (TESM)[43] approach was also intended to magnify short-duration speech cues that had low levels. Improvements in consonant and word recognition were observed with TESM. Additional improvements of about 9 to 11% were seen for half of the participants on sentence recognition in noise at 10 dB signal-to-noise ratio (S/N).

Other issues concerning dynamic range control involve the speed of compression and loudness balancing. Stone and Moore[44] noted that the oft-used fast-action compression could reduce the ability of implantees to perceive amplitude modulations due to decreased modulation depth. Fast-action compression also increases comodulation across frequency channels, which could increase the likelihood of perceptual grouping of speech and noise,[45] decreasing the ability of implantees to segregate sounds. Cochlear implant simulations presented to normal-hearing listeners showed improvement in sentence recognition in noise of ~5%. McDermott et al[46] noted that loudness summation is not considered when fitting implants. Typically, the threshold and maximum comfortable loudness level are set for each electrode individually. The summed loudness, however, when all electrodes are active can be much greater, depending on the pulse rate, the number of electrodes active, and on the individual listeners. The "SpeL" processing scheme was designed to match the loudness in implant users that normal hearing users would hear acoustically.[46] Initial results have shown that SpeL improves audibility, but it has not yet been shown to improve speech recognition.[47]

The spectral resolving power of implant users is also limited. Fishman et al,[48] Dorman et al,[49] and Friesen et al,[50] for example, found that despite having up to 22 processing channels, speech understanding does not improve significantly with more than about eight channels. Although eight channels is sufficient for good speech understanding in quiet conditions,[51] more channels are needed for good speech understanding in noisy conditions[50] and for good music perception.[52,53] Several attempts have been made to increase the number of functional channels. These include the use of modiolar-hugging implants and the use of bipolar electrode configurations, which can decrease current spread within the cochlea. Neither of the approaches has yet to have a significant impact on clinical outcomes.[13,54,55] One reason might be the compromised nerve survival of implant users.[56–58] Ambitious work is being conducted to address this problem with investigations of nerve growth factors[59–61] and hair cell regeneration.[62–64] Although progress is encouraging, the amount of time required for development and approval of such future biological treatments is unknown. One approach with current technology involves improving the place coding of low frequencies using "current steering" by altering the current level balance between neighboring electrodes.[65] Such adjustments lead to pitch changes and were shown to improve F0 discrimination ability.

The lack of ability of cochlear implants to pass the temporal fine structure of acoustic waves to the auditory nerve is yet another limitation. The ability to segregate speech from noise,[66] perceive tonal speech,[67] and hear musical melodies[52,68] all rely heavily on temporal fine structure. Further, temporal fine structure is a critical element of binaural hearing in which interaural time differences are critical.[69,70] For example, a cocktail party, with numerous competing speakers, is a serious problem for implant users. Implant listeners cannot easily pick out one speaker from another. The ability to segregate different fundamental frequencies (F0) is one critical element that helps listeners separate one speaker from another.[71,72] Such information is encoded in the periodicity or pitch of the temporal fine structure.[73] Delivery of temporal fine structure information could provide cues to speaker segregation based on periodicity. Binaural unmasking resulting from interaural time differences (ITDs) can provide additional benefit in a cocktail party situation.[74] With bilateral implantation, temporal fine structure information could further improve speech understanding in noise with spatial separation. Zeng et al[75] have shown, using cochlear implant simulations, that encoding frequency modulations can improve speech understanding in noise. Frequency modulations could be delivered with temporal fine structure.

There are three current processing strategies that could improve electrical delivery of temporal fine structure without greatly increasing channel interaction: (1) high pulse rates, >2000 pps; (2) combined acoustic and electric stimulation; and (3) use of a low-level, high rate conditioning stimulus. High pulse rates and combined acoustic and electric stimulation have already been implemented clinically. Use of a conditioning stimulus appears promising, but is still experimental.

Slower pulse rates used in SPEAK and ACE lead to highly synchronized firing of the auditory nerve. In the auditory nerve of a normal-hearing person, firing is not precisely synchronized, especially at low levels. Pulse rates greater than 2000 pps increase the probability of stochastic firing of nerves,[21,76] decreasing the degree of synchronization. Each time a nerve fires, it undergoes a short refractory

period during which it will not fire again. The refractory periods of nerves vary. At a slower pulse rate, all the nerves will recover and fire synchronously at the next pulse. If the rate is increased beyond ~2000 pps, however, some nerves will be in the refractory period while others are not; thus a stochastic firing pattern could be introduced, making the electrically stimulated nerve respond more like an acoustically stimulated nerve.

The Clarion II processor (Advanced Bionics; Valencia, CA) can implement faster rates of stimulation, so a high resolution (HiResolution) strategy was introduced,[25] employing many of the same principles as the CIS but using faster pulse rates. Frijns et al[77] found that HiResolution led to better speech understanding in noise. The effectiveness of high rates varied with the number of electrodes stimulated. If the optimum number of electrodes was selected, nearly all users showed an improved ability to understand speech in noise. More dramatic results were documented by Koch et al,[78] demonstrating improvements using Hearing in Noise Test (HINT) sentences presented at 10 dB S/N among listeners who had poor or average speech understanding ability. Most likely due to a ceiling effect, participants who were the best with slow pulse rates did not show much improvement with HiResolution; however, these listeners did report subjective benefit. The results with HiResolution show additional incremental improvements in speech understanding in noise, possibly because of improved encoding of temporal fine structure.

Combined electric and acoustic stimulation provides another approach to transmit temporal fine structure. Combined stimulation has been effective in patients who have some residual hearing and viable hair cells for stimulation.[66,79] The fine structure is encoded in the normal way, via hair cell transmission. Combined stimulation can be achieved by using a hearing aid in one ear and an implant in the other,[66,80] or by using a hearing aid and implant in the same ear with a short electrode array.[79] Unfortunately, there are many patients with highly limited or nonexistent residual hearing. For these people, combined stimulation will be of no benefit.

Use of a "conditioning" or "desynchronizing" stimulus might also enhance transmission of temporal fine structure. A conditioning stimulus is a high-rate and low-level pulse train intended to encourage spontaneous activity in the nerve.[76] The stimulus is designed to lightly activate the auditory nerve at all times, re-creating spontaneous activity like a normally functioning auditory nerve. Physiologic studies[81] have shown that the use of a conditioner creates a more normal pattern of auditory nerve responses. Early psychophysical work with a conditioner has shown that the conditioner increases the dynamic range.[82] These results are consistent with the presence of increased spontaneous activity in the auditory nerve. When implementing sound processing with a conditioner, less compression is required. Boike and Souza[83] have shown that in hearing aids, increasing the dynamic range within a patient improves speech perception. The same might be true with an implant.

A conditioning stimulus can be added to any other processing scheme, for example, ACE, HiResolution, or SAS. Initial studies have shown that a conditioning stimulus provides significant and sometimes substantial benefit for understanding speech in noise for about one third of the patients who have tested the strategy. Conditioning was implemented in eight patients at the Leiden University Medical Center who were unilaterally implanted. A 5000-pps conditioner was applied to every other electrode in the electrode array. A 1000-pps/ch CIS was used on the nonconditioned electrodes. When fitting, the patients would hear the level of the conditioner initially, but they would adapt within a few minutes, so they did not chronically hear the conditioner. Of seven patients who completed the trial, two had remarkable performance with the conditioner, showing a 4-dB average improvement of speech reception threshold (SRT) in noise. In quiet conditions, speech understanding improved from 80 to 100% in both people. Three participants preferred the conditioner, but did not show objective benefit after 1 month. The remaining two listeners did not like the conditioner and returned to their clinical strategy. All listeners who continued to use the strategy after the initial fitting reported improved sound quality with the conditioner.

More recently, additional trials were conducted at the University of Iowa with continued encouraging results. Again, about one third of the participants had marked improvements in speech understanding in noise. One person, with the conditioner, had an SRT in babble noise of −9 dB, remarkable for an implant user and comparable to the SRT of person with a mild hearing loss. Two others showed significant objective improvements for speech understanding in noise, with SRTs improving from 5 to 19 dB. Three others preferred the conditioning strategy but did not show objective benefit, and three more did not like the conditioner and switched to their original strategy.

The conditioner has also been applied to two bilateral implant users. One of these patients did not like conditioning and opted for the clinical strategy. The second patient had highly asymmetric abilities. When the conditioner was added to the worse ear, this person's ability to understand speech increased dramatically. The patient's SRT in noise was +9 dB without the conditioner and −9 dB with the conditioner, an improvement of 18 dB. After 6 months of experience with the conditioner in one ear (with both implants operating) City University of New York (CUNY) sentence scores in noise (S/N = 10 dB) improved from less than 60 to 95%.

Thus, the conditioning approach shows substantial benefit in some patients, some benefit in others, and no benefit in still others. The reasons why some people glean substantial benefit and others do not are not yet known.

Further research is required to determine these reasons and to determine the extent to which a conditioner can impact clinical outcomes. Clinical trials are required before the conditioning approach becomes commercially available.

◆ Conclusion

The first cochlear implants were single-channel devices that demonstrated the clinical viability of electrical stimulation of the auditory nerve. Users of single-channel devices had the benefit of acoustic awareness, but were usually poor at understanding speech. Later, multichannel devices were employed using simultaneous and successive electrical stimulation of the auditory nerve. Initial work included attempts to extract speech parameters from the acoustic stimulus. As a general rule, delivery of more speech information yielded a better clinical outcome. Later work showed that interleaved "peak-picking" strategies were more successful. These are currently implemented in the Med-El "*n*-of-*m*" strategy and in Cochlear Corporation's SPEAK and ACE strategies. The primary limitation with these sound processors is the inability of users to recognize speech in noise, tonal speech, and musical melodies. These limitations likely result from the inability of the sound processors to transmit sufficient spectral resolution and temporal fine structure. Although physiologic limitations have slowed progress toward improving spectral resolution, approaches for improving the encoding of temporal fine structure have been implemented. HiResolution processing has been shown to improve speech understanding in noise. Additionally, for patients with some residual hearing, combined acoustic and electric stimulation has been shown to provide significant benefit. Future work includes the use of a conditioning stimulus to encourage more normal auditory nerve firing patterns. Although still experimental, a conditioning stimulus has provided improvements in about two thirds of cochlear implantees tested.

Acknowledgments

This work was supported by the VM Bloedel Hearing Research Center and National Institutes of Health (NIH) grant DC00242. Dr. Clifford Hume provided helpful comments on the text.

References

1. Zeng F-G. Temporal pitch in electric hearing. Hear Res 2002;174:101–106
2. Hochmair ES, Hochmair-Desoyer IJ, Burian K. Investigations towards and artificial cochlear. Int J Artif Organs 1979;2:255–261
3. Hochmair ES, Hochmair-Desoyer IJ. Percepts elicited by different speech coding strategies. Ann N Y Acad Sci 1983;405:268–279
4. Hochmair-Desoeyer IJ, Hochmair ES, Stiglbrunner H. Psychoacoustic temporal processing and speech understanding in cochlear implant patients. In: Schindler R, Merzenich M, eds. Cochlear Implants. New York: Raven Press, 1985:291–304
5. Tyler RS. Open-set recognition with the 3 m/Vienna single-channel cochlear implant. Arch Otolaryngol Head Neck Surg 1988;114:1123–1126
6. von Bekesy G. Experiments in Hearing. New York: McGraw-Hill, 1960
7. Pisoni DB, Remez RE, eds. The Handbook of Speech Perception. Malden, MA, Oxford, UK, Victoria, Australia: Blackwell, 2005
8. Tong YC, Clark GM, Seligman PM, Patrick JF. Speech processing for a multiple-electrode cochlear implant hearing prosthesis. J Acoust Soc Am 1980;68:1897–1899

9. Clark GM, Tong YC, Martin LF. A multiple-channel cochlear implant. An evaluation using open-set CID sentences. Laryngoscope 1981;91:628–634

10. Dowell RC, Clark GM, Seligman PM, Brown AM. Perception of connected speech without lipreading, using a multichannel hearing prosthesis. Acta Otolaryngol 1986;102:7–11

11. Blamey P, Dowell R, Clark GM. Acoustic parameters measured by a formant-estimating speech processor for a multiple-channel cochlear implant. J Acoust Soc Am 1987;82:38–47

12. Dowell RC, Seligman PM, Blamey P, Clark GM. Evaluation of a two-formant speech processing strategy for a multichannel cochlear prosthesis. Ann Otol Rhinol Laryngol 1987;96(suppl 128):132–134

13. von Wallenberg EL, Battmer RD. Comparative speech recognition results in eight subjects using two different coding strategies with the Nucleus 22 channel cochlear implant. Br J Audiol 1991;25:371–380

14. Dowell RC, Dawson PW, Dettman SJ, et al. Multichannel cochlear implantation in children: a summary of current work at the University of Melbourne. Am J Otol 1991;12(suppl):137–143

15. Skinner MW, Holden LK, Holden TA, et al. Performance of postlinguistically deaf adults with the Wearable Speech Processor (WSP III) and Mini Speech Processor (MSP) of the Nucleus Multi-Electrode Cochlear Implant. Ear Hear 1991;12:3–22

16. Eddington DK. Speech discrimination in deaf subjects with cochlear implants. J Acoust Soc Am 1980;68:885–891

17. Merzenich MM, Rebscher SJ, Loeb GE, Byers CL, Schindler RA. The UCSF cochlear implant project. Adv Audiol 1984;2:119–144

18. Dorman MF, Hannley MT, Dankowski K, Smith L, McCnadless G. Word recognition by 50 patients fitted with the Symbion multichannel cochlear implant. Ear Hear 1989;10:44–49

19. Boex C, Balthasas Cd, Kos M-I, Pelizzone M. Electrical field interactions in different cochlear implant systems. J Acoust Soc Am 2003;114:2049–2057

20. Shannon RV. Multichannel electrical stimulation of the auditory nerve in man. I. Basic psychophysics. Hear Res 1983;11:157–189

21. White MW, Merzenich MM, Gardi JN. Multichannel cochlear implants. Channel interactions and processor design. Arch Otolaryngol 1984;110:493–510

22. Wilson BS, Finley CC, Lawson DT, Wolford RD, Eddington DK, Rabinowitz WM. Better speech recognition with cochlear implants. Nature 1991;352:236–238

23. Loizou P. Mimicking the human ear: an overview of signal-processing strategies for converting sound into electrical signals in cochlear implants. IEEE Signal Process Mag 1998;15:101–130

24. Stollwerck LE, Goodrum-Clarke K, Lynch C, et al. Speech processing strategy preferences among 55 European CLARION cochlear implant users. Scand Audiol Suppl 2001;52:36–38

25. Frijns JHM, Briaire JJ, Laat JAPMd, Grote JJ. Initial evaluation of the Clarion CII cochlear implant: Speech perception and neural response imaging. Ear Hear 2002;23:184–197

26. Osberger MJ, Fisher L. New directions in speech processing: patient performance with simultaneous analog stimulation. Ann Otol Rhinol Laryngol 2000;185:70–73

27. Battmer RD, Zilberman Y, Haake P, Lenarz T. Simultaneous analog stimulation (SAS)–continuous interleaved sampler (CIS) pilot comparison study in Europe. Ann Otol Rhinol Laryngol Suppl 1999;177:69–73

28. Zwolan T, Kileny PR, Smith S, Mills D, Koch D, Osberger MJ. Adult cochlear implant patient performance with evolving electrode technology. Otol Neurotol 2001;22:844–849

29. Wilson BS, Finley CC, Farmer JC, et al. Comparative studies of speech processing strategies for cochlear implants. Laryngoscope 1988;98:1069–1077

30. McDermott HJ, McKay CM, Vandali AE. A new portable sound processor for the University of Melbourne/Nucleus Limited multielectrode cochlear implant. J Acoust Soc Am 1992;91:3367–3371

31. McKay CM, McDermott HJ, Vandali AE, Clark GM. A comparison of speech perception of cochlear implantees using the Spectral Maximum Sound Processor (SMSP) and the MSP (MULTIPEAK) processor. Acta Otolaryngol 1992;112:752–761

32. David EE, Ostroff JM, Shipp D, et al. Speech coding strategies and revised cochlear implant candidacy: an analysis of post-implant performance. Otol Neurotol 2003;24:228–233

33. King AJ, Kacelnik O, Mrsic-Flogel TD, Schnupp JW, Parsons CH, Moore DR. How plastic is spatial hearing? Audiol Neurootol 2001;6:182–186

34. Kiefer J, Hohl S, Stuerzebecher E, Pfennigdorff T, Gstoettner W. Comparison of speech recognition with different speech coding strategies (SPEAK, CIS and ACE) and their relationship to telemetric measures of compound action potentials in the Nucleus CI 24M cochlear implant system. Audiology 2001;40:32–42

35. Skinner MW, Holden LK, Whitford LA, Plant KL, Psarros C, Holden TA. Speech recognition with the Nucleus 24 SPEAK, ACE and CIS speech coding strategies in newly implanted adults. Ear Hear 2002;23:207–223

36. Vandali AE, Whitford LA, Plant KL, Clark GM. Speech perception as a function of electrical stimulation rate: Using the Nucleus 24 cochlear implant system. Ear Hear 2000;21:608–624

37. Loizou PC, Poroy O, Dorman M. The effect of parametric variations of cochlear implant processors on speech understanding. J Acoust Soc Am 2000;108:790–802

38. Loizou PC, Stickney G, Mishra L, Assmann P. Comparison of speech processing strategies used in the Clarion implant processor. Ear Hear 2003;24:12–19

39. Moore BCJ. Coding of sounds in the auditory system and its relevance to signal processing and coding in cochlear implants. Otol Neurotol 2003;24:243–254

40. James CJ, Blamey PJ, Martin L, Swanson B, Just Y, Macfarlane D. Adaptive dynamic range optimization for cochlear implants: a preliminary study. Ear Hear 2002;23:49S–58S

41. Wieringen AV, Carlyon RP, Long CJ, Wouters J. Pitch of amplitude-modulated irregular-rate stimuli in acoustic and electric hearing. J Acoust Soc Am 2003;114:1516–1528

42. Geurts L, Wouters J. Enhancing the speech envelope of continuous interleaved sampling processors for cochlear implants. J Acoust Soc Am 1999;105:2476–2484

43. Vandali AE. Emphasis of short-duration acoustic speech cues for cochlear implant users. J Acoust Soc Am 2001;109:2049–2061

44. Stone MA, Moore BCJ. Effect of the speech of a single-channel dynamic range compressor on intelligibility in a competing speech task. J Acoust Soc Am 2003;114:1023–1034

45. Hall JW 3rd, Grose JH. Comodulation masking release and auditory grouping. J Acoust Soc Am 1990;88:119–125

46. McDermott HJ, McKay CM, Richardson LM, Henshall KR. Application of loudness models to sound processing for cochlear implants. J Acoust Soc Am 2003;114:2190–2197

47. McDermott HJ, Sucher CM, McKay CM. Speech perception with a cochlear implant sound processor incorporating loudness models. Acoustic Res Letters Online 2005;6:7–13

48. Fishman KE, Shannon RV, Slattery WH. Speech recognition as a function of the number of electrodes used in the SPEAK cochlear implant speech processor. J Speech Lang Hear Res 1997;40:1201–1215

49. Dorman MF, Loizou PC, Fitzke J, Tu Z. The recognition of sentences in noise by normal-hearing listeners using simulations of cochlear-implant signal processors with 6–20 channels. J Acoust Soc Am 1998;104:3583–3585

50. Friesen LM, Shannon RV, Baskent D, Wang X. Speech recognition in noise as a function of the number of spectral channels: comparison of acoustic hearing and cochlear implants. J Acoust Soc Am 2001;110:1150–1163

51. Shannon RV, Zeng F-G, Kamath V, Wygonski J, Ekelid M. Speech recognition with primarily temporal cues. Science 1995;270:303–304

52. Smith ZM, Delgutte B, Oxenham AJ. Chimaeric sounds reveal dichotomy in auditory perception. Nature 2002;416:87–90

53. Pfingst BE, Franck KH, Xu L, Bauer EM, Zwolan TA. Effects of electrode configuration and place of stimulation on speech perception with cochlear prostheses. J Assoc Res Otolaryngol 2001;2:87–103

54. Kileny PR, Zwolan TA, Telian SA, Boerst A. Performance with the 20 +2L lateral wall cochlear implant. Am J Otol 1998;19:313–319

55. Zwolan TA, Kileny PR, Ashbaugh C, Telian SA. Patient performance with Cochlear Corporation "20 + 2" implant: bipolar versus monopolar activation. Am J Otol 1996;17:717–723

56. Nadol JB, Xu WZ. Diameter of the cochlear nerve in deaf humans: implications for cochlear implantation. Ann Otol Rhinol Laryngol 1992;101:988–993

57. Hinojosa R, Lindsay JR. Profound deafness: associated sensory and neural degeneration. Arch Otolaryngol 1980;106:193–209

58. Otte J, Schunknecht HF, Kerr AG. Ganglion cell populations in normal and pathological human cochleae: implications for cochlear implantations. Laryngoscope 1978;88:1231–1246

59. Nakaizumi T, Kawamoto K, Minoda R, Raphael Y. Adenovirus-mediated expression of brain-derived neurotrophic factor protests spiral ganglion neurons from ototoxic damage. Audiol Neurootol 2004;9:135–143

60. Shinohara T, Bredberg G, Ulfendahl M, et al. Neurotrophic factor intervention restores auditory function in deafened animals. Proc Natl Acad Sci U S A 2002;99:1657–1660

61. Miller JM, Chi DH, O'Keeffe LJ, Kruszka P, Raphael Y, Altschuler RA. Neurotrophins can enhance spiral ganglion cell survival after inner hair cell loss. Int J Dev Neurosci 1997;15:631–643

62. Izumikawa M, Minoda R, Kawamoto K, et al. Auditory hair cell replacement and hearing improvement by Atoh1 gene therapy in deaf mammals. Nat Med 2005;11:271–276

63. Parker MA, Cotanche DA. The potential use of stem cells for cochlear repair. Audiol Neurootol 2004;9:72–80

64. Stone JS, Rubel EW. Cellular studies of auditory hair cell regeneration in birds. Proc Natl Acad Sci U S A 2000;97:11714–11721

65. Geurts L, Wouters J. Better place-coding of the fundamental frequency in cochlear implants. J Acoust Soc Am 2004;115:844–852

66. Kong Y-Y, Stickney GS, Zeng F-G. Speech and melody recognition in binaurally combined acoustic and electric hearing. J Acoust Soc Am 2005;117:1351–1361

67. Xu L, Pfingst BE. Relative importance of temporal envelope and fine structure in lexical-tone perception (L). J Acoust Soc Am 2003;114:3024–3027

68. Kong Y-Y, Cruz R, Jones JA, Zeng F-G. Music perception with temporal cues in acoustic and electric hearing. Ear Hear 2004;25:173–185

69. Middlebrooks JC, Green DM. Sound localization by human listeners. Annu Rev Psychol 1991;42:135–159

70. Wightman FL, Kistler DJ. The dominant role of low frequency interaural time differences in sound localization. J Acoust Soc Am 1992;91:1648–1661

71. Summerfield Q, Assmann PF. Perception of concurrent vowels: effects of harmonic misalignment and pitch-period asynchrony. J Acoust Soc Am 1991;89:1364–1377

72. Culling JF, Darwin CJ. Perceptual separation of simultaneous vowels: within and across-formant grouping by F0. J Acoust Soc Am 1993;93:3454–3467

73. Faulkner A, Rosen S, Smith C. Effects of the salience of pitch and periodicity information on the intelligibility of four-channel vocoded speech: Implications for cochlear implants. J Acoust Soc Am 2000;108:1877–1887

74. Zurek PM. Binaural advantages and directional effects in speech intelligibility. In: Studebaker GA, Hochberg I, eds. Acoustical Factors Affecting Hearing Aid Performance, 2nd ed. Needham Heights, MA: Allyn and Bacon, 1993

75. Zeng F-G, Nie K, Stickney GS, et al. Speech recognition with amplitude and frequency modulations. Proc Natl Acad Sci U S A 2005;102:2293–2298

76. Rubinstein JT, Wilson BS, Finley CC, Abbas PJ. Pseudospontaneous activity: stochastic independence of auditory nerve fibers with electrical stimulation. Hear Res 1999;127:108–118

77. Frijns JHM, Klop WMC, Bonnet RM, Briaire JJ. Optimizing the number of electrodes with high-rate stimulation of the Clarion CII cochlear implant. Acta Otolaryngol 2003;123:138–142

78. Koch DB, Osberger MJ, Segel P, Kessler D. HiResolution™ and conventional sound processing in the HiResolution™ Bionic Ear: using appropriate outcome measures to assess speech recognition ability. Audiol Neurootol 2004;9:214–223

79. Gantz BJ, Turner CW. Combining acoustic and electric hearing. Laryngoscope 2003;113:1726–1730

80. Tyler RS, Parkinson AJ, Wilson BS, Witt S, Preece JP, Noble W. Patients utilizing a hearing aid and a cochlear implant: speech perception and localization. Ear Hear 2002;23:98–105

81. Litvak L, Delgutte B, Eddington D. Improved neural representation of vowels in electric stimulation using desynchronizing pulse trains. J Acoust Soc Am 2003;114:2099–2111

82. Hong RS, Rubinstein JT. High-rate conditioning pulse trains in cochlear implants: dynamic range measures with sinusoidal stimuli. J Acoust Soc Am 2003;114:3327–3342

83. Boike KT, Souza PE. Effect of compression ratio on speech recognition and speech-quality ratings with wide dynamic range compression amplification. J Speech Lang Hear Res 2000;43:456–468

5

Possibilities for a Closer Mimicking of Normal Auditory Functions with Cochlear Implants

Blake S. Wilson,
Reinhold Schatzer, and
Enrique A. Lopez-Poveda

Recent advances in electrode and stimulus design have increased the level of control that implants can exert over spatial and temporal patterns of responses in the auditory nerve. The advances include perimodiolar placements of electrodes, use of high-rate carriers or high-rate conditioner pulses, and current steering to produce "virtual channels" or intermediate sites of stimulation between adjacent electrodes. All but the last of these are reviewed in Wilson et al (2003a). Virtual channels and their construction are described in Wilson et al (1994b), and later in this chapter.

The higher levels of neural control might be exploited to provide a closer mimicking with implants of the signal processing that occurs in the normal cochlea. In particular, the subtleties of the normal processing might be represented at the auditory nerve using high-rate carriers, spatially selective electrodes, virtual channels, or combinations of these.

Present processing strategies for implants, such as the *continuous interleaved sampling* (CIS) strategy shown in the top panel of **Fig. 5–1**, provide only a very crude approximation to the normal processing. For example, a bank of linear band-pass filters is used instead of the highly nonlinear and coupled filters that would model the behavior of the basilar membrane (BM) and associated structures (e.g., the outer hair cells) in the intact cochlea. In addition, a single nonlinear mapping function is used in the CIS and other strategies to produce the overall compression (from the dynamic range of sound pressure variations to the dynamic range of stimuli for single neurons) that the

normal system achieves in multiple steps. The compression in CIS and other processors is instantaneous, whereas compression at the synapses between inner hair cells (IHCs) and single fibers of the auditory nerve in the normal cochlea is noninstantaneous, with large adaptation effects.

Such differences between normal processing and what current implants provide may limit the perceptual abilities of implant patients. For example, Deng and Geisler (1987), among others, have shown that nonlinearities in filtering at the BM and associated structures greatly enhance the neural representation of speech sounds presented in competition with noise. Similarly, findings of Tchorz and Kollmeier (1999) have indicated the importance of adaptation at the IHC/neuron synapse in representing temporal events or markers in speech, especially for speech presented in noise. Reception of sounds more complex than speech, for example, symphonic music, may require the full interplay and function of the many processing steps in the normal auditory periphery.

A thorough discussion of the intricacies of signal processing in the normal cochlea is presented in Wilson et al (2003a). This discussion also includes a detailed description of how current processing strategies for implants fail to reproduce or replicate many aspects of the normal processing.

This chapter suggests a general approach for moving implants toward normal processing and describes the first steps in developing this approach. In addition, preliminary data are presented that show promise for the approach and some of the tested variations.

48

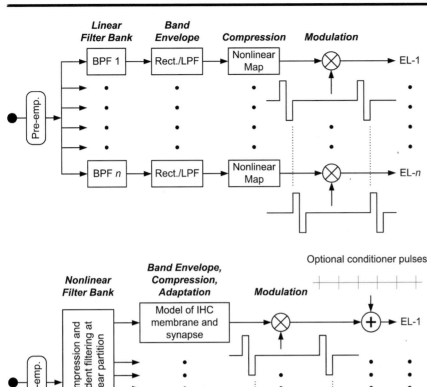

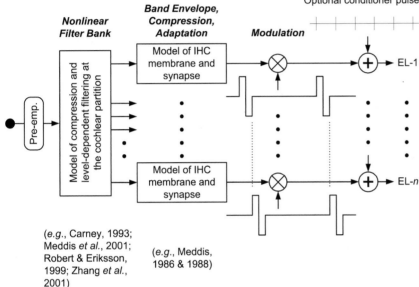

Figure 5–1 Two approaches to speech processor design. *Top panel*: A block diagram of a standard continuous interleaved sampling (CIS) design. *Bottom panel*: A block diagram of a new approach aimed at providing a closer mimicking of processing in the normal cochlea. Possible models that could be utilized in a "closer-mimicking" processor are listed beneath the corresponding blocks. BPF, band-pass filter; EL, electrode; IHC, inner hair cell; LPF, low-pass filter; Pre-emp., preemphasis filter; Rect., rectifier. [*Top panel*: adapted from Wilson BS, Finley CC, Lawson DT, Wolford RD, Eddington DK, Rabinowitz WM. (1991). Better speech recognition with cochlear implants. Nature 352:236–238, with permission of the Nature Publishing Group.]

◆ A General Approach for Closer Mimicking

A block diagram of the overall approach just mentioned is presented in the bottom panel of **Fig. 5–1**. The idea is to use better models of the normal processing, whose outputs may be fully or largely conveyed through the higher levels of neural control now available with implants.

Comparison of the top and bottom panels in **Fig. 5–1** shows that in the new structure a model of nonlinear filtering is used instead of the bank of linear filters, and a model of the IHC membrane and synapse is used instead of an envelope detector and nonlinear mapping table. Note that the mapping table is not needed in the new structure, because the multiple stages of compression implemented in the models should provide the overall compression required for mapping the wide dynamic range of processor inputs onto stimulus levels appropriate for neural activation. (Some scaling may be needed, but the compression functions should be at least

approximately correct.) The compression achieved in this way would be much more analogous to the way it is achieved in normal hearing.

Conditioner pulses or high carrier rates may be used if desired, to impart spontaneous-like activity in auditory neurons and stochastic independence among neurons (Rubinstein et al, 1999; Wilson et al, 1997). This can increase the dynamic range of auditory neuron responses to electrical stimuli, bringing it closer to that observed for normal hearing using acoustic stimuli. Stochastic independence among neurons also may be helpful in representing rapid temporal variations in the stimuli at each electrode, in the collected (ensemble) responses of all neurons in the excitation field (e.g., Parnas, 1996; Wilson et al, 1997).

Spontaneous activity and stochastic independence among neurons are among the attributes of normal hearing that are not reproduced using standard strategies and parameter choices for cochlear implants. Reinstating these attributes to the extent possible may be helpful.

The approach illustrated in the bottom panel of **Fig. 5–1** is intended as a move in the direction of closer mimicking. It does not include feedback control from the central nervous system, and it does not include a way to stimulate fibers close to an electrode differentially, the latter of which would be required to mimic the distributions of thresholds and dynamic ranges of the multiple neurons innervating each IHC in the normal cochlea. However, it does have the potential to reproduce or approximate other important aspects of the normal processing, including: (1) details of filtering at the BM and associated structures, and (2) noninstantaneous compression and adaptation at the IHCs and their synapses.

◆ Implementations of "Closer-Mimicking" Processors

Studies are underway in our laboratories to evaluate various implementations of processors based on the general approach outlined above. We are proceeding in steps, including: (1) substitution of a bank of dual-resonance, nonlinear (DRNL) filters (Lopez-Poveda and Meddis, 2001; Meddis et al, 2001) for the bank of linear filters used in a standard CIS processor; (2) substitution of the Meddis IHC model (Meddis, 1986, 1988) for the envelope detector and for some of the compression ordinarily provided by the nonlinear mapping table in a standard CIS processor; and (3) combinations of (1) and (2) and fine-tuning of the interstage gains and amounts of compression at various stages. Work thus far has focused on implementation and evaluation of processors using DRNL filters (step 1). For those processors, the envelope detectors and nonlinear mapping tables are retained, but the amount of compression provided by the tables is greatly reduced as substantial compression is provided by the DRNL filters. The DRNL filters have many parameters whose adjustment may affect performance. We have started with a set of parameter values designed to provide approximately uniform compressions at the most responsive frequencies (nominal "center frequencies") of the different filters. This choice departs from the highly nonuniform compression across frequencies described in Lopez-Poveda and Meddis (2001), but corresponds to more recent findings (Lopez-Poveda et al, 2003; Williams and Bacon, 2005).

We also have begun to explore effects produced by manipulations in the parameters from the above starting point. For example, we have adjusted parameters to produce a broader tuning for each of the filters, so that their responses overlap at least to some extent across channels.

In general, the frequency responses of the DRNL filters are much sharper than those of the Butterworth filters used in standard CIS processors, at least for six to 12 channels of processing and stimulation and at least for low-to-moderate input levels. Thus, if one simply substitutes DRNL filters for the Butterworth filters without alteration, then substantial gaps will be introduced in the represented spectra of lower-level inputs to the filter bank. Such a "picket fence" effect might degrade performance, even though other aspects of DRNL processing may be beneficial.

◆ Initial Studies with Dual-Resonance, Nonlinear Filters and "*n*-to-*m*" Approaches

Studies to date have included evaluation of DRNL-based processors with broadened filters, as noted above. In addition, we have tested *n*-to-*m* constructs, in which more than one channel of DRNL processing is assigned to each stimulus site. In one variation, the average of outputs from the multiple channels is calculated and then that average is used to determine the amplitude of a stimulus pulse for a particular electrode. Each DRNL channel includes a DRNL filter, an envelope detector, and a lookup table for compressive mapping of envelope levels onto pulse amplitudes. Thus, the average is the average of mapped amplitudes for the number of DRNL channels assigned to the electrode. We call this the "average *n*-to-*m* approach," in which *m* is the maximum number of electrodes available in the implant and in which *n* is the total number of DRNL channels, an integer multiple of *m*. In another variation, the maximum among outputs from the channels for each electrode is identified and then that maximum is used to determine the amplitude of the stimulus pulse. We call this the "maximum *n*-to-*m* approach." Both approaches are designed to retain the sharp tuning of DRNL filters using the standard (starting) parameters, while minimizing or eliminating the "picket fence" effect.

These *n*-to-*m* approaches are illustrated in **Fig. 5–2**. As shown, the spectral gaps or "picket fence" effect produced by assigning only one DRNL filter (or channel) to each stimulus site (top panel) is reduced or largely eliminated with the average *n*-to-*m* or maximum *n*-to-*m* approaches (middle and bottom panels).

Results from tests with seven subjects indicate that the *n*-to-*m* approaches can be helpful (Schatzer et al, 2003). In particular, use of these approaches produced significant increases in speech reception scores in some cases, compared with processors that simply assigned the output of each DRNL channel to a single corresponding stimulus site. [These subjects all used bilateral Med-El (Innsbruck, Austria) implants, with a maximum of eight or 12 stimulus sites on each side, depending on the particular implant device, either the Combi 40 with eight sites or the Combi 40+ with 12 sites.] Improvements for speech reception in noise were generally larger than improvements for speech reception in quiet conditions. In a few cases where comparisons were made, the maximum *n*-to-*m* approach was better than the average *n*-to-*m* approach. The best of the DRNL processors using an *n*-to-*m* approach produced speech reception scores that were as good as, but not better than, control CIS processors using *m* channels (with standard Butterworth filters) and *m* sites of stimulation.

We regarded this as an encouraging result, an immediate matching of performance with a new processing strategy, with very little or no experience in using the new strategy. In many prior studies, we and others (e.g., Tyler et al, 1986) have found that such an initial equivalence can be followed by much better performance with the new strategy, once subjects gain some experience with the new strategy.

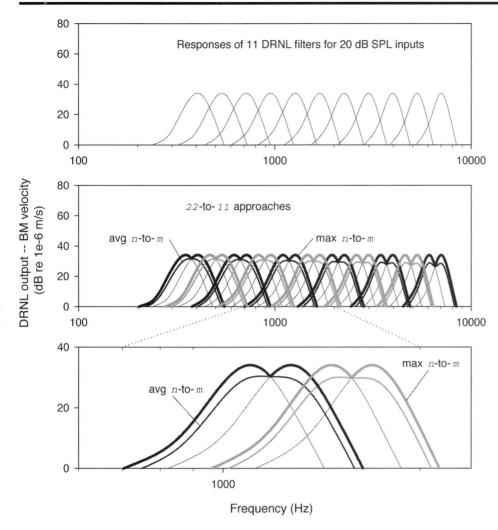

Figure 5–2 Illustration of *n*-to-*m* approaches for combining dual-resonance, nonlinear (DRNL) channel outputs. Only the DRNL filter outputs are shown here for simplicity. In actual processor implementations, effects of envelope detection and compressive mapping would be included, as described in the text. *Top panel*: A 1-to-1 assignment of filter outputs to 11 intracochlear electrodes. *Middle panel*: Average (medium lines) and maximum (thick lines) *22-to-11* approaches for combining the outputs of 22 DRNL filters (thin lines) and directing the combinations to 11 electrodes. *Bottom panel*: An expanded display that includes only four of the filters and the average and maximum combinations of their outputs. BM, basilar membrane; SPL, sound pressure level. (Note that the y-axis scale also is expanded in the bottom panel.)

At the same time, we recognized several possibilities for improvement in the design of processors using DRNL filters that might produce even higher levels of initial performance. Those possibilities included: (1) further adjustment and testing of the many parameter values in DRNL filters; (2) combination or selection of DRNL filter outputs, rather than the DRNL channel outputs, in designs using *n*-to-*m* approaches; and (3) using the same number of filters as stimulus sites, but with a high number of stimulus sites.

The first of these possibilities recognizes that the parametric space within and across DRNL filters is quite large. We have just begun to explore this space.

The second possibility recognizes that considerable distortions and complexities may be produced in combining or selecting signals that have been altered by a highly nonlinear mapping function, in addition to the nonlinearities of the DRNL filters. Combination or selection of the filter outputs, prior to envelope detection and (further) nonlinear processing, might be better than combination or selection following all of these operations.

The third possibility might retain the likely advantages of DRNL filters (that may result from compression and nonlinear tuning, as in normal hearing) while not discarding or distorting information as is inherent in the *n*-to-*m*

approaches. The spectral gap problem would be handled through the use of a high number of stimulus sites, rather than with one of the *n*-to-*m* approaches.

◆ Combined Use of Dual-Resonance, Nonlinear Filters and Virtual Channels

In more recent studies (Wilson et al, 2003b), we compared three basic processor designs in tests with a user of the Ineraid device (previously manufactured by Symbion, Inc., of Salt Lake City, UT, and then by Smith & Nephew Richards, Inc., of Bartlett, TN; this device is no longer manufactured), which includes a percutaneous connector and six intracochlear electrodes. The designs included a processor using 24 DRNL channels mapped to the six electrodes using a maximum *24-to-6* approach, as described above and in greater detail in Schatzer et al, 2003. The parameter choices used for the DRNL filters included a set to provide a flat frequency response across the spectrum spanned by all the filters, as also described in Schatzer et al. The spectrum was from 350 to 7000 Hz. This processor is referenced in the remainder of this chapter as the "cp CIS" processor ("cp" refers to a DRNL filter bank that is designed to provide a close replication of responses to sound at the *cochlear partition*). Other aspects of the processor, such as the interlacing of stimuli across electrodes, are the same as in the standard CIS strategy (this strategy is described in greater detail in Wilson et al, 1991).

The two other processor designs employed virtual channels as a way to increase the number of discriminable stimulus sites beyond the number of actual electrodes. This concept was introduced by our team in the early 1990s (Wilson et al, 1992, 1993, 1994a,b), and has since been investigated by others (Donaldson et al, 2004; Litvak et al, 2003; Poroy and Loizou, 2001). In the reports by Donaldson et al and Litvak et al, the term *current steering* is used instead of the term *virtual channels* to reference the same concept.

A series of diagrams illustrating the construction of virtual channels is presented in **Fig. 5–3**. With virtual channels (or current steering), adjacent electrodes may be stimulated simultaneously to shift the perceived pitch in any direction with respect to the percepts elicited with stimulation of one of the electrodes only. Results from studies with implant subjects indicate that pitch can be manipulated through various choices of simultaneous and single-electrode conditions (e.g., Wilson et al, 1993). If, for instance, the apical-most electrode of the Ineraid array (electrode 1) is stimulated alone (**Fig. 5–3A**), subjects have reported a low pitch. If the next electrode in the array (electrode 2) is stimulated alone (**Fig. 5–3B**), a higher pitch is reported. An intermediate pitch can be produced for all Ineraid subjects studied to date by stimulating the two electrodes together with identical, in-phase pulses (**Fig. 5–3C**). Finally, by reversing the phase of one of the simultaneous pulses, pitch percepts higher or lower than those produced by stimulation of either electrode alone can be produced. For example, a pitch lower than that elicited by stimulation of electrode 1 only can be produced by simultaneous presentation of a (generally smaller) pulse of opposite polarity at electrode 2 (**Fig. 5–3D**). The availability of pitches other than those elicited with stimulation of single electrodes only may provide additional discriminable sites along (and beyond) the length of the electrode array. Such additional sites may support additional, perceptually separable, channels of stimulation and reception. We call these additional channels "virtual channels," and processors that use them *virtual channel interleaved sampling* (VCIS) processors.

The two additional processor designs included in the comparisons of the present studies used a VCIS approach to provide 21 discriminable sites of stimulation with Ineraid (Cochlear Corporation, Englewood, CO) subject SR3's array of six intracochlear electrodes. The approach is illustrated in **Fig. 5–4**, in which stimulus site 1 is produced by stimulation of electrode 1 only, stimulus site 2 by simultaneous stimulation of electrodes 1 and 2 with a pulse amplitude of 75% for electrode 1 and of 25% for electrode 2, and so on. Results from pitch-ranking tests, using a two-alternative, forced choice (2AFC) procedure, indicated that each of the 21 sites thus formed produced a distinct pitch for SR3, that is, a pitch that is significantly different from those produced by stimulation of the neighboring site(s).

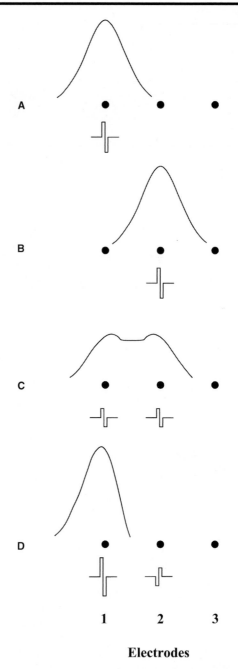

1   2   3

Electrodes

Figure 5–3 Schematic illustrations of neural responses for various conditions of stimulation with single and multiple electrodes. The top curve in each panel is a hypothetical sketch of the number of neural responses, as a function of position along the cochlea, for a given condition of stimulation. The condition is indicated by the pulse waveform(s) beneath one or more of the dots, which represent the positions of three adjacent electrodes. These different conditions of stimulation elicit distinct pitches for implant patients, as described in the text.

We note that even this fine resolution may not fully exploit SR3's perceptual abilities. In pilot studies, we also evaluated pitch ranking with 10% steps in current ratios for electrodes 1 and 2, and for electrodes 5 and 6, as opposed to the 25% steps used in the tests mentioned above. SR3 was able to rank these closely spaced sites, with the 10% changes in current

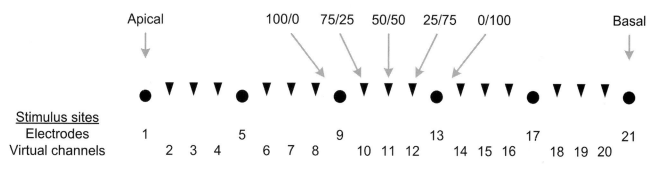

Figure 5–4 Diagram of stimulus sites used in speech processor designs for tests with subject SR3. The filled circles represent sites of stimulation at each of the six intracochlear electrodes in the Ineraid implant. The inverted triangles represent additional sites produced with simultaneous stimulation of adjacent electrodes, at the indicated ratios of pulse amplitudes for the two electrodes. These additional sites are called "virtual channels." Pitch ranking of the 21 sites was conducted using a 2AFC procedure (Wilson et al, 2003b), in which two sites were stimulated successively in random order and the subject indicated whether the second sound heard was lower or higher in pitch than the first. The results showed that the pitch elicited by stimulation of each site was significantly different from the pitch elicited by stimulation of its immediately adjacent site(s). The rank ordering of pitches ranged from low to high without exception for increases in site number as specified in the bottom part of the figure.

ratios, four out of four times for all pairings. (The tests with the 25% steps included seven comparisons for each pairing; this is the minimum number for statistical significance. Thus, the findings from the tests with 10% steps must be regarded as preliminary.)

Although 21 sites were produced by processors using the VCIS approach in the present studies, more sites may be possible, for SR3 and perhaps for other subjects as well. This expectation is consistent with the pilot data just mentioned and with the results reported by Litvak et al (2003). In that latter study, the pitch elicited with simultaneous stimulation of two adjacent electrodes in the Clarion CII implant (this implant is manufactured by Advanced Bionics Corp., Sylmar, CA; the electrodes in this implant are 1 mm apart, as opposed to the 4 mm spacing in the Ineraid implant) was compared with the pitch elicited by stimulation of the apical electrode in the pair only. For simultaneous stimulation, the proportion of pulse amplitudes was varied in small steps between a relatively high current for the apical electrode to a relatively high current for the basal electrode. Eighteen subjects were tested. The fraction of current needed for the basal electrode to produce a significantly different pitch from stimulation of the apical electrode alone ranged from 1 to 67%, depending on the subject. The average across subjects was 19%, smaller than the 25% steps in current ratios used in the present VCIS implementations, with the Ineraid electrode array (with a spacing between adjacent electrodes four times that of the Clarion array).

The two other processors tested with SR3 included a "standard" VCIS processor as previously described (e.g., Wilson et al, 1994b) and a processor that used DRNL filters instead of the linear Butterworth filters used in the standard design. These additional processors, called "std VCIS" and "cp VCIS," respectively, were identical in all other respects except for: (1) the exponent used in the mapping table for each channel, and (2) an interstage gain just prior to the mapping table. In general, the exponent used with cp processors is far higher than the exponent used with standard processors. The higher exponent produces a less compressive mapping

function, which provides an overall compression with cp processors that is similar to the overall compression with standard processors. The different interstage gains between the processors are used to provide approximately equal inputs to the mapping table, with quite different banks of "front-end" filters for the two processors.

Results from the principal comparisons in the tests with SR3 are presented in **Figs. 5–5** and **5–6**. The processors

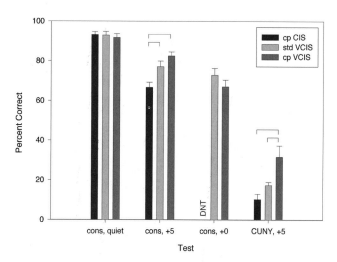

Figure 5–5 Processor comparisons in tests with Ineraid subject SR3. The processors included a max 24-to-6 processor using DRNL filters (cp CIS), a 21-site VCIS processor using Butterworth filters (std VCIS), and a 21-site VCIS processor using DRNL filters (cp VCIS). Means and standard errors of the means are shown. The tests included identification of medial consonants in quiet and in noise, and recognition of the City University of New York (CUNY) sentences presented in competition with noise. The signal-to-noise ratios (S/Ns) for the consonant tests included +5 and 0 dB, and S/N for the sentence tests was +5 dB. Analyses of the variance indicated significant differences among the scores for the consonant test using the S/N of +5 dB, and for the sentence test, also using the S/N of +5 dB. The brackets indicate the results of post hoc multiple comparisons for those tests, using the Holm-Sidak method. Bars sharing a bracket are significantly different at (at least) the $p < .05$ level. DNT is an abbreviation for "did not test."

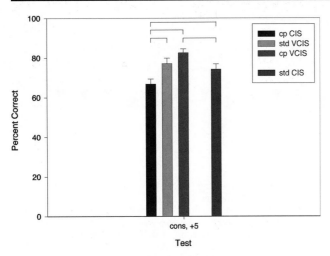

Figure 5–6 Comparison of a standard CIS processor (std CIS) with the experimental processors included in **Fig. 5–5**. The standard CIS processor used six channels of processing and six sites of stimulation. Means and standard errors of the means are shown. An analysis of the variance (ANOVA) indicated significant differences among the scores for the only test administered for all four types of processor, consonant identification at the S/N of +5 dB. The brackets indicate the results of post hoc multiple comparisons following the ANOVA, using the Holm-Sidak method. Bars sharing a bracket are significantly different at (at least) the $p < .05$ level.

included a maximum *24-to-6* processor using DRNL filters (cp CIS), a 21-site VCIS processor using Butterworth filters (std VCIS), and a 21-site VCIS processor using DRNL filters (cp VCIS). The tests included identification of 24 consonants in an /a/-consonant-/a/ context and recognition of the City University of New York (CUNY) sentences. The consonants were presented in quiet or in competition with CCITT (speech spectrum) noise at the signal-to-noise ratios (S/Ns) of +5 or 0 dB. The sentences were presented in competition with CCITT noise at the S/N of +5 dB. All tests were conducted with hearing alone and without feedback as to correct or incorrect responses. Further details about the tests and processor implementations are presented in Wilson et al (2003b).

Speech reception scores for the three processor conditions and all tests are presented in **Fig. 5–5**. Analyses of the variance (ANOVAs) indicated significant differences among the scores for the consonant test using the S/N of +5 dB ($F[2,27] = 10.4$, $p < .001$), and for the sentence test, also using the S/N of +5 dB ($F[2,9] = 8.8$, $p = .008$). The two scores for the consonant test using the S/N of 0 dB are not significantly different ($t[18] = 1.2$, $p = .237$). Post hoc comparisons using the Holm-Sidak method indicated the following significant differences among the scores for the consonant test at the S/N of +5 dB: cp VCIS is better than cp CIS, and std VCIS also is better than cp CIS. Post hoc comparisons using the same method indicated the following significant differences among the scores for the sentence test, also at the S/N of +5 dB: cp VCIS is better than cp CIS, and cp VCIS is better than std VCIS.

Scores for consonant identification in quiet are greater than 90% correct for each of the processors. Ceiling effects may have limited the power of this test to demonstrate possible differences among processors.

Following completion of the above tests, we wondered how these experimental processors might compare with a standard CIS processor using only six channels of processing and six sites of stimulation. At the end of SR3's visit, a six-channel CIS processor was evaluated using the consonant test at the S/N of +5 dB. The standard CIS processor used the same pulse rate, pulse duration, overall frequency range, and characteristics of the envelope detectors as the experimental processors. The exponent for the mapping function used in the standard CIS processor was the same as that used for the std VCIS processor.

The results from the test with the standard CIS processor (std CIS), along with the prior results for the experimental processors, are presented in **Fig. 5–6**. An ANOVA indicated significant differences among the scores for the different processors ($F[3,36] = 6.7$, $p = .001$). Post hoc comparisons using the Holm-Sidak method indicated the following significant differences: cp VCIS is better than cp CIS and std VCIS is better than cp CIS (as before), and cp VCIS is better than std CIS, and std CIS is better than cp CIS. The cp VCIS processor is the best in these comparisons, and the score obtained with it is significantly better than the scores obtained with the cp CIS or std CIS processors.

◆ Discussion of Findings to Date

The findings reviewed above are consistent with the idea that a relatively high number of (discriminable) stimulus sites may be needed for effective use of DRNL filters in a speech processor for cochlear implants. When a high number of sites is available, possible advantages of DRNL filters may be immediately apparent, as suggested by the present results.

Other strategies, which map a high number of DRNL channel outputs to a small number of stimulus sites (the maximum *n-to-m* or average *n-to-m* approaches), may not be as effective. Combinations or selection of outputs must produce distortions with either approach. However, use of outputs from the DRNL filters, as opposed to the DRNL channels (which include the envelope detectors and nonlinear mapping function), may reduce distortions and thereby improve the performance of *n-to-m* approaches. We plan to evaluate this possibility in future studies.

Among the processors tested with subject SR3, the cp VCIS processor produced the best performance overall and in addition was the clear winner according to the subject's anecdotal comments. She asked us to "keep this one," a rare comment for this highly experienced subject. (This subject also has quite-high levels of performance with her standard CIS processor, which she has used in her daily life for many years.)

As noted above, more than 21 sites may be available using the VCIS approach with SR3 and perhaps other subjects. Future studies should address this possibility. In addition, alternative ways to provide a high number of sites should be investigated. Two such possibilities are to use DRNL processing in conjunction with the Nucleus electrode array (Cochlear Ltd., Sydney, Australia), with 22 intracochlear electrodes and up to 22 discriminable pitches for some subjects (e.g., Zwolan et al, 1997), or in conjunction with bilateral cochlear implants, that may provide a higher number of discriminable stimulus sites than either unilateral implant alone (e.g., Lawson et al, 2001).

An even greater number of sites might be produced with a combination of an array with a high number of electrodes and the VCIS approach. Of course, this would require simultaneous stimulation of adjacent electrodes to form the virtual channels. In addition, the number of discriminable virtual channels (or sites) is likely to depend on the inter-electrode spacing. The number may be higher with a wide spacing (e.g., the 4 mm of the Ineraid implant) than with a narrow spacing (e.g., the 0.75 mm spacing of the Nucleus implants). The number of discriminable steps for a given type of electrode array also will without a doubt depend on the subject, as has been shown by Poroy and Loizou (2001) for the Ineraid array and by Donaldson et al (2004) and Litvak et al (2003) for the Clarion "HiFocus" array.

At present, four implant systems would support the construction of virtual channels in combination with an electrode array with a high number of contacts. They are the Clarion CII and HiResolution 90K systems, the new PULSAR device from Med-El, and an experimental version of the Nucleus device that includes a percutaneous connector and the "Contour" electrode array (Cochlear Ltd., Sydney, Australia). The HiResolution 90K has a smaller implanted receiver/stimulator than the Clarion CII device but is otherwise identical to the CII. The HiFocus electrode array used with these systems includes 16 intracochlear contacts spaced at 1-mm intervals. The electrode array used with the PULSAR includes 12 sites of stimulation spaced at 2.4-mm intervals. The Contour array has 22 contacts spaced at 0.75-mm intervals, and also has a curved shape designed to bring the contacts into close proximity to the inner wall of the scala tympani (Balkany et al, 2002). Such apposition to the inner wall may increase the spatial specificity of stimulation by single electrodes compared with other placements of the electrode array. All four devices support simultaneous stimulation of multiple electrodes.

An important question for future research is how to maximize the number of discriminable sites with cochlear implants. This might be done with a particular type of electrode array, for example, one with a high number of contacts in close proximity to the inner wall of the scala tympani, or it might be done using the VCIS approach in conjunction with a particular type of electrode array or with any of a variety of arrays. Alternatively, a dense array of electrodes implanted directly within the auditory nerve may support an especially high number of discriminable sites. [Such intramodiolar implants are under development; see progress reports for National Institutes of Health (NIH) projects N01-DC-1–2108 and N01-DC-5–0005, available at http://www.nidcd.nih.gov/funding/programs/npp, and also Badi et al, 2003, and Hillman et al, 2003.]

The present results suggest that a high number of sites, in combination with DRNL processing, may be an especially effective way to represent speech information with cochlear implants. Clearly, studies with additional subjects are needed to evaluate the generality of these initial findings with only one subject. In addition, use of different types of electrode arrays, perhaps in combination with virtual channels, may be better than the present use of the Ineraid array in combination with three virtual channels between each pair of adjacent electrodes.

◆ Future Directions

Our immediate plans include further studies with Ineraid subjects to: (1) evaluate the generality of the findings with SR3, using the same processor (and virtual channel) conditions; (2) determine whether more than three discriminable positions may be available between adjacent electrodes of the Ineraid implant; (3) determine the range of variation across subjects (and choices of adjacent electrodes within subjects) in the maximum number of discriminable positions that can be produced using virtual channels; and (4) evaluate n-to-m approaches that combine or select DRNL filter outputs as opposed to DRNL channel outputs. In these studies, we also plan to investigate in greater detail the parameter space within and across DRNL filters.

In addition to these studies with Ineraid subjects, studies are now underway with four subjects who have been implanted with the experimental version of the Nucleus device. These latter studies will allow evaluation of DRNL processing in conjunction with a high number of stimulus sites, using the 22 electrodes of the Contour array, or using those electrodes in combination with the VCIS approach.

We regard the present findings as encouraging but preliminary. We plan further studies.

◆ Conclusion

The first steps in implementing a general approach for providing a closer mimicking of normal auditory functions with cochlear implants have been taken. Findings to date have been encouraging. Processors using n-to-m approaches have in general supported speech reception performance that is immediately on a par with that of the standard CIS processors used in everyday life by the subjects. For the one tested subject, a processor using DRNL filters in combination with virtual-channel stimulation supported significantly better performance than the standard CIS processor, especially for speech reception in noise. Further studies are needed to evaluate the generality of these preliminary findings and to optimize the incorporation of DRNL filters in speech processor designs. In addition, substitution of the IHC membrane and synapse model for the standard envelope detector needs to be evaluated separately and in combination with a DRNL filter bank.

Acknowledgments

This chapter is based in part on a special guest address given by the first author at the VIII International Cochlear Implant Conference, held in Indianapolis, Indiana, May 10 to 13, 2004. Portions of the text were updated or adapted from Wilson et al (2003a,b, 2005). The described studies and preparation of the chapter were supported by NIH project N01-DC-2–1002, "Speech Processors for Auditory Prostheses." Support for travel expenses for subjects visiting us from Europe was kindly provided by the Med-El GmbH, in Innsbruck, Austria. We thank Dewey Lawson, Xiaoan Sun, Robert Wolford, and Marian Zerbi for enlightening discussions and technical assistance.

References*

Badi AN, Kertesz TR, Gurgel RK, Shelton C, Normann RA. (2003). Development of a novel eighth-nerve intraneural auditory neuroprosthesis. Laryngoscope 113:833–842

Balkany TJ, Eshraghi AA, Yang N. (2002). Modiolar proximity of three perimodiolar cochlear implant electrodes. Acta Otolaryngol 122:363–369

Carney LH. (1993). A model for the responses of low-frequency auditory-nerve fibers in cat. J Acoust Soc Am 93:401–417

Deng L, Geisler CD. (1987). A composite auditory model for processing speech sounds. J Acoust Soc Am 82:2001–2012

Donaldson G, Kreft H, Litvak L, Mishra L, Overstreet E. (2004). Steering current through simultaneous electrode activation in the Clarion II: place-pitch resolution. Poster presented at the VIII International Cochlear Implant Conference, Indianapolis, IN, May 10–13

Hillman T, Badi AN, Normann RA, Kertesz T, Shelton C. (2003). Cochlear nerve stimulation with a 3-dimensional penetrating electrode array. Otol Neurotol 24:764–768

Lawson DT, Wolford RD, Brill SM, Schatzer R, Wilson BS. (2001). Speech processors for auditory prostheses: further studies regarding benefits of bilateral cochlear implants. Twelfth Quarterly Progress Report, NIH project N01-DC-8–2105, Neural Prosthesis Program, National Institutes of Health, Bethesda, MD†

Litvak LM, Overstreet E, Mishra L. (2003). Steering current through simultaneous activation of intracochlear electrodes in the Clarion CII cochlear implant: frequency resolution. Poster presented at the 2003 Conference on Implantable Auditory Prostheses, Pacific Grove, CA, August 17–22

Lopez-Poveda EA, Meddis R. (2001). A human nonlinear cochlear filterbank. J Acoust Soc Am 110:3107–3118

Lopez-Poveda EA, Plack CJ, Meddis R. (2003). Cochlear nonlinearity between 500 and 8000 Hz in listeners with normal hearing. J Acoust Soc Am 113:951–960

Meddis R. (1986). Simulation of mechanical to neural transduction in the auditory receptor. J Acoust Soc Am 79:702–711

Meddis R. (1988). Simulation of auditory-neural transduction: further studies. J Acoust Soc Am 83:1056–1063

Meddis R, O'Mard LP, Lopez-Poveda EA. (2001). A computational algorithm for computing nonlinear auditory frequency selectivity. J Acoust Soc Am 109:2852–2861

Parnas BR. (1996). Noise and neuronal populations conspire to encode simple waveforms reliably. IEEE Trans Biomed Eng 43:313–318

Poroy O, Loizou PC. (2001). Pitch perception using virtual channels. Poster presented at the 2001 Conference on Implantable Auditory Prostheses, Pacific Grove, CA, August 17–22

Robert A, Eriksson JL. (1999). A composite model of the auditory periphery for simulating responses to complex tones. J Acoust Soc Am 106:1852–1864

Rubinstein JT, Wilson BS, Finley CC, Abbas PJ. (1999). Pseudospontaneous activity: stochastic independence of auditory nerve fibers with electrical stimulation. Hear Res 127:108–118

Schatzer R, Wilson BS, Wolford RD, Lawson DT. (2003). Speech processors for auditory prostheses: signal processing strategy for a closer mimicking of normal auditory functions. Sixth Quarterly Progress Report, NIH project N01-DC-2–1002, Neural Prosthesis Program, National Institutes of Health, Bethesda, MD†

Tchorz J, Kollmeier B. (1999). A model of auditory perception as a front end for automatic speech recognition. J Acoust Soc Am 106:2040–2050

Tyler RS, Preece JP, Lansing CR, Otto SR, Gantz BJ. (1986). Previous experience as a confounding factor in comparing cochlear-implant processing schemes. J Speech Hear Res 29:282–287

Williams EJ, Bacon SP. (2005). Compression estimates using behavioral and otoacoustic emission measures. Hear Res 201:44–54

Wilson BS, Finley CC, Lawson DT, Wolford RD, Eddington DK, Rabinowitz WM. (1991). Better speech recognition with cochlear implants. Nature 352:236–238

Wilson BS, Finley CC, Lawson DT, Zerbi M. (1997). Temporal representations with cochlear implants. Am J Otol 18:S30–S34

Wilson BS, Lawson DT, Müller JM, et al. (2003a). Cochlear implants: some likely next steps. Annu Rev Biomed Eng;5:207–249

Wilson BS, Lawson DT, Zerbi M. (1994a). Speech processors for auditory prostheses: evaluation of VCIS processors. Sixth Quarterly Progress Report, NIH project N01-DC-2–2401, Neural Prosthesis Program, National Institutes of Health, Bethesda, MD†

Wilson BS, Lawson DT, Zerbi M, Finley CC. (1992). Speech processors for auditory prostheses: virtual channel interleaved sampling (VCIS) processors—initial studies with subject SR2. First Quarterly Progress Report, NIH project N01-DC-2–2401, Neural Prosthesis Program, National Institutes of Health, Bethesda, MD†

Wilson BS, Lawson DT, Zerbi M, Finley CC. (1994b). Recent developments with the CIS strategies. In: Hochmair-Desoyer IJ, Hochmair ES, eds. Advances in Cochlear Implants. Vienna: Manz, pp. 103–112

Wilson BS, Schatzer R, Lopez-Poveda EA, Sun X, Lawson DT, Wolford RD. (2005). Two new directions in speech processor design for cochlear implants. Ear Hear 26:73S–81S

Wilson BS, Wolford RD, Schatzer R, Sun X, Lawson DT. (2003b). Speech processors for auditory prostheses: combined use of dual-resonance nonlinear (DRNL) filters and virtual channels. Seventh Quarterly Progress Report, NIH project N01-DC-2–1002, Neural Prosthesis Program, National Institutes of Health, Bethesda, MD†

Wilson BS, Zerbi M, Lawson DT. (1993). Speech processors for auditory prostheses: identification of virtual channels on the basis of pitch. Third Quarterly Progress Report, NIH project N01-DC-2–2401, Neural Prosthesis Program, National Institutes of Health, Bethesda, MD†

Zhang X, Heinz MG, Bruce IC, Carney LH. (2001). A phenomenological model for the responses of auditory-nerve fibers: I. Nonlinear tuning with compression and suppression. J Acoust Soc Am 109:648–670

Zwolan TA, Collins LM, Wakefield GH. (1997). Electrode discrimination and speech recognition in postlingually deafened adult cochlear implant subjects. J Acoust Soc Am 102:3673–3685

*The National Institutes of Health (NIH) progress reports (†) are available at http://www.rti.org/capr/caprqprs.html or http://www.nidcd.nih.gov/funding/programs/npp.

6

Selection of Cochlear Implant Candidates

Teresa A. Zwolan

In the United States, the Food and Drug Administration (FDA), a consumer protection and health agency, has historically had great influence on cochlear implant candidacy. This agency oversees the selling, distribution, and marketing of drugs, medical devices, and other products. Importantly, the FDA determines if the specific wording used in device labeling, including information regarding indications for its use, is appropriate. Prior to receiving approval, device manufacturers must provide the FDA with details of their product, including a description of its function, results of clinical trials on specific groups of patients, information on adverse effects, and details on the materials that comprise the product. The FDA reviews the information and determines if it considers the product to be safe and effective for widespread use. The information provided by the FDA is a guideline for professionals. Thus, the determination of implant candidacy is ultimately based on the best knowledge and judgment of the managing physician. This may result in implantation of patients who do not meet candidacy requirements specified on the product's label. Such "off-label" uses of cochlear implants are infrequent, as many insurance companies may refuse payment if a device is not indicated for the recipient based on FDA guidelines. According to the FDA's Web site, "If physicians use a product for an indication not in the approved labeling, they have the responsibility to be well informed about the product, to base its use on firm scientific rationale and on sound medical evidence, and to maintain records of the product's use and effects." Information regarding past and present candidacy guidelines for cochlear implant devices available in the United States is provided in **Appendix 6–1**.

Numerous clinical trials have been conducted by the FDA since cochlear implants were first introduced, and numerous supplements have been submitted to the FDA as these devices have undergone technological improvements. Changes in candidacy have primarily included implanting persons with increasing amounts of residual hearing, implanting persons with increasing amounts of preoperative open-set speech perception skills, implanting children at younger ages, and implanting greater numbers of persons with abnormal cochleae. The primary reason that selection criteria have changed is that patients with implants are obtaining increasing amounts of open-set speech recognition with the available devices. Although this increased performance is largely due to the technological advancements that have occurred in the field, it may also be due, at least in part, to the fact that patients with greater amounts of residual hearing and greater amounts of residual speech recognition skills are receiving cochlear implants.

◆ Pre- and Postoperative Assessment and Evaluation

The preoperative evaluation is an extremely important part of the implant process. The primary purpose of the preoperative evaluation is to determine if the patient is medically and audiologically suitable for a cochlear implant. Additionally, information obtained during the preimplant evaluation process can be compared with postoperative performance to evaluate patient progress and to evaluate device efficacy. Test procedures commonly included in the preoperative test battery for determining implant candidacy are described in the following sections.

Medical Evaluation

During the preoperative medical evaluation, the physician obtains a complete medical history and performs a physical examination. The surgeon attempts to identify the cause of the hearing loss if it is not known, determines if treatment options other than a cochlear implant are more suitable for the patient, and determines if the cochlear implant candidate's general health is suitable for implantation. Additional information regarding surgical decisions that may affect candidacy for a cochlear implant may be found in other chapters in this book. Postoperatively, patients should be seen biannually by their implant surgeon for routine evaluations. They should also be seen by the surgeon if any otologic problems arise or if problems with the electrode array are noted by the audiologist.

Cochlear Imaging

Computed tomography (CT) or magnetic resonance imaging (MRI) of the temporal bone are routinely performed as part of the preoperative evaluation process and provide an image of the structure of the cochlea and help identify any cochlear anomalies. The results of such testing may be used to determine the most appropriate ear for implantation. Although severe anomalies and/or cochlear ossification may affect insertion depth, placement of the electrode array, or type of device selected, they do not necessarily preclude the patient from implantation (Balkany et al, 1996; Eisenman et al, 2001; Tucci et al, 1995). Postoperatively, imaging studies may be used to evaluate device placement and to determine if changes have occurred regarding the location of the electrode array within the cochlea. Additional information regarding imaging and its role in patient selection and evaluation may be found in Chapter 7.

Audiological Evaluation

The primary purpose of the preoperative audiological evaluation is to determine the type and severity of hearing loss. Typically, this evaluation will include determination of unaided air and bone conduction thresholds, unaided speech discrimination, speech reception threshold (SRT) (if possible), speech detection threshold (SDT), otoacoustic emissions (OAEs), and immittance testing to include tympanometry and acoustic reflexes.

Candidacy Guidelines Regarding Audiometric Test Results

In the early clinical trials, only persons who demonstrated a bilateral profound sensorineural hearing loss [pure tone average (PTA) greater than or equal to 90 dB HL] were considered to be candidates for a cochlear implant. Past and present candidacy guidelines for cochlear implant devices available in the United States are provided in **Appendix 6–1**. Present guidelines are more lenient than guidelines used in the past and allow for persons with slightly better hearing (particularly in the low frequencies) to be considered for a cochlear implant. Additionally, these indications vary slightly among the currently available devices. For example, guidelines for the Nucleus Freedom with Contour Advance indicate that postlinguistically deafened adults who are candidates for the implant typically have "moderate to profound hearing loss in the low frequencies and profound ($\geq$90 dB HL) hearing loss in the mid-to-high speech frequencies." Guidelines for the Clarion HiResolution Bionic Ear System (Advanced Bionics; Valencia, CA) indicate that adults should have "severe to profound, bilateral sensorineural hearing deafness ($\geq$70 dB HL)," while indications for the Med-El Pulsar CI^{100} (Innsbruck, Austria) states "a pure tone average of 70 dB or greater at 500 Hz, 1000 Hz, and 2000 Hz."

Guidelines for children are often stricter than those for adults and may vary depending on the age of the child. For example, recommended guidelines for the Nucleus Freedom implant with Contour Advance indicate that children who are less than 24 months of age should demonstrate a bilateral profound hearing loss, whereas children 24 months of age or older only need to demonstrate a severe to profound hearing loss bilaterally. Indications for children for the HiResolution Bionic Ear System and for the Med-El Pulsar CI^{100} indicate that all children 12 months of age through 17 years should demonstrate a profound, bilateral sensorineural hearing loss.

Electrophysiologic Testing

Several implant centers include electrophysiologic tests in their preoperative test battery. Tests such as the auditory brainstem response (ABR) verify audiometric test results, help identify patients with auditory dyssynchrony, and help rule out the possibility of functional deafness. Such testing is particularly important when testing young children.

In some clinics, the electrophysiologic measure of electric auditory brainstem response (EABR) testing (Kileny & Zwolan, 2004; Kileny et al, 1994) is routinely performed with children who are less than 2 years of age, when a child presents with cochlear malformations, or when the preferred ear for implantation demonstrates no residual hearing. Such testing can be helpful to verify electrical stimulability of the auditory system, and is particularly useful when questions arise regarding the presence or stimulability of the VIIIth nerve in the ear to be implanted.

Hearing Aid Evaluation

The primary purpose of the preoperative hearing aid evaluation (HAE) is to evaluate the patient's performance with appropriate amplification. This procedure has two primary components: evaluation of the patient's detection skills and evaluation of the patient's aided speech perception skills. The first step in the HAE should include an evaluation of the patient's personal amplification to determine if the aid meets manufacturer's specifications. Second, the suitability of the device should be evaluated. Some patients' hearing loss may have progressed since the hearing aid was originally obtained, making it inappropriate for their current hearing loss. Additionally, improvements may have occurred in hearing aid technology that may increase the benefit the patient is able to receive from a different type of amplification. This can be particularly true if the patient has never experienced digital hearing aid technology. If the patient's hearing aid does not meet manufacturer's specifications for performance, or if the aid is not suitable for the patient's degree and severity of loss, an appropriate hearing aid must be fitted to the patient prior to performing the preoperative evaluation.

Typically, the HAE includes determination of aided warble tone sound-field detection thresholds at 250, 500, 1000, 2000, 3000, and 4000 Hz; determination of the aided most comfortable loudness (MCL) level, uncomfortable loudness level (ULCL), aided SDT, and aided SRT; and speech perception testing. These procedures should be performed with each ear aided separately as well as in binaural aided condition.

Once aided responses have been obtained, it is important to compare these responses to those expected with a cochlear implant. On average, patients with cochlear implants demonstrate sound-field warble tone thresholds that fall between 25 and 40 dB HL for the test frequencies of 250 to 4000 Hz. The aided detection thresholds obtained by a patient with hearing aids can be compared with the levels obtained by patients with implants to determine if the patient's detection skills will likely improve with a cochlear implant. When making such a comparison, it is important to inform patients that aided detection thresholds represent simple detection and provide no information regarding the discriminability of the sounds presented at the various test frequencies.

Postoperatively, it is important to evaluate the implant users' ability to detect warble tones in a sound field. Such testing provides information regarding their detection skills and verifies that a particular program is appropriate. Additionally, sound field thresholds obtained with the cochlear implant can identify problem areas and can be used to guide programming of the speech processor.

Candidacy Guidelines Regarding Appropriateness of Amplification

As the criteria for implantation have become more lenient, it has become increasingly important for clinicians to ensure that all measures have been taken to determine if the implant candidate will benefit from appropriate amplification. Example procedures that can be used to determine if the hearing aid characteristics are appropriate for the implant candidate's degree and configuration of hearing loss include the computer-assisted Phase IV Hearing Aid Selection and Evaluation Program (Mason & Popelka, 1982).

When evaluating candidacy for a cochlear implant, it is important to consider the amount of time the candidate has used appropriate amplification. This is particularly true with children, prelingually deafened adults, and adults and children who demonstrate some open-set speech recognition skills, as experience with amplification can greatly influence auditory detection and speech recognition skills.

Candidacy Guidelines Regarding Trial with Amplification

Guidelines regarding the need for hearing aid use prior to cochlear implantation are usually provided in the indications for use in children but are not provided for adults, as it is assumed that adults will have had adequate experience with hearing aids. If they do not have such experience, such as in the case of sudden hearing loss, a hearing aid trial is essential. In the past, guidelines for children required longer trials with amplification than are recommended today. For example, a minimum 6-month trial with appropriate amplification and rehabilitation was recommended to ascertain the potential for aided benefit with the Nucleus 22 device. Currently, the recommended duration of a hearing aid trial varies slightly among devices that have most recently received FDA approval. Current guidelines for the Nucleus Freedom with Contour Advance and Med-El Pulsar CI[100] device recommend a 3- to 6-month hearing aid trial for children without previous hearing aid experience. Candidacy guidelines for the Clarion HiResolution Bionic Ear System for children more specifically recommend a 6-month trial for children 2 through 17 years of age, and at least 3 months in children 12 through 23 months of age. For all three devices, the minimum duration of hearing aid use is waived if there is radiological evidence of cochlear ossification.

Speech and Language Evaluation

The purpose of the preoperative speech and language evaluation is to determine if the child demonstrates developmental language and/or articulation disorders, to describe the child's communicative status with respect to normative models of language development, and to help define appropriate expectations for speech and language skills following intervention with a cochlear implant. The preoperative evaluation provides an opportunity to develop preliminary goals, objectives, and treatment approaches. Similar to speech perception materials, the specific tests used in the speech and language evaluation are dependent on the child's age and language level. Postoperatively, children with cochlear implants should continue to participate in regularly scheduled speech and language evaluations. Like speech perception measures, postoperative speech and language evaluations help determine which speech cues are or are not being perceived by the child, provide information that may aid in programming the child's device, and help determine auditory therapy goals.

Psychological Evaluation

The psychological evaluation is primarily performed with pediatric patients but may be necessary with adults who present with concerns regarding cognitive status or mental function. With children, a preoperative evaluation should include assessment of cognitive abilities to determine if factors other than hearing impairment may be hindering the child's auditory development. Additionally, the presence of a cognitive impairment could greatly influence the child's ability to develop spoken language skills with a cochlear implant. Thus, identification of such problems is necessary for counseling parents regarding the expected outcomes for their child. Importantly, parents of very young children should be informed that some psychological deficits (i.e., autism) often cannot be identified until the child is 2 years of age or older. As many children receive an implant prior to their second birthday, parents should be warned of the possibility that their child's performance with the device may be affected by future identification of a cognitive impairment.

During recent years, greater numbers of children are being evaluated for a cochlear implant who present with a disability in addition to their hearing loss (Donaldson et al, 2004). This has increased the need for preoperative psychological evaluations. The results of such evaluations help determine if the child will be able to utilize the auditory signal, influencing the decision of whether or not to provide the child with a cochlear implant. Importantly, the input of the psychologist is essential when counseling parents about expectations for performance and when determining if referrals to other professionals are necessary prior to and after the child receives an implant.

Speech Perception Testing

The primary purpose of speech perception testing is to evaluate performance with an appropriate hearing aid and to determine if the patient's speech perception skills will likely improve with a cochlear implant. Accurate documentation of preoperative speech perception skills is important as such data will determine if the intervention was appropriate and successful for the patient and will also influence future expansion of cochlear implant candidacy. Postoperatively, speech perception testing is important as it helps verify programming of the patient's device, helps identify cues that are or are not being perceived by the implant user, and provides a measure of internal device efficacy, information regarding the implant user's rehabilitative needs, and information that will be useful in determining future selection criteria.

Speech perception testing should be performed in a sound field using recorded test materials whenever possible (this is often not feasible, however, when testing small children). In the past, the most frequently recommended presentation level for speech perception test materials was 70 dB sound pressure level (SPL). This level has been used in numerous clinical trials. Skinner et al (1997) recommended that cochlear implant candidates and recipients be evaluated with speech tests presented at 60 dB SPL. They state that such a level represents a normal conversational level while a presentation level of 70 dB SPL represents a raised-to-loud vocal level. Recently, Firszt et al (2004) demonstrated that Clarion, Med-El, and Nucleus recipients performed similarly on sentence and word tests when stimuli were presented at 60 and 70 dB SPL. Additionally, subjects continued to demonstrate substantial open-set speech perception when stimuli were presented at the softer level of 50 dB SPL. They concluded that candidacy criteria should be based on speech recognition tests presented at 60 and/or 50 dB SPL, as such levels reflect the listening challenges that individuals encounter in natural communication situations. Because of this, many future studies will present stimuli at levels softer than the previously used level of 70 dB SPL.

During speech perception testing, patients should utilize appropriate amplification preoperatively and should utilize their speech processor set to a normal use setting postoperatively. In both instances, they should be tested in a sound-treated room that contains minimal visual and auditory distractions. The presentation level should be calculated using a calibration microphone placed at a reference point located at the center of the listener's head. Test materials should be presented a single time only, and feedback should not be provided. Caution should be taken to ensure that test materials are used a single time only, as this will reduce the likelihood that learning will influence the patient's test score.

With adult patients, the speech perception evaluation should include assessment of the ability to understand phonemes and words when presented in isolated monosyllables, an assessment of the ability to perceive words when presented in the context of a sentence, and a measure of lipreading ability. Monosyllabic word tests most commonly used by implant centers today include the Northwestern University (NU-6) Monosyllabic Words Test (Tillman & Carhart, 1966) and the Consonant-Nucleus-Consonant (CNC) Monosyllabic Words Test (Peterson & Lehiste, 1962). Sentence materials mot often used in clinics today include the Hearing in Noise Test (HINT) (Nilsson et al, 1994) and City University of New York (CUNY) sentences (Boothroyd et al, 1985). As many patients present preoperatively with an ability to understand some words and sentences, they can additionally be tested in noise to determine the effect that such noise has on performance. The recommended presentation level for background noise is a +10 signal-to-noise ratio.

To measure lipreading ability, sentence materials may be presented via live voice or via video display, and stimuli should be presented in three different ways. First, sentences should be presented in a "hearing alone" mode to evaluate open-set speech recognition skills. Second, stimuli should be presented in a "hearing plus vision" mode. Lastly, sentences should be presented in a "lipreading alone" mode. Subtraction of the lipreading alone score from the lipreading plus hearing score provides a measure of the amount of lipreading enhancement the patient receives from the hearing aid or cochlear implant. The lipreading alone score is particularly important in the preoperative evaluation as it provides the clinician with an idea of how well the patient will comprehend the vast amount of information that will be provided regarding cochlear implantation. If testing indicates the patient is a poor lipreader, the clinician should utilize means other than verbal communication (e.g., written communication) to ensure that the patient understands all of the information provided. Additional information regarding speech perception tests commonly used with adults in pre- and postoperative cochlear implant evaluations may be found in **Table 6–1**.

William Luxford of the House Ear Institute led a committee composed of participants from various professional organizations and from cochlear implant manufacturers to develop the Minimum Speech Test Battery for Adult Cochlear Implant Users (Luxford, 2000). The primary purpose of the battery was to provide centers with test materials for

Table 6–1 Speech Perception Tests Commonly Used with Adults in Pre- and Postoperative Cochlear Implant Evaluation

Test	Reference
CID Everyday Sentences	Silverman & Hirsh (1955)
Consonant-Nucleus-Consonant (CNC) Test	Peterson & Lehiste (1962)
Hearing in Noise Test (HINT)	Nilsson et al (1994)
Minimal Auditory Capabilities (MAC) Battery	Owens et al (1981)
Northwestern University Auditory Test No. 6	Tillman & Carhart (1966)

evaluation of the pre- and postoperative speech recognition performance of implant users, irrespective of the type of implant or speech processing strategy, so that individual and group comparisons may be made within and across implants and encoding strategies. Many cochlear implant centers utilize this test battery in their clinical practice as a tool for determination of implant candidacy.

The speech perception evaluation is also a particularly important part of the pre- and postoperative process for children. Rather than utilization of a single test, batteries of tests that measure a variety of speech perception skills should be used with children, as such tests are more sensitive to individual differences in performance. Preoperatively, such tests determine if the child is receiving auditory information with the current amplification and helps determine if speech perception skills will likely improve with a cochlear implant. Postoperatively, such tests provide information regarding the speech cues that are or are not being perceived by the child, may aid in programming his/her device, and may help determine auditory therapy goals.

The specific tests used in pre- and postoperative evaluations of children vary greatly as they are dependent on the child's age and linguistic and cognitive ability. In general, pediatric speech perception tests can be categorized into three primary types: (1) closed-set tests that measure prosodic cue, speech feature, or word perception; (2) open-set word and sentence tests that provide an estimate of the child's ability to communicate in the real world; and

(3) objective report scales, such as the Meaningful Auditory Integration Scale (MAIS) (Robbins et al, 1991), which uses parental reports to evaluate the child's listening skills in the daily environment. Speech perception tests commonly used with children in pre- and postoperative cochlear implant evaluations are listed in **Table 6–2**.

Candidacy Guidelines Regarding Speech Perception Ability

In the early clinical trials, only patients who demonstrated no open-set speech recognition skills were considered to be candidates for a cochlear implant. When the first clinical trials to evaluate the Nucleus device were initiated, adult and pediatric patients were required to demonstrate no open-set speech recognition skills (Mecklenburg et al, 1991). The clinical trial to evaluate the Nucleus 22 device in severely hearing impaired adults was the first FDA-guided study that indicated it was appropriate to implant individuals with some open-set speech recognition skills. This clinical trial was initiated in 1988 and was completed in 1995. Candidates for this study were divided into two phases. Phase I included patients who demonstrated scores less than or equal to 25% correct on Central Institute for the Deaf (CID) Everyday Sentences (in the nonimplant ear), less than or equal to 10% on CID Everyday Sentences in the implant ear, and less than or equal to 30% correct when tested in a binaural aided condition. Phase II subjects included those who scored less than or equal to 25% correct on CID Everyday Sentences in either the implant or nonimplant ear and less than or equal to 30% correct when tested binaurally.

The FDA studies conducted since then have always included patients with some open-set speech recognition skills. Although all three devices recommend use of recorded sentences to evaluate aided benefit in adults, the scores used to define limited benefit vary slightly. For example, indications for the Nucleus Freedom with Contour Advance define limited benefit from amplification as a score ≤50% correct in the ear to be implanted and ≤60% in the best-aided listening condition. Indications for the HiResolution Bionic

Table 6–2 Speech Perception Tests Commonly Used with Children in Pre- and Postoperative Cochlear Implant Evaluations

Test	References
Bamford-Kowal-Bench (BKB) Sentences	Bench et al (1979)
Early Speech Perception Test, Low Verbal Version	Moog & Geers (1990)
Early Speech Perception Test, Standard Version	Moog & Geers (1990)
Glendonald Auditory Screening Procedure (GASP)	Erber (1982)
Lexical Neighborhood Test (LNT)	Kirk et al (1995)
Ling Sound Test	Ling (1989)
Meaningful Auditory Integration Scale	Robbins et al (1991)
Meaningful Auditory Integration Scale for Use with Infants and Toddlers (IT-MAIS)	Zimmerman-Philips et al 1998
Minimal Pairs	Robbins et al (1988)
Monosyllable-Trochee-Spondee (MTS) Test	Erber & Alencewicz (1976)
Multisyllabic Lexical Neighborhood Test (MLNT)	Kirk et al (1995)
Northwestern University Children's Perception of Speech (NU-CHIPS) Test	Elliott & Katz (1980)
Phonetically Balanced Kindergarten Word List (PBK-50)	Haskins (1949)
Word Intelligibility by Picture Identification (WIPI)	Ross & Lerman (1971)

Ear System define limited benefit as a score $\leq 50\%$, whereas the Med-El Pulsar CI[100] device recommends a test score $\leq 40\%$ correct on such measures. It is important to keep in mind that these scores are recommended guidelines. Thus, some patients who have received cochlear implants have demonstrated scores that are better than the above-mentioned recommendations. Additional factors that go into a decision regarding implant candidacy include the patient's willingness or ability to use amplification, the effect that reduced speech recognition has on the patient's ability to function in occupational and social settings, as well as the patient's ability to tolerate the amplified signal.

Selection criteria for children, which have also been expanded to include candidates with minimal open-set speech perception skills, vary among currently approved devices. FDA-approved indications for use of all three devices state that in younger children, limited benefit is defined as lack of progress in the development of simple auditory skills in conjunction with appropriate amplification and participation in intensive aural rehabilitation over a 3- to 6-month period. All three manufacturers recommended that hearing aid benefit be quantified in young children using measures such as the MAIS (Robbins et al, 1991) or the Early Speech Perception (ESP) test (Moog & Geers, 1990). With older children, all three manufacturers recommend use of the open-set Multisyllabic Lexical Neighborhood Test (MLNT) (Kirk et al, 1995) or Lexical Neighborhood Test (LNT) (Kirk et al, 1995), depending on the child's cognitive and linguistic skills. Like the adults, the particular score used to define lack of benefit varies. For the Nucleus Freedom with Contour Advance, lack of aided benefit is defined as a score less than or equal to 30% correct, whereas the Clarion HiResolution Bionic Ear System and the Med-El Pulsar CI[100] define this as a score $\leq 20\%$ on such measures.

◆ Additional Factors that Might Affect Candidacy

Age at Implantation

There has been a growing trend to decrease the age at which children receive a cochlear implant. Many investigators have argued that doing so will provide children with greater access to auditory information, which is crucial for development of speech and language skills (Hoffman, 1997; Osberger, 1997). Implantation of children less than 2 years of age requires special skills on the part of the implant team. First, determination of implant candidacy poses a special challenge, as evaluation of the child's speech and language and speech perception skills is difficult. Second, postoperative follow-up is complicated by the fact that most children in this age group are unable to provide a conditioned response, which is routinely used to program and set the device. Thus, there is an increasing need to develop and evaluate objective measures that will aid in the selection, evaluation, and postoperative treatment of such young children.

Although FDA recommended criteria indicate that cochlear implants are appropriate for children 12 months of age or older for all of the available devices, several investigators in the United States have implanted children who were less than 12 months of age at the time of surgery. Preliminary results obtained with such young children indicate that cochlear implant surgery is safe in children aged 7 to 12 months with appropriate anesthetic and postoperative support (James & Papsin, 2004), and that many children who underwent implantation as infants developed language skills commensurate with those of their hearing peers (Hammes et al, 2002).

Candidacy Guidelines Related to Age

The first clinical trial to evaluate a multichannel cochlear implant in children was the Nucleus 22 device. The candidacy guidelines for this trial indicated that appropriate candidates could be as young as 2 years of age. The first clinical trial to include children less than 2 years of age as candidates was for the Clarion device. In its clinical trial, this device could be used with children as young as 18 months of age if x-rays demonstrated evidence of ossification. All of the devices currently approved by the FDA indicate that cochlear implants are appropriate for children 12 months of age and older.

Auditory Neuropathy/Dyssynchrony

Auditory neuropathy (AN) is a term used to describe an auditory disorder characterized by recordable otoacoustic emissions or cochlear microphonic, absent, or atypical auditory brainstem responses, and speech recognition skills that are poorer than would be expected based on the audiogram (Rapin & Gravel, 2003). Because of these factors, determination of candidacy for a cochlear implant in patients with AN can be difficult. Often, such patients meet candidacy criteria based on their poor speech recognition skills but may fail to meet criteria based on their audiometric thresholds (i.e., their hearing is "too good"). Determination of cochlear implant candidacy of such individuals is additionally complicated by two important factors. First, some patients with AN have demonstrated recovery or improvement of detection and speech recognition skills over time (Neault, 2003). Second, many children who present with AN also present with additional medical diagnoses that may affect expected outcomes for performance (O'Sullivan, 2004; Rance et al, 1999).

Several investigators have reported that cochlear implant recipients with AN demonstrate postoperative outcomes that are similar to those obtained by more traditional cochlear implant recipients (Buss et al, 2002; Mason et al, 2003; Peterson et al, 2003; Sininger & Trautwein, 2002). These investigators also indicate, however, that the outcomes vary from patient to patient, similar to the results obtained by cochlear implant patients in general. Thus, determination of candidacy for a cochlear implant for a child with AN should be determined on a case-by-case basis. One factor that should receive strong consideration is the child's development (or lack of development) of spoken language skills as the presence of a severe language delay demonstrates a need for intervention.

Children with Additional Disabilities

Previously, children were excluded from participating in early cochlear implant clinical trials if they presented with any type of cognitive delay. More recently, however, children with additional disabilities, such as cognitive and noncognitive delays, are routinely receiving cochlear implants. Pyman et al (2000) performed a retrospective analysis of data on 75 consecutively implanted children up to 5 years of age and found that children with motor and/or cognitive delays were significantly slower than other children in the development of speech perception skills after implantation. Other authors have reported similar findings, but have additionally indicated that provision of a cochlear implant can improve the life quality of profoundly deaf subjects with associated disabilities, increasing their listening and communication skills, their self-sufficiency (Filipo et al, 2004), and their ability to interact with others (Donaldson et al, 2004).

Recipients with Medicare and Medicaid Insurance

Medicare is the U.S. national health insurance program that provides health insurance to citizens age 65 and over, to those who have permanent kidney failure, and to certain individuals under 65 with disabilities. The Centers for Medicare and Medicaid Services (CMS) administers the Medicare program and works with the states to administer Medicaid, the State Children's Health Insurance Program (SCHIP), and health insurance portability standards. Large numbers of cochlear implant candidates receive their health care coverage from Medicare, Medicaid, or SCHIP. Financial coverage of a cochlear implant for such individuals is greatly influenced by CMS's national coverage determinations (NCDs), which specify the conditions under which recipients are covered for a cochlear implant.

Prior to 2005, the CMS NCD stated that adults must demonstrate test scores of 30% or less on sentence recognition scores from tape-recorded tests in the patient's best listening condition, and that cochlear implants in children are not covered until the child is 2 years old and then only where deafness is demonstrated by the inability to improve on age-appropriate closed-set word identification tasks with amplification. This policy was based on previous FDA-approved labeling.

In July 2004, Cochlear Corporation (Sydney, Australia) made a formal request for revision of CMS coverage language to reflect current FDA-approved indications and candidacy standards accepted by the cochlear implant medical community. As a result, CMS reviewed its policies and on April 4, 2005, released a decision stating, "The evidence is adequate to conclude that cochlear implantation is reasonable and necessary for treatment of bilateral pre- or postlinguistic, sensorineural, moderate-to-profound hearing loss in individuals who demonstrate limited benefit from amplification. Limited benefit from amplification is defined by test scores of ≤40% correct in the best-aided listening condition on tape recorded tests of open-set sentence cognition." Their decision also included the following: "The evidence is sufficient to conclude that a cochlear implant is reasonable and necessary for individuals with hearing test scores of >40% and ≤60% only when the provider is participating in and patients are enrolled in either an FDA-approved category B IDE [Investigational Device Exemption] clinical trial, a trial under the CMS Clinical Trial Policy, or a prospective, controlled comparative trial approved by CMS as consistent with the evidentiary requirements for National Coverage Analyses and meeting specific quality standards." Additional information regarding CMS coverage language for cochlear implants can be obtained from the CMS Web site: http://www.cms.hhs.gov/.

◆ Conclusion

Selection of candidates for cochlear implantation is a process that has evolved greatly over the past several years. Current candidacy guidelines indicate that it is appropriate to provide cochlear implants to persons with increasing amounts of residual hearing, to persons with increasing amounts of preoperative open-set speech perception skills, and to children as young as 12 months of age. These changes are largely due to the fact that individuals are obtaining remarkable results with cochlear implants.

Technological advances and enhanced surgical techniques will certainly contribute to continued improvements in the field of cochlear implants. Careful documentation of factors that have been used to determine candidacy and reliable and consistent documentation of postoperative performance are needed if the selection criteria used to determine candidacy are to continue to evolve at an appropriate pace.

Appendix 6–1   Candidacy Guidelines for Food and Drug Administration (FDA)-Approved Devices Currently Available in the United States

Device Name	Device Manufacturer	Population Approved for	Year of FDA Approval	Indications
Clarion	Advanced Bionics Corporation	Postlingually deafened adults	1996	Eighteen years of age or older. Profound, bilateral sensorineural deafness (greater than or equal to 90 dB). Postlingually deafened. Lack of benefit from appropriately fitted hearing aids. In adults, lack of benefit with hearing aids is defined as scoring 20% or less on tests of open-set sentence recognition (CID sentences).
Clarion	Advanced Bionics Corporation	Children	1997	Two through 17 years of age. If x-rays demonstrate evidence of ossification, children as young as 18 months may be implanted. Profound bilateral, sensorineural deafness ≥90 dB. Undergone or be willing to undergo a hearing aid trial with appropriately fitted hearing aids. Lack of benefit from appropriately fitted hearing aids. In younger children, lack of benefit from hearing aids is defined as a failure to attain basic auditory milestones such as a child's inconsistent response to his/her name in quiet or to environmental sounds (Meaningful Auditory Integration Scale). In older children, lack of aided benefit is defined as scoring 0% on open-set word recognition (Phonetically Balanced Kindergarten Test: Word List) administered with monitored live voice (70 dB SPL). Both younger and older children should demonstrate only minimal ability on age appropriate open-set sentence measures and a plateau in auditory development.
Clarion	Advanced Bionics Corporation	Severely and profoundly hearing impaired adults	2000	Adults 18 years of age or older with no previous implant experience. Patients should have a sensorineural hearing loss of a severe or greater degree in both ears, defined as a pure tone average (500, 1000, and 2000 Hz) of 70 dB HL or greater. Patient must have used an appropriate hearing aid for at least 2 months. The audiologist must determine if the hearing aid characteristics are appropriate for the patient's degree and configuration of hearing loss using criteria specified by. Patient must demonstrate marginal benefit with appropriately fitted hearing aids, deafened by a Hearing in Noise Test (HINT) sentence score of less than or equal to 40% correct (two lists) in the best aided condition. Patient must also demonstrate a score ≤30% correct on the Consonant-Nucleus-Consonant (CNC) words test in the nonimplant ear and ≤20% correct on the CNC test in the ear to be implanted.
Clarion HiResolution™ Bionic Ear System: HiRes 90K™ receiver and HiFocus® or HiFocus Helix electrode array	Advanced Bionics Corporation	Adults and children	2003	Adults 18 years of age or older. Severe-to-profound, bilateral sensorineural hearing loss (70 dB HL). Postlingual onset of severe or profound hearing loss. Limited benefit from appropriately fit hearing aids, defined as scoring 50% or less on a test of open-set sentence recognition (HINT sentences). Children 12 months of age through 17 years of age. Profound, bilateral sensorineural deafness ≥90 dB HL). Use of appropriately fitted hearing aids for at least 6 months in children 2 through 17 years of age, or at least 3 months in children 12 through 23 months of age. The minimum duration of hearing aid use is waived if x-rays indicate ossification of the cochlea. Little or no benefit from appropriately fit hearing aids. In younger children (<4 years of age), lack of benefit is defined as a failure to reach developmentally appropriate auditory milestones (such as spontaneous response to name in quiet or to environmental sounds) measured using the Infant-Toddler Meaningful Auditory Integration Scale or Meaningful Auditory Integration Scale or ≤20% correct on a simple open-set word recognition test (Multisyllabic Lexical Neighborhood Test) administered using monitored live voice (70 dB SPL). In older children (≥4 years of age), lack of hearing aid benefit is defined as scoring ≤12% on a difficult open-set word recognition test (Phonetically Balanced Kindergarten Test) or ≤30% on an open-set sentence test (Hearing in Noise Test for Children) administered using recorded materials in the sound field (70 dB SPL).

Device	Company	Year	Population	Description
Nucleus 22	Cochlear Corporation	1985	Postlinguistically deafened adults	Intended for use in patients 18 years of age or older who have bilateral, postlinguistic, sensorineural hearing impairment and obtain limited benefit from appropriate binaural hearing aids. Limited benefit from amplification is defined by test scores of 30% correct or less in the best-aided listening condition on tape-recorded tests of open-set speech recognition. These patients typically have low-frequency residual hearing in the moderate-to-profound range and profound ($\geq$90 dB HL) hearing loss in the mid-to-high speech frequencies.
Nucleus 22	Cochlear Corporation	1990	Children	Intended for use in patients 2 through 17 years of age who have bilateral profound sensorineural deafness and achieve little or no benefit from a hearing (or vibrotactile) aid, as demonstrated by the inability to improve on an age appropriate closed-set word identification task. Families and (if possible) candidates should be well motivated and possess appropriate expectations.
Nucleus 22		1995	Severely hearing impaired adults	Once FDA approval was received for this population, Cochlear Corporation changed to its current wording in its indications for use with postlinguistically deafened adults.
Nucleus 22		1995	Prelinguistically and perilinguistically deafened adults	Intended for use in prelinguistically and perilinguistically deafened adults who are 18 years of age or older and who have profound sensorineural deafness and are unable to benefit from appropriate amplification by a hearing aid.
Nucleus 24		1998	Postlinguistically deafened adults	The Nucleus 24 Cochlear Implant System is intended for use in individuals 18 years of age or older who have a bilateral, postlinguistic, sensorineural hearing impairment and obtain limited benefit from appropriate binaural hearing aids. These individuals typically have moderate to profound hearing loss in the low frequencies and profound ($\geq$90 dB HL) hearing loss in the mid-to-high speech frequencies. Limited benefit from amplification is defined by test scores of 40% correct or less in the best-aided listening condition on tape-recorded tests of open-set speech recognition.
Nucleus 24		1998	Prelinguistically and perilinguistically deafened adults	The Nucleus 24 is intended for use in prelinguistically and perilinguistically deafened individuals, 18 years of age or older, who have profound sensorineural deafness and do not benefit from appropriate hearing aids.
Nucleus 24	Cochlear Corporation	1998	Children	The Nucleus 24 is intended for use in children 18 months through 17 years of age who have bilateral profound sensorineural deafness and demonstrate little or no benefit from appropriate binaural hearing aids. In younger children, little or no aided benefit is defined as lack of progress in the development of simple auditory skills in conjunction with appropriate amplification and participation in intensive aural rehabilitation over a 3- to 6-month period. It is recommended that limited benefit be quantified on a measure such as the Meaningful Auditory Integration Scale or the Early Speech Perception test. In older children, lack of aided benefit is deafened as less than 20% correct on the open-set Multisyllablic Lexical Neighborhood Test (MLNT) or Lexical Neighborhood Test (LNT), depending on the child's cognitive and linguistic skills. A 3- to 6- month hearing aid trial is required for children without previous hearing aid experience.

(*Continued*)

Appendix 6–1 Candidacy Guidelines for Food and Drug Administration (FDA)-Approved Devices Currently Available in the United States *(Continued)*

Device Name	Device Manufacturer	Population Approved for	Year of FDA Approval	Indications
Nucleus 24 Contour cochlear implants CI24R (CS), CI24R (CA), CI24RE (CA) and Nucleus Freedom implant with Contour Advance Electrode CI24RE (CA)	Cochlear Corporation	Adults and children	1998 (24 system)	*Adults:* The Nucleus 24 Contour cochlear implant system, hereinafter referred to as the Nucleus 24 Contour, is intended for use in individuals 18 year of age or older who have bilateral, pre-, peri-, or postlinguistic, sensorineural hearing impairment and obtain limited benefit from appropriate binaural hearing aids. These individuals typically have moderate to profound hearing loss in the low frequencies and profound ($\geq$90 dB HL) hearing loss in the middle to high speech frequencies. Limited benefit from amplification is defined by test scores of 50% correct or less in the ear to be implanted (60% or less in the best-aided listening condition) on tape-recorded tests of open set sentence recognition. *Children:* The Nucleus 24 Contour is intended for use in children 12 to 24 months of age who have bilateral profound sensorineural deafness and demonstrate limited benefit from appropriate binaural hearing aids. Children 2 years of age or older may demonstrate severe to profound hearing loss bilaterally. In younger children, limited benefit is defined as lack of profess in the development of simple auditory skills in conjunction with appropriate amplification and participation in intensive aural habilitation over a 3- to 6- month period. It is recommended that limited benefit be quantified on a measure such as the Meaningful Auditory Integration Scale or the Early Speech Perception test. In older children, limited benefit is defined as $\leq$30% correct on the open set Multisyllabic Neighborhood Test (MLNT) or Lexical Neighborhood Test (LNT), depending the child's cognitive and linguistic skills. A 3- to 6-month hearing aid trial is recommended for children without previous aided experience.
Nucleus Freedom implant with Contour Advance™ Electrode CI24RE (CA)	Cochlear Corporation	Adults and children	2005	*Adults:* The Nucleus Freedom implant with Contour Advance™ Electrode cochlear implant system is intended for use in individuals 18 year of age or older who have bilateral, pre-, peri-, or postlinguistic, sensorineural hearing impairment and obtain limited benefit from appropriate binaural hearing aids. These individuals typically have moderate to profound hearing loss in the low frequencies and profound ($\geq$90 dB HL) hearing loss in the middle to high speech frequencies. Limited benefit from amplification is defined by test scores of 50% correct or less in the ear to be implanted (60% or less in the best-aided listening condition) on tape recorded tests of open set sentence recognition.

Children:

The Nucleus Freedom implant with Contour Advance Electrode cochlear implant system is intended for use in children 12 to 24 months of age who have bilateral profound sensorineural deafness and demonstrate limited benefit from appropriate binaural hearing aids. Children 2 years of age or older may demonstrate severe to profound hearing loss bilaterally. In younger children, limited benefit is defined as lack of progress in the development of simple auditory skills in conjunction with appropriate amplification and participation in intensive aural habilitation over a 3- to 6-month period. It is recommended that limited benefit be quantified on a measure such as the Meaningful Auditory Integration Scale or the Early Speech Perception test. In older children, limited benefit is defined as ≤30% correct on the open-set MLNT or LNT, depending n the child's cognitive and linguistic skills. A 3- to 6-month hearing aid trial is recommended for children without previous aided experience.

	Med-El	2001	Adults and children
Med-El Combi 40 +			

The Med-El Combi 40+ Cochlear Implant System, hereinafter referred to as the Combi 40+, is intended to provide the opportunity to detect and recognize auditory information through electrical stimulation of the auditory nerve for severe to profoundly hearing-impaired individuals who obtain little or no benefit from conventional acoustic amplification in the best-aided condition.

Adults:

Adults 18 years of age or older who have bilateral, sensorineural hearing impairment and obtain limited benefit from appropriately fitted binaural hearing aids. These individuals typically demonstrate bilateral severe to profound sensorineural hearing loss determined by a pure tone average of 70 dB or greater at 500 Hz, 1000 Hz, and 2000 Hz. Limited benefit from amplification is defined by test scores of 40% correct or less in best-aided listening condition on DC recorded tests of open-set sentence recognition (HINT sentences).

Children:

Children aged 12 months to 17 years 11 months must demonstrate a profound, bilateral sensorineural hearing loss with thresholds of 90 dB or greater at 1000 Hz. In younger children, little or no benefit is defined by lack of progress in the development of simple auditory skills in conjunction with appropriate amplification and participating intensive aural habilitation over a 3- to 6-month period. In older children, lack of aid benefit is defined as <20% correct on the MLNT or LNT, depending on the child's cognitive ability and linguistic skills. A 3- to 6-month hearing aid trial is required for children without previous experience with hearing aids. Radiological evidence of cochlear ossification may justify a shorter trial with amplification.

	Med-El	2005	Adults and children
Med-El Pulsar CI[100]			

The Med-El Pulsar CI[100] Cochlear Implant System is intended to provide the opportunity to detect and recognize auditory information through electrical stimulation of the auditory pathways for those severe to profoundly hearing-impaired individuals who obtain little or no benefit from conventional acoustic amplification in the best-aided condition.

Adults:

Adults 18 years of age or older who have a severe to profound, bilateral, sensorineural hearing loss and obtain limited benefit from appropriately fitted binaural hearing aids. Note: This hearing loss may be evidenced by a bilateral pure tone average of 70 dB or greater at 500, 1000, and 2000 Hz and by a best-aided score of <40% correct on open-set HINT sentences.

Children:

Children 12 months of age and older who demonstrate a profound, bilateral sensorineural hearing loss with thresholds of 90 dB or greater at 1000 Hz, and obtain little to no benefit from appropriately fitted binaural hearing aids. Note: This hearing loss in younger children may be evidenced by a lack of progress in simple auditory skill development, despite appropriate amplification and aural habilitation, over a 3- to 6-month period. This hearing loss in older children may be evidenced by a score of <20% correct on the MLNT or LNT.

References

Balkany T, Gantz BJ, Steenerson RL, Cohen NL. (1996). Systematic approach to electrode insertion in the ossified cochlea. Otolaryngol Head Neck Surg 114:4–11

Bench J, Kowal A, Bamford J. (1979). The BKB (Bamford-Kowal-Bench) sentence lists for partially-hearing children. Br J Audiol 13:108–112

Boothroyd A, Hanin L, Hnath T. (1985). A sentence test of speech perception: reliability, set equivalence, and short term learning (Internal report RCI 10). New York: City University of New York

Buss E, Labadie RF, Brown CJ, Gross AJ, Grose JH, Pillsbury HC. (2002). Outcome of cochlear implantation in pediatric auditory neuropathy. Otol Neurotol 23:328–332

Donaldson AI, Heavner KS, Zwolan TA. (2004). Measuring progress in children with autism spectrum disorder who have cochlear implants. Arch Otolaryngol Head Neck Surg 130:666–671

Eisenman DJ, Ashbaugh CA, Zwolan TA, Arts HA, Telian SA. (2001). Implantation of the malformed cochlea. Otol Neurotol 22:834–841

Elliott LL, Katz D. (1980). Development of a new children's test of speech discrimination (Technical manual). St. Louis, MO: Auditec

Erber NP. (1982). Auditory Training. Washington, DC: Alexander Graham Bell Association for the Deaf

Erber NP, Alencewicz CM. (1976). Audiologic evaluation of deaf children. J Speech Hear Disord 41:256–267

Filipo R, Bosco E, Mancini P, Ballantyne D. (2004). Cochlear implants in special cases: deafness in the presence of disabilities and/or associated problems. Acta Otolaryngol Suppl 552:74–80

Firszt JB, Holden LK, Skinner MW, et al. (2004). Recognition of speech presented at soft to loud levels by adult cochlear implant recipients of three cochlear implant systems. Ear Hear 25:375–387

Hammes DM, Novak MA, Rotz LA, Willis M, Edmondson DM, Thomas JF. (2002). Early identification and cochlear implantation: critical factors for spoken language development. Ann Otol Rhinol Laryngol Suppl 189:74–78

Haskins HA. (1949). A phonetically balanced test of speech discrimination for children. Unpublished master's thesis, Northwestern University, Evanston, IL

Hoffman RA. (1997). Cochlear implant in the child under two years of age: skull growth, otitis media, and selection. Otolaryngol Head Neck Surg 117(3 pt 1):217–219

James AL, Papsin BC. (2004). Cochlear implant surgery at 12 months of age or younger. Laryngoscope 114:2191–2195

Kileny PR, Zwolan TA. (2004). Perioperative, transtympanic electric ABR in paediatric cochlear implant candidates. Cochlear Implants International 5(suppl 1):23–25

Kileny PR, Zwolan TA, Zimmerman-Phillips S, Telian SA. (1994). Electrically evoked auditory brainstem response in pediatric patients with cochlear implants. Arch Otolaryngol Head Neck Surg 120:1083–1090

Kirk KI, Pisoni DB, Osberger MJ. (1995). Lexical effects on spoken word recognition by pediatric cochlear implant users. Ear Hear 16:470–481

Ling D. (1989). Foundations of spoken language for hearing impaired children. Washington, DC: Alexander Graham Bell Association for the Deaf

Luxford W. (2000). Minimum speech test battery for adult cochlear implant patients. In: Waltzman S, Cohen N, eds. Cochlear Implants. New York: Thieme

Mason JC, De Michele A, Stevens C, Ruth RA, Hashisaki GT. (2003). Cochlear implantation n patients with auditory neuropathy of varied etiologies. Laryngoscope 113:45–49

Mason D, Popelka GA. (1982). User's Guide for Phase IV Hearing Aid Selection and Evaluation Program. Central Institute for the Deaf, St. Louis, MO

Mecklenburg DJ, Demorest ME, Staller SJ. (1991). Scope and design of the clinical trial of the Nucleus multichannel cochlear implant in children. Ear Hear 12(suppl):10S–14S

Moog JS, Geers AE. (1990). Early speech perception test for profoundly hearing-impaired children. St. Louis: Central Institute for the Deaf

Neault M. (2003). Auditory dys-synchrony of infancy: implications for implantation. Presentation at the Ninth Symposium On Cochlear Implants in Children. April 24–26, Washington, DC

Nilsson M, Soli SD, Sullivan JA. (1994). Development of the Hearing in Noise Test for the measurement of speech reception thresholds in quiet and in noise. J Acoust Soc Am 95:1085–1099

Osberger MJ. (1997). Cochlear implantation in children under the age of two years: candidacy considerations. Otolaryngol Head Neck Surg 117(3 pt 1):145–149

O'Sullivan MB. (2004). Cochlear implants in special populations. Presentation at the University of Michigan Spring Workshops for Educators and other Professionals. Traverse City, MI, June

Owens E, Kessler DK, Telleen CC, Schubert ED. (1981). The minimal auditory capabilities (MAC) battery. Hearing Aid J 9:32

Peterson A, Shallop J, Driscoll C, et al. (2003). Outcomes of cochlear implantation in children with auditory neuropathy. J Am Acad Audiol 14:188–201

Peterson GE, Lehiste I. (1962). Revised CNC lists for auditory tests. J Speech Hear Disord 1962;27:62–70

Pyman B, Blamey P, Lacy P, Clark G, Dowell R. (2000). The development of speech perception in children using cochlear implants: effects of etiologic factors and delayed milestones. Am J Otol 21:57–61

Rance G, Beer DE, Cone-Wesson B, et al. (1999). Clinical findings for a group of infants and young children with auditory neuropathy. Ear Hear 20:238–252

Rapin I, Gravel J. (2003). "Auditory neuropathy": physiologic and pathologic evidence calls for more diagnostic specificity. Int J Pediatr Otolaryngol 67:707–728

Robbins AM, Renshaw JJ, Berry SW. (1991). Evaluating meaningful auditory integration in profoundly hearing impaired children. Am J Otol 12(suppl):144–150

Robbins AM, et al. (1988). Minimal Pairs Test. Indianapolis, IN: Indiana University School of Medicine

Ross M, Lerman J. (1971). Word Intelligibility by Picture Identification. Pittsburgh, PA: Stanwix House, Inc

Silverman SR, Hirsh IJ. (1955). Problems related to the use of speech in clinical audiometry. Ann Otol Rhinol Laryngol 64:1234–1244

Sininger YS, Trautwein P. (2002). Electrical stimulation of the auditory nerve via cochlear implants in patients with auditory neuropathy. Ann Otol Rhinol Laryngol Suppl 189:29–31

Skinner MW, Holden LK, Holden TA, Demorest MI, Fourakis MS. (1997). Speech recognition at simulated soft, conversational, and raised-to-loud vocal efforts by adults with cochlear implants. J Acoust Soc Am 101:3766–3782

Tillman TW, Carhart R. (1966). An expanded test for speech discrimination utilizing CNC monosyllabic words. Northwestern University Auditory Test No. 6. USAF School of Aerospace Medicine Technical Report. Brooks Air Force Base, TX

Tucci DL, Telian SA, Zimmerman-Phillips S, Zwolan TA, Kileny PR. (1995). Cochlear implantation in patients with cochlear malformations. Arch Otolaryngol Head Neck Surg 121:833–838

Zimmerman-Philips S, McConkey-Robbins A, Osberger MJ. (1998). Assessing device benefit in infants and Toddlers. Poster presentation at the 7th Symposium on Cochlear Implants in Children, Iowa City, Iowa, June 4–7

7

Principles of Cochlear Implant Imaging

Andrew J. Fishman and
Roy A. Holliday

Radiographic imaging plays a major role in cochlear implantation with regard to preoperative candidacy evaluation, intraoperative monitoring, postoperative evaluation, as well as research and experimental techniques. At a minimum, successful cochlear implantation requires that electrical impulses be delivered to a surviving spiral ganglion cell population, and that these impulses be transmitted to a functioning auditory cortex by an existent neural connection. Accordingly, imaging the auditory pathway of the implant candidate is necessary to screen for morphological conditions that preclude or complicate the implantation process. Increasing resolution of computed tomography (CT) and magnetic resonance imaging (MRI) technology has provided the clinician with more detailed information about the integrity of the auditory pathway. As technologies evolve, a clear understanding of what information can be obtained as well as the limitations of various imaging modalities is essential to proper candidacy evaluation, and selection of the ear to be implanted in complex cases.

Also important is the effect that the presence of a cochlear implant has on future imaging of the head and neck region of an implantee. In the past, the presence of a cochlear implant was considered to be a major contraindication to MRI.[1] Because it is now possible to obtain useful images with advances in CT and MRI technology, the issue of device MRI compatibility has opened up a new area of investigation.

◆ Preoperative Imaging

Preoperative imaging is instrumental in determining the feasibility and facility of cochlear implantation. Analysis is performed in a stepwise approach, answering the following three questions: Are there cochleovestibular anomalies that preclude implantation? Is there evidence of luminal obstruction? Are there additional findings that may complicate the surgery or subsequent patient management? This section is not intended to review principles or techniques of image acquisition, but rather to provide a platform for discussion between the implant team and the radiologist.

Are There Cochleovestibular Anomalies that Preclude Implantation?

Approximately 20% of patients with congenital sensorineural hearing loss (SNHL) have radiographically identifiable morphological abnormalities of the inner ear.[2] In general, inner ear malformations can be associated with a wide range of hearing sensitivity.[3] These patients can manifest progression of hearing loss, though many may retain useful hearing into adult life. As a general rule, however, the more severe the deformity, the worse the hearing.[3] Due to the variability and progressive nature of hearing loss in these disorders, most large implant centers are likely to evaluate patients with a variety of malformations. Given the current technology, the minimum requirement for cochlear implantation is the presence of an implantable cavity in proximity to stimulable neural elements whose projections connect to the auditory cortex. Accordingly, the first question that must be answered is the following: Are there any cochleovestibular anomalies that preclude implantation?

Embryology

To fully appreciate the wide variety of possible cochleovestibular malformations, it is helpful to first review the embryogenesis of the inner ear.[3,4] We will consider separately the formation of the membranous labyrinth, the bony otic capsule, and the cochleovestibular nerves and ganglia.

The development of the combined cochlear and vestibular membranous labyrinthine system begins with the formation of the otic placode as an ectodermal thickening that forms on the surface of the neural tube in the third gestational week. The otic placode invaginates from the surface and forms the otocyst in the fourth gestational week. The otocyst develops three infolds in the fifth week. The resultant pouches represent the primordial endolymphatic sac and duct, the utricle and semicircular canals, and the saccule and cochlea. Beginning in the sixth week, the cochlear duct grows from its primordial bud beginning from the basal region spiraling apically to reach its full 2.5 to 2.75 turns by the eighth to tenth week. The neuroepithelial end organs continue to develop beyond this period with the organ of Corti completing its formation in the 25th week.

The semicircular canals begin their formation as three small, folded evaginations on the primordial vestibular appendage. They develop as disk-like outpouchings whose centers eventually compress and fuse to ultimately form the semicircular duct structure. By the sixth week of gestational life, this compression and fusion has taken place in first the superior and then the posterior canals. The three canals continue to enlarge and complete their formation to full adult size in sequence beginning with the superior around the 20th week, and followed by the posterior and finally the lateral semicircular canals. Interestingly, the endolymphatic sac and duct are the first to appear and the last to complete their development.

The osseous otic capsule eventually forms from a morphologically fully developed cartilage precursor model via 14 centers of ossification, beginning around the 15th gestational week, and is completed during the 23rd gestational week. The cartilage model and underlying membranous labyrinth continue to grow in the region of the posterior and lateral semicircular canals, while other structures, which have previously attained their final shape and size, have begun ossifying. The cochleovestibular nerves and ganglia develop in concert with the membranous labyrinth and cochleovestibular end organs. They are of neural crest origin and migrate between the epithelial layer and basement membrane of the otic vesicle during the fourth gestational week.

Cochlear Malformations

There is much confusion in the literature regarding the nomenclature of cochlear morphologic anomalies especially regarding the term *Mondini malformation*. In 1791, Carlo Mondini presented his findings on an anatomical dissection of a young deaf boy.[5] According to his writings, prior reports of human deafness were attributed to abnormalities of the external auditory canal and eustachian tube, tympanic membrane, middle ear and ossicles, or compression of the auditory nerve. During his dissection on the posterior face of the petrous bone, he discovered significant vestibular aqueduct enlargement and commented that the usual bony lip that "protects the vestibular aqueduct" was missing and was substituted by a membranous plate of dura. He noted that the vestibule was not deformed but was of greater than usual size. He also noted an increase in the size of the elliptical recess though it was normal in shape. He commented that the semicircular canals appeared normal and that the positions of their openings into the vestibule were unremarkable. In observing the medial opening of the vestibular aqueduct, he commented that it was quite enlarged and was larger than the size of the common crus. The cochlea was described as possessing only 1.5 turns and ending in a cavity corresponding to the last spiral turn. He also described an incompletely formed interscalar septum. The more contemporary term *incomplete partition* is commonly used to describe this classic anomaly and denotes this specific aspect of the deformity.[3,6] In this historic subject, the deformity was bilateral.

Because of its relative frequency as well as its historic significance, the term *Mondini malformation* is commonly used to describe all forms of cochlear morphological abnormalities and not just the incomplete partition. The term *Mondini dysplasia* was used by Schuknecht[7] in an in-depth analysis of the histopathology and clinical features of cochlear anomalies. Schuknecht's treatise described a variety of malformations including one patient with "the normal 2.5 turns but measur[ing] only 23 mm in length (normal: 32 mm)" and another with "Mondini dysplasia limited to the vestibular system," as well as several patients with cochleae possessing 1.5 turns, and other variant morphologies of both the cochlear duct and vestibular system. Schuknecht histologically described these malformations as isolated findings or in association with the Klippel-Feil, Pendred, and DiGeorge syndromes. His work detailed the clinical nature of these disorders as being unilateral or bilateral, and associated with acoustic and vestibular dysfunction that is variable in severity, static, or progressive.

Phelps[8] reserves the term *Mondini deformity* for cochleae whose basal turns are normal and possess a deficiency of the interscalar septum of the distal 1.5 coils. He differentiates these cochleae from those termed *dysplastic* owing to their widened basal turn being in wide communication with a dilated vestibule. According to Phelps the significance is in the clinical absence of a spontaneous cerebrospinal fluid (CSF) leak and meningitis in patients with his strict definition of Mondini deformity as opposed to those patients with dysplasia who did manifest these complications in a series of 20 patients studied.

Since the writings of Mondini, several investigators have documented a variety of inner ear malformations. Though not the first to describe or name these malformations, Jackler et al[3] in 1987 proposed a classification system for the congenitally malformed inner ear based on the theory that a variety of deformities result from arrested development at different stages of embryogenesis. The authors clearly stated that their classification could not describe all observable abnormalities but was meant to serve as a framework upon which other describable anomalies could be added, which by their supposition would have resulted from aberrant, rather than arrested, development.

This body of work warrants mention as it is often cited and serves well as an initial systematic basis for the interpretation of images. Jackler et al formulated their classification system upon review of polytomes and CT scans of 63 patients with 98 congenitally malformed ears, and provided the following categorization (**Table 7–1**). The disorders identified as having normal cochleae were subdivided out solely for the purposes of Jackler's classification scheme. It is important to recognize that disorders of the vestibule, semicircular canals, and vestibular aqueduct are also often found in conjunction with cochlear malformations. Inner ear deformities tend to occur bilaterally in 65%.[3] When bilateral, there is a 93% chance that they will be similar, though various combinations of morphological classes have been documented.[3]

Table 7–1   Classification of Cochleovestibular Anomalies[3]

Absent or malformed cochleae
1. Complete labyrinthine aplasia
2. Cochlear aplasia
3. Cochlear hypoplasia
4. Incomplete partition
5. Common cavity
Normal cochleae
1. Vestibule: lateral semicircular canal dysplasia
2. Enlarged vestibular aqueduct

Complete labyrinthine aplasia, also called Michel deformity, could result from arrest prior to formation of the otocyst, resulting in complete absence of inner ear development.[3] This is the rarest among the above classified malformations (**Fig. 7–1**).

Cochlear aplasia is defined as an absent cochlea with an intact but often variably deformed vestibular labyrinth. This is the second rarest cochlear malformation noted by Jackler et al, representing ~3% of identified cochlear malformations.

The term *cochlear hypoplasia* has been used to describe a range of abnormalities from a rudimentary cochlear diverticulum to an incompletely formed cochlear bud of several millimeters (**Fig. 7–2**). This group comprised 15% of cases from Jackler et al; it was thought to represent arrested

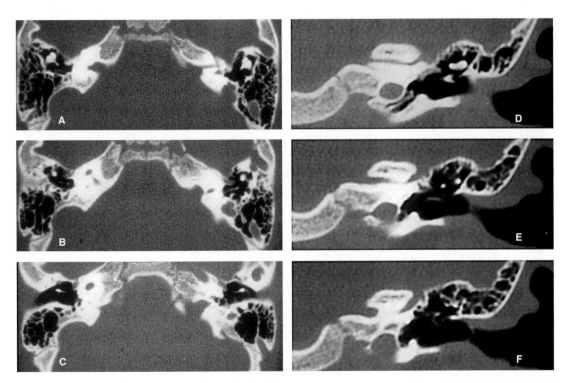

Figure 7–1   Computed tomography (CT) scan of a patient with a common cavity deformity on the right and complete cochleovestibular aplasia on the left. Axial sections **(A,B,C)** are depicted from superior to inferior. **(A)** A narrow internal auditory canal (IAC) on the left containing only a facial nerve. **(B)** The IAC on the right communicating with the common cavity. Coronal sections through the left temporal bone **(D,E,F)** demonstrate the absence of the otic capsule with only the carotid and facial nerve canals visible in the region. **(D)** The tensor tympani muscle. This patient was successfully implanted in the right ear.

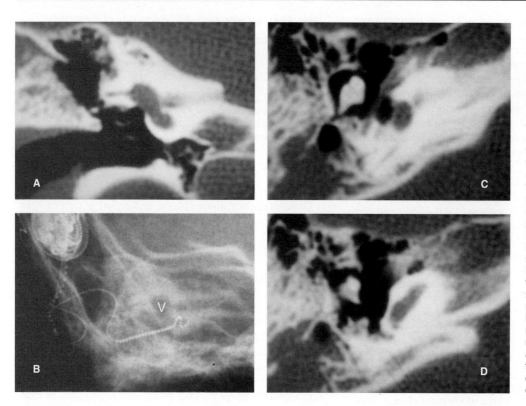

Figure 7–2 CT scan of a patient with bilateral cochlear hypoplasia. Images are shown from the right temporal bone that was successfully implanted. **(A)** A coronal section through the vestibule demonstrates the relatively normal formation of the vestibular apparatus as well as the presence of an oval window. **(B)** An intraoperative transorbital plain radiograph of the multichannel electrode array implanted in this patient. This is the expected appearance of the array placed into this small cavity. Note that the morphology is quite similar to the coronal section **(A)**. V, vestibule; marked for reference. **(C)** The oval window and ossicles are also seen in axial image. These are useful surgical landmarks because they allow for the formation of a topographic roadmap when implanting abnormal cochleae. **(D)** Only the proximal basal turn of the cochlea is present. The middle or apical turns are absent.

development during the sixth gestational week, and may be associated with either a normal or malformed vestibule and semicircular canals.

Incomplete partition is a term used by Jackler et al in their study, and it is pointed out that this is the closest to the malformation originally described by Mondini. This is the most commonly described cochlear abnormality, making up 55% of the study described. It is thought to represent arrest in development during the seventh gestational week, a time at which the cochlea would have completed 1 to

1.5 turns.[3] Radiographically, these cochleae possess only 1.5 turns comprised of a basal turn leading to the appearance of a confluent middle and apical turn, which may also be viewed and described as incomplete partitioning by a deficient interscalar septum.[3,6] These cochleae may also manifest varying degrees of abnormalities of the vestibular system and endolymphatic duct and sac (**Fig. 7–3**).

The term *common cavity* is used to denote confluence of the cochlea and vestibule into a common rudimentary cavity that usually lacks an internal architecture and is

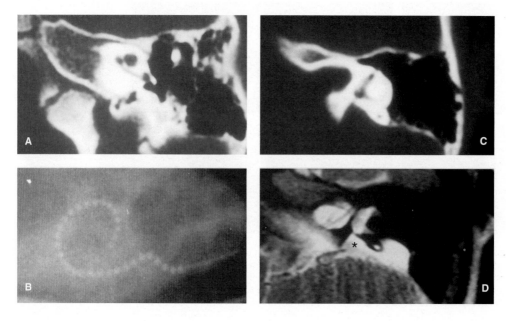

Figure 7–3 Images from a patient with bilateral incomplete partition. **(A)** Axial CT scan clearly depicts an intact basal turn and confluent middle and apical turns. **(B)** Note that a multichannel electrode array was implanted nearly a full turn with a few stiffening rings remaining outside the cochleostomy. This patient also has a wide vestibular aqueduct as seen in the axial CT image **(C)** as well as in the T2-weighted magnetic resonance imaging (MRI) **(D)** marked by (*). Intraoperatively, egress of cerebrospinal fluid (CSF) was easily controlled with packing of fascia around the array at the cochleostomy.

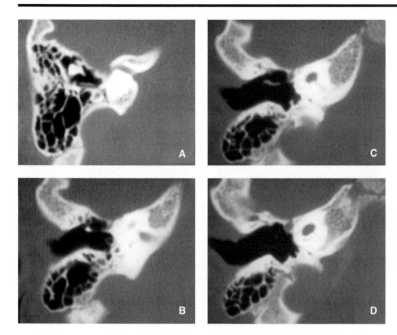

Figure 7–4 Axial CT scan of the right temporal bone from the patient in **Fig. 7–1**. Sections are depicted from superior to inferior (**A–D**). Note the labyrinthine facial nerve passing anteriorly and superiorly to the common cochleovestibular chamber. (**A**) In this patient the semicircular canals are absent. The bony cochlear aqueduct is visible (**C,D**).

often associated with abnormally formed semicircular canals. This is the second most common abnormality described, and made up 26% of the Jackler et al study (**Fig. 7–4**).

The classification scheme proposed by Jackler et al is not all-inclusive. There are varieties of disorders that may be encountered that defy classification, as the authors well noted. A very narrow internal auditory canal of a diameter 2 to 2.5 mm or less on either conventional or CT has been reported in association with a normal inner ear as well as a variety of inner ear malformations.[9–12] It has been reported unilaterally and bilaterally, in association with a variety of other congenital anomalies and as an isolated disorder. The clinical significance of this finding on a preimplant evaluation is that there is a high likelihood that it indicates the presence of only a facial nerve and the absence of the cochleovestibular nerve. A CT scan demonstrating an internal auditory canal of less than 2 to 2.5 mm is considered by many authors to be an absolute contraindication to cochlear implantation.[9,10,13] Evaluation of the contents of the internal auditory canal using MRI scanning may be warranted in selected patients, as increased experience is being gained with high-resolution scanning techniques.

There is also a particular form of X-linked deafness that has been both radiographically described and genetically identified.[10,14,15] It is seen in some severely deaf males who have a deficiency of bone between the lateral end of bulbous internal auditory canal and the basal turn of the cochlea.[10] It has been detailed by both CT and MRI and it entails the clinical implication that there is an obvious large communication between the CSF-containing internal auditory canal and the cochlea. This situation also causes concern because a multichannel electrode array may inadvertently be introduced into the internal canal at the time of implantation.

In summary, the specific terminology used is less important than the detail in which reported cases are described with regard to radiographic and histologic features of each element of the inner ear: specific cochlear morphology, size and relation to the vestibule, patency of the bony modiolus, and the nature of inner ear aqueducts. With adequate patient evaluation and knowledge, clinicians can avoid jumping to conclusions regarding the association of these various clinical features with hearing, implantation outcome, and complications.

Patient Evaluation

Initial radiologic evaluation of the cochlear implant candidate is typically performed with high-resolution CT scanning. Patients with a malformed inner ear or narrow internal auditory canal may undergo supplemental MRI. An MRI of inner ear malformations requires different parameters than those commonly employed in the evaluation of adult hearing loss. The acquisition of appropriate images requires higher resolution and greater-strength magnets.[16,17] Intravenous contrast is rarely used. An MRI is obtained in a patient with an inner ear anomaly to identify both the nonosseus partitioning of the malformed cochlea and the neural structures contained within the internal auditory canal (**Fig. 7–5**). CT and MRI studies are only macroscopic evaluations of the cochleovestibular apparatus; form does not necessarily imply function. Evidence of the existence of a stimulable auditory neural pathway, either by documentation of prior or residual hearing or by utilization of promontory stimulation testing, predicts a more favorable outcome (**Figs. 7–6** and **7–7**).

A few cochleovestibular anomalies preclude implantation. Complete labyrinthine aplasia would be an absolute contraindication for implantation on the affected side. The determination of cochlear aplasia should involve the careful differentiation from a common cavity deformity by a combination of MRI and promontory stimulation in selected patients to evaluate the possible presence of an adjacent stimulable cochlear nerve ganglion cell population.

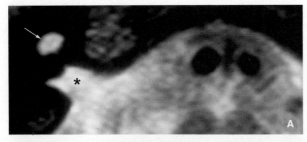

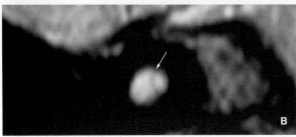

Figure 7–5 T2-weighted MRI demonstrating nonosseous partitioning of a common cavity. These images are from the inner ear shown in **Fig. 7–4**. **(A)** Note the bright signal from fluid seen in the internal auditory canal (∗) and the cochleovestibular chamber in the axial section. There are low signal intensity septations visible within the common cavity on both the axial **(A)** and coronal **(B)** images that are not seen on CT scanning (white arrows).

The failure to identify a cochlear nerve by high-resolution MRI would also contraindicate implantation regardless of the presence of an implantable cavity.

With careful patient selection and preoperative planning, utilization of the various imaging and electrophysiologic testing modalities available, and consultation with experienced device programmers, implantation has been successfully done on many patients with a variety of cochlear malformations.[18–25]

Is There Evidence of Luminal Obstruction?

In the absence of morphological contraindications to implantation, the next question that must be answered is the following: Is there any evidence of luminal obstruction? Inner ear inflammation, abnormalities of bone metabolism, or trauma may ultimately result in luminal obstruction either by ingrowth of fibrous scar tissue or pathologic neo-ossification. The etiology that is most commonly encountered, especially in pediatric cochlear implant candidates, is postmeningitic labyrinthitis ossificans. Other postinflammatory causes include suppurative labyrinthitis secondary to otitis media or cholesteatoma, and hematogenous infections (septicemia, mumps, Rubella, or other viral infections). Metabolic bone disorders include otosclerosis and Paget's

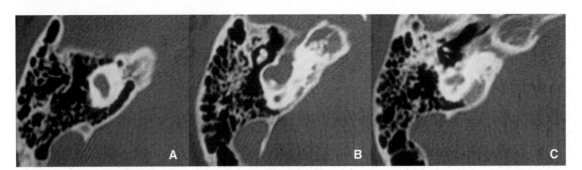

Figure 7–6 Axial CT scan images in another patient with a common cavity deformity. Michel's aplasia was present on the contralateral side. The sections **(A–C)** are depicted from superior to inferior. **(B)** Note the formation of rudimentary semicircular canals. **(C)** The internal auditory canal becomes apparent. This patient demonstrated

some preoperative subjective auditory sensations and language development. Promontory stimulation, as well, indicated the presence of auditory perception. She was successfully implanted with a multichannel device, and currently derives significant benefit from implant use.

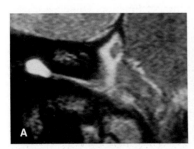
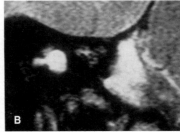
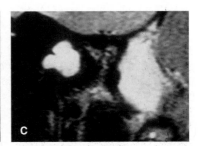

Figure 7–7 T2-weighted coronal MRI of the inner ear depicted in **Fig. 7–6**, depicted from anterior to posterior. **(A)** Note the narrow internal auditory canal leading to the fluid containing common cochleovestibular cavity. **(B,C)** The formation of rudimentary semicircular canals that also contain fluid.

disease. Common posttraumatic causes include labyrinthect-omy and temporal bone fractures. Wegener's granulomatosis and autoimmune inner diseases such as Cogan's syndrome have also been reported to result in labyrinthine ossification.[26-29]

Bacterial meningitis is the most common cause of acquired severe SNHL in children.[30] Some degree of hearing loss has been reported in retrospective analyses to develop in 7 to 29% of survivors of meningitis.[31,32] Deafness may follow bacterial meningitis in children in 2 to 7% of cases, with 1.5% being severe and bilateral.[30,33] The organisms commonly responsible for postmeningitic deafness are *Haemophilus influenzae* and *Streptococcus pneumoniae*. *Neisseria meningitidis* is also a causative organism, though it is thought to result in a lower incidence of postinfectious deafness.[33,34] Though most series report *H. influenzae* as the leading causative organism in most meningitic deafness, it is of note that a greater proportion of children surviving pneumococcal meningitis (33%) develop hearing loss, as opposed to *H. influenzae* type b (9%) or meningococcal meningitis (5%).[30,32,35] Pneumococcal meningitis that presents a gram-positive exotoxin is additionally associated with severe ossification, whereas the ossification associated with *Haemophilus* is generally less severe owing to the effects of endotoxins, which may be diminished by corticosteroids.[30,33] Some degree of cochlear neo-ossification may be encountered intraoperatively in as high as 70% of patients deafened by meningitis.[36] In series including all deafness etiologies, some degree of basal turn cochlear neo-ossification has been reported in ~15% of adult patients, and as high as 28 to 35% of pediatric patients.[37-39]

Pathophysiology of Labyrinthine Ossification

The cochlear aqueduct is a bony channel that connects the subarachnoid space of the posterior cranial fossa to the scala tympani. It opens adjacent to the round window and is lined with a loose network of fibrous tissue termed the "periotic duct," which is an extension of the arachnoid.[40] This is thought to be the site of origin of the inflammatory process into the inner ear in cases of meningitis. Other possible routes include the internal auditory canal and modiolus, the middle ear windows secondary to otitis media, lateral canal fistulization secondary to chronic inflammatory processes, trauma, and hematogenous spread.[41,42] When encountered, ossification is nearly always most severe in the region of the round window and proximal scala tympani in the basal turn, adjacent to the opening of the cochlear aqueduct.[29] The middle and apical turns are less commonly affected, and the scala vestibuli is often spared.[18] Because most cases of labyrinthitis ossificans are partial and the extent of obstruction commonly manifests asymmetrically within an individual patient, preoperative imaging plays an essential role in selecting the side to implant.[43] Total cochlear ossification may occur, and is more commonly seen in children than adults.[18,44]

Cochlear ossification following meningitis is associated with a severe loss of cochlear hair cells as well as a decreased spiral ganglion cell population.[45] There is no clearly predictable relationship between the extent of ossification and the number of injured spiral ganglion cells.[46] Hinojosa et al[47] studied the temporal bones of deaf patients with labyrinthitis ossificans and found that the remaining neuronal cell population ranged from 6310 to 28,196 with a mean of 17,152. This is in comparison to the total cochlear neuronal population of ~35,500 in the human infant.[48] Linthicum et al[49] studied the postmortem effects of implants on neuronal population and found that benefit may occur with as few as 3300 neurons. Cochlear ossification does not contraindicate cochlear implantation per se; it does, however, complicate electrode insertion.[50]

There are several theories regarding the pathogenesis of labyrinthine neo-ossification. Druss[51] described in 1936 two types of new bone: metaplastic bone, which originates from ingrown fibrous scar or connective tissue, and osteoplastic bone, which originates from the adjacent otic capsule after disruption of the endosteum. Postlabyrinthitis ossification is thought to occur via the metaplastic process. During the initial acute stage of infection, bacteria within the perilymphatic spaces induce an acute inflammatory reaction characterized by leukocyte infiltration as well as fibroblast proliferation.[52] Labyrinthine fibrosis is considered to be the early stage of ossification and may occur within weeks of initial infection.[29,52,53] Ossification eventually ensues and this is termed the osseous or late stage of labyrinthitis ossificans. According to Sugiura and Paparella,[52,54] undifferentiated mesenchymal cells originating in the endosteum, modiolar spaces, and basilar membrane likely differentiate into fibroblasts and either subsequently or directly into osteoblasts, and form local or diffuse osseous deposits.

Several authors have postulated that the pathogenesis of metaplastic bone formation may be related to disruptions of cochlear blood supply, which has been demonstrated both experimentally and observed histologically in the temporal bones of patients having undergone a variety of surgical procedures.[26,55-59] This theory has been claimed to be supported by cell cultures experiments performed by Gorham and Test[60] in which low oxygen tension favors bone formation, whereas high oxygen tension favors osteoclastic resorption. Additional investigators have commented on the similar findings between the ossification of vascular occlusion and that of suppurative labyrinthitis.[52,54]

The two types of neo-ossification were further characterized in histologic studies performed by Kotzias and Linthicum[26] on human temporal bones with a variety of pathologic processes including patients who had undergone a variety of neurotologic procedures. The metaplastic form is characterized by high cellularity and the relative absence of eosinophilia. There are no osteoblasts on the surface. Though its margins are indistinct, it is confined to the lumen of the cochlea. The osteoplastic form occurs only when there has been disruption of the endosteum such as occurs during trauma or a surgical defect. It is characterized by less cellularity and increased eosinophilia, and is characteristically lamellar in form, with clear margins and osteoblasts on the surface and not clearly distinct from the endosteal layer.

The postmeningitic neo-ossification is thought to occur via the metaplastic process with the ectopic bone being typically chalky white whereas the native otic capsule bone is generally ivory in hue.[36] The difference in color and the neo-ossified bone's being confined to the lumen of the cochlea aid in differentiating it from the native otic capsule during drilling of the ossified cochlea in the implantation procedure.

Advanced otosclerosis may, in rare cases, cause luminal obstruction that is usually limited to the round window or first few millimeters of the scala tympani.[13,26,29] It has been suggested by Kotzias and Linthicum[26] that the otosclerotic process may damage the endosteal layer, resulting in the osteoplastic form of neo-ossification. Green et al[29] histologically identified foci of otosclerosis within the areas of neo-ossification. All their specimens, as well, demonstrated the pathology to be limited to the first 6 mm of the basal turn in the scala tympani. The pattern of ossification induced by trauma is less predictable.[13]

Evaluation of Cochlear Patency by Computed Tomography Scanning

Multiple authors have reported discrepancies between the CT scan interpretation of cochlear patency and the findings at implant surgery. This is likely due in part to the thicker image slices available at the time these studies were performed, as well as the early stage of experience of the image interpreters. Early fibro-ossific changes that were not identified on CT scanning are frequently encountered during surgery in postmeningitic patients. This would be especially likely when there is little ossification within the fibrous matrix.[31,43,61] The time course for metaplastic ossification is quite variable but is thought to begin with fibrosis as early as 8 days to a few weeks after the initial insult.[26,29,52,53,55] The ultimate time frame and extent of eventual osseous deposition is quite variable. It has been reported to be detected as early as 2 months postmeningitis in humans by CT scanning.[53] Evidence of ongoing ossification has also been detected to be present histologically in human temporal bones as late as 30 years past the initial insult.[29]

The reported accuracy of high-resolution CT scan identification of cochlear ossification has ranged from 53% to greater than 90%.[13,36,62–64] A review of these studies is useful because they detail the pattern and likelihood of ossification found among various deafness etiologies as well as the potential pitfalls of CT scan interpretation with regard to particular regions of the cochlea. In 1987, Jackler et al[63] compared CT scan interpretations with intraoperative findings on 35 cochlear implant patients (17 adults and 18 children) with a variety of deafness etiologies. The group included one adult and seven children deafened by meningitis, making up 23% of the study population. CT scans were performed on a General Electric (GE) 8800 (Fairfield, CT) system with 1.5-mm contiguous axial sections processed using a bone algorithm. Axial scans were taken parallel to the infraorbital-meatal line, and coronal scans were tilted 105 degrees from this plane. The authors reported their CT scan data as either patent or ossified (partial or complete) and detailed the location (round window, basal turn, middle turn, apical turn).

All patients deafened by meningitis had some degree of ossification found at the time of surgery; however, only five of eight had a preoperative CT interpretation suggesting ossification, with the remaining three interpreted as normal. This yielded a 38% false-negative rate among patients deafened by meningitis. However, looking at the specific case data presented, it is apparent that among the three instances of postmeningitic false-negative CT interpretation, two had partial ossification limited to the round window and the third had soft tissue in the round window region, and that all the cases of basal turn involvement were correctly identified by CT.

When all etiologies were considered, there were an additional three false-negative CT interpretations making a total of six of 13, or a 46% false-negative rate. This included one patient with Cogan's syndrome who had ossification found in the round window and basal turn, and one patient with trauma and basal turn ossification, as well as one patient with prior malignant otitis externa who had undetected complete cochlear soft tissue obliteration. All the children with congenital deafness (10) or ototoxicity (one) and all the adults with progressive familial, viral, syphilis, Meniere's disease, and unknown etiologies had patent readings on CT scan and no ossification noted at the time of surgery. The effects that these findings had on insertion and outcome is difficult to ascertain as the 18 children in the study were implanted with a House/3M (St. Paul, MN) single-channel device, and no performance data are provided. This is especially true in light of the fact that the great majority of patients today are implanted with long multichannel arrays.

Seicshnaydre et al[64] in 1992 compared preoperative CT interpretation with intraoperative findings on 31 children who received a Nucleus multichannel cochlear implant (Cochlear Corporation; Englewood, CO). They reported that scanning was done utilizing a high-resolution bone algorithm with slice thicknesses of 1 to 1.5 mm in the axial and coronal plane. They analyzed their data differently from the previous study. They considered four categories with regard to ossification: normal, narrowed basal turn, bony lip at round window, and ossified cochlea. They also subdivided their cases into postmeningitic and nonmeningitic etiologies. A look at their specific data reveals the difficulty in interpreting the more subtle findings of narrowed basal turn and abnormalities of the round window. Among patient whose CT scans were interpreted as positive for narrowing or the basal turn, 71% were true positives and 29% were false-positive interpretations after confirmation at surgery. Of note is that all the false-positive cases were in nonmeningitic cases. As for abnormalities of the round window, there was an 80% false-positive rate of interpretation in nonmeningitic cases, whereas all the meningitic cases were correctly interpreted.

Seidman et al[36] in 1994 performed a retrospective comparison of preoperative CT scan radiologic reports and findings during cochlear implant surgery. CT scans were performed on a GE 9800 system with a slice thickness of 1.5 mm nonoverlapping and utilizing a high-resolution bone algorithm. The authors' analysis included 32 patients deafened by meningitis. Although 22 (69%) patients were found to have intraoperative evidence of ossification, only seven were properly identified preoperatively. Ten patients were correctly identified as patent, while 15 were falsely identified as patent yielding a 60% (15 of 25) false-negative rate for

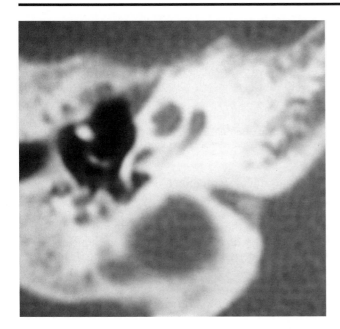

Figure 7–8 CT scan of a patient bilaterally deafened by meningitis demonstrates osseous obstruction limited to the proximal basal turn. Though the middle and apical turns appear patent on CT, further evaluation with MRI is warranted to further assess the possibility of luminal fibrosis. Note that the relationship between the round window and cochlear aqueduct are nicely demonstrated in this section.

preoperative CT scan interpretation of cochlear ossification among postmeningitic patients in this study. Interestingly, the authors also reported one false-positive CT interpretation in a patient with osteogenesis imperfecta with a high-resolution CT scan suggesting cochlear otospongiotic changes and luminal occlusion.

Langman and Quigley[65] in 1996 reported a sensitivity of 100% and specificity of 86% for the identification of cochlear obstruction using CT scans taken at 1.5-mm contiguous slices on a GE 9800 scanner; however, as the authors pointed out, only 14% of the patients in their study were deafened by meningitis. They did not report data specific to etiology.

In summary, it has been our observation as well as reported in the literature that advances in CT scan technology and radiologist experience have improved the ability to predict luminal obstruction on the basis of CT scan, as current technology allows for the routine acquisition of 1-mm slice thicknesses.[13,62] A subset of these patients, particularly those deafened by meningitis, may benefit from MRI to help distinguish the early fibrous phases of labyrinthitis ossificans from a patent fluid-filled lumen, as both may appear gray on CT scans.[33,66–68] The evaluation of cochlear patency is initially performed by high-resolution CT scanning. Ossified obstruction can reliably be identified involving the basal segment in isolation or extending distally into the middle and apical turns. Involvement limited to the basal segment on CT may be further evaluated by MRI so that a patent fluid-filled distal lumen may be differentiated from soft tissue obliteration as this may influence surgical planning (**Figs. 7–8** to **7–11**).

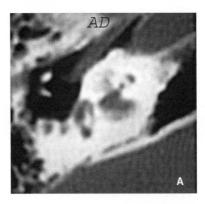

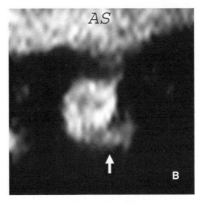

Figure 7–9 (A) This patient bilaterally deafened by meningitis demonstrated osseus obliteration of the cochlea extending into the middle and apical turns on the right side (AD). The left cochlea appeared patent by CT scan; however, the left (AS) coronal MRI **(B)** demonstrates the presence of intermediate signal within the basal turn (white arrow), which is suggestive of luminal fibrosis.

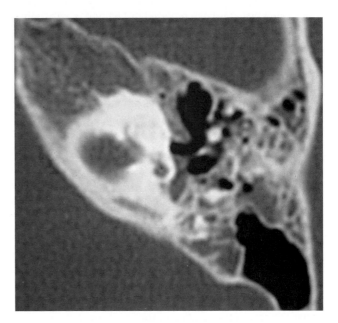

Figure 7–10 CT scan of a patient bilaterally deafened by meningitis demonstrates extensive osseous obliteration involving all turns of the cochlea. The opposite side appeared patent. Note the unusual bulbous appearance of the internal auditory canal, which is demonstrated on the T2-weighted MRI in **Fig. 7–11**.

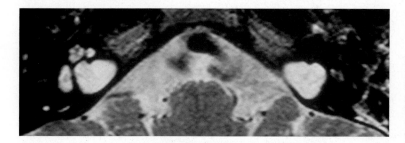

Figure 7–11 MRI of the patient depicted in **Fig. 7–10**. Note the bilaterally abnormal bulbous morphology of the internal auditory canals as demonstrated by the bright signal from CSF fluid on this T2-weighted image. A bright fluid signal is also present in the lumen of the right cochlea but absent on the left side, which demonstrated extensive osseous obliteration on CT scan.

Are There Additional Findings that May Complicate the Surgery or Subsequent Patient Management?

The initial objectives of preoperative sectional imaging are the determination of cochlear morphology and luminal patency. Additional useful information may be derived that can optimize safety and facility of surgery, as well as influence subsequent patient management. Proper surgical planning must involve careful review of sectional images so that potential complications may be anticipated and properly managed. Preoperative imaging often provides valuable information that would not preclude implantation, but rather helps assess which would be the technically easier ear to implant.

Vascular Anatomy

Aberrant middle ear vascular anatomy that might complicate mastoidectomy and facial recess approach to the cochleostomy may be anticipated by the routine acquisition of preoperative CT scanning. An extreme anterior displacement of the sigmoid sinus with approximation against the posterior canal wall has been reported in 1.6% and a high-riding jugular bulb may be present in 6% of the general population.[69] It is rare (though possible) that a jugular bulb or diverticulum may overlie the round window niche or promontory (**Fig. 7–12**). The distance between the round window and carotid artery may be determined in cases where a drill-out procedure is planned. Abnormal course or dehiscence of the carotid canal may also be detected.

Facial Nerve

Preoperative CT scanning is especially useful in identifying the position of the aberrant facial nerve that may be associated with cochlear malformations. It has been well documented in such cases that the course of the facial nerve may be quite unusual and at increased risk of injury during implantation surgery.[18,70,71] By careful preoperative mapping of the course of the facial nerve canal, such patients may be safely and successfully implanted (**Fig. 7–13**). Careful review of the position of the facial nerve is also warranted as well in patients without cochlear malformations, as there may be dehiscences of the intratympanic portion that may be encountered during the approach to the cochleostomy site.

In some patients with otosclerosis, the presence of spongiotic bone between the apical turn of the cochlea and the pregeniculate facial nerve canal permits unwanted stimulation of the facial nerve during implant use.[72] Careful analysis of the CT study helps to anticipate that certain electrodes will require deprogramming (**Fig. 7–14**).

Mastoid and Tympanic Cavity

The mastoid air cell system and tympanic cavity should also be included in the analysis of preoperative CT studies. The degree of mastoid pneumatization is especially useful information when operating on very young children. Though considered fully developed at birth, the depth of the facial recess as well as its degree of pneumatization may be anticipated.

Radiographic findings in conjunction with clinical severity may be considered in side selection as well as determination of the most appropriate course of therapy for patients with associated chronic ear disease. Chronic ear disease need not be an absolute contraindication for cochlear implantation if carefully selected patients are managed with staged procedures. Traditional canal-wall-up surgery or a more extensive exenteration with a blind sac and oversew type

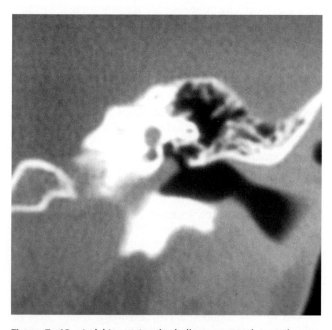

Figure 7–12 A dehiscent jugular bulb may extend onto the promontory, potentially interfering with the drilling of a cochleostomy.

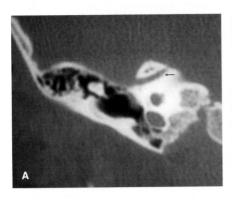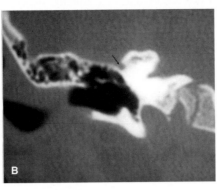

Figure 7–13 Coronal CT scan of a patient with a common cavity deformity. **(A)** The facial nerve passing superiorly over the common cochleovestibular chamber (arrow). **(B)** A more posterior section, demonstrating that the facial nerve travels along the tegmen. Intraoperatively, the nerve was identified in its descending portion and followed superiorly to the tegmen in the antral region. Here, it formed its second genu with the tympanic portion that coursed along the tegmen tympani. Preoperative knowledge of this anomalous course was felt to enhance the surgical safety of cochlear implantation in this patient.

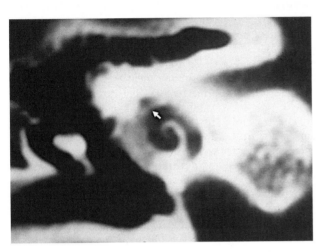

Figure 7–14 CT scan of a patient with otosclerosis. Note the otospongiotic changes present adjacent to the labyrinthine portion of the facial nerve in this coronal section (white arrow). Such pathology could predispose the patient to facial nerve stimulation by the electrodes in this region.

operation can be performed in more severe cases. Subsequent implantation can be performed in a stable, well-protected, well-healed fat-obliterated mastoid cavity.

The usual landmarks for performing mastoidectomy and facial recess may be distorted or absent in patients with cochlear abnormalities. Careful review of CT images is essential to safely performing surgery on these patients. There are often associated morphological abnormalities of the vestibular system and ossicular chain.[3] Overall, the lateral semicircular canal is considered the most frequently malformed inner ear structure, which is speculated to be due to its late embryonic formation.[2,3,73,74]

The Cochlear Aqueduct

There is a consensus that the cochlear aqueduct plays a role in the pathologic process of labyrinthine ossification. Its role in the pathogenesis of spontaneous and intraoperative CSF fistula is less clear. Gushers during stapedectomy have been traditionally hypothesized to be associated with enlargements of the cochlear aqueduct. Jackler and Hwang[75] doubted that the cochlear aqueduct plays a significant role in the etiology of CSF fistula. Radiographic reports of cochlear

aqueduct enlargement are rare.[76] Jackler and Hwang recommended that radiographic enlargement should be reported as a diameter exceeding 2 mm in its narrowest mid–otic capsule portion. They pointed out that the lateral otic capsule portion of the cochlear aqueduct is consistently narrow despite variability in the medial opening into the subarachnoid space, and is filled with a complex mesh of loose connective tissue.[75,77]

Traditional arguments implicating the cochlear aqueduct as the source of CSF fistula assert that despite the presence of the tissue mesh, there is a contiguous lumen.[75,78] Jackler and Hwang, however, suggest that there is no correlation between the clinical scenario of perilymphatic gusher and demonstrable radiographic enlargements of the cochlear aqueduct, casting doubt on even the existence of radiographically demonstrable enlargements of the lateral otic capsule portion of the cochlear aqueduct reported in the literature.[75] Others have argued that even slight increases in the diameter may cause increases in flows, which may be at measurements smaller than can be detected on CT.[79] It has been rebutted, however, that this argument does not take into account the baffling effect of the membranous mesh.[75]

It is plausible, nonetheless, that the cochlear aqueduct may account for the "oozer" but not the "gusher" seen on entering the vestibule during stapes surgery.[80] It is also possible that a similar pathogenesis may exist when easily controllable pulsatile perilymph is encountered during implant surgery at the time of cochleostomy. Its potential management should be anticipated if the presence of an abnormally enlarged cochlear aqueduct is seen on a preoperative CT scanning of the implant candidate.

There is at least one case report from 1982 in the literature of a 15-year-old boy with normal hearing who had a CSF fistula between the posterior fossa and middle ear via an enlarged cochlear aqueduct that was demonstrated by both metrizamide and Pantopaque contrast cisternography performed using conventional polytomography and CT scanning.[81] Middle ear exploration reportedly revealed CSF leaking through a defect in the round window that was patched. Two years later, during neurosurgical exploration via craniotomy for the treatment of recurrent CSF rhinorrhea and pneumococcal meningitis, it was reported that a tube of arachnoid was passing through a bony defect at the level of the cochlear aqueduct. This was thought to be successfully obliterated with muscle, with subsequent resolution of the

CSF rhinorrhea and meningitis. The patient was reported as having otherwise normal inner ears and preservation of hearing.

A more-likely-to-be-encountered and well-documented etiology for CSF leakage is through defective partitioning between the internal auditory canal (IAC) fundus and the malformed inner ear.[75,81,82] This was documented as well by Park et al[81] in two other patients managed for recurrent meningitis and CSF fistula with demonstrable cochlear malformations. Both were children with unilateral deafness and inner ear malformations. One had a unilateral incomplete partition or classic Mondini deformity and the other had bilateral dilated enlargements of the cochlea and vestibule.

The Vestibular Aqueduct

The association of enlargement of the vestibular aqueduct and congenital SNHL is well recognized.[7,23,83–87] Radiographically, it may occur in conjunction with other identifiable inner ear anomalies as previously discussed, or as an isolated finding on CT or MRI[86–92] (**Figs. 7–3** and **7–15**). Radiographic enlargement has been reported using different imaging modalities and criteria, but is generally considered to exist when the aqueduct's diameter is greater than 1.5 to 2.0 mm at its midpoint, measured between the common crus and the external aperture into the posterior fossa.[86,93–96]

The large vestibular aqueduct syndrome is traditionally considered to be a distinct clinical entity in patients with radiographic evidence of enlargement of the vestibular aqueduct.[86,87] Hearing loss is typically bilateral and progressive, with stepwise decrements often associated by episodes of relatively minor head trauma. Enlargement of the vestibular aqueduct is considered as well to be a relatively common

finding in children with congenital SNHL.[75,86,87] Some authors regard it as the single most common radiographic finding among patients with congenital SNHL.[75]

The major traditional hypothesis regarding the pathogenesis of this anomaly involves aberrant or arrested development of the endolymphatic duct and sac system, which is based on the observation that in early embryogenesis the duct is shorter, straighter, and proportionally much broader than in later maturity.[86] As more experience has been gained with MRI scanning, the defect is currently being described and studied as one involving the entire endolymphatic duct and sac system.[88–92]

There is also some evidence supporting a familial component to the disorder.[97] Some work is being done to investigate its genetics basis as well as its association with other known syndromes.[94,98] There are a variety of speculative etiologies of the hearing loss associated with this disorder based mostly on clinical, radiographic, and surgical observations as well as some analyses of endolymphatic chemical composition. Among them are damage secondary to transduction of intracranial CSF pressures, reflux of protein-rich hyperosmolar endolymph from the endolymphatic sac into the cochlea through the widely patent duct, as well as inherent functional abnormalities of the endolymphatic sac system leading to abnormal intracochlear fluid composition and dynamics.[86,92,93,95,99] Published analyses utilizing high-resolution CT scanning have demonstrated associated modiolar defects in patients with large vestibular aqueducts, engendering further speculation as to the etiology of the associated hearing loss and CSF leaks.[95,96]

The clinical significance of radiographic enlargements of the vestibular aqueduct and endolymphatic duct and sac system in the cochlear implant candidate is twofold. It may serve both as a diagnosis and as an indicator of the potential for the need to manage an intraoperative CSF leak at the time of cochleostomy. Despite this risk, many such patients have been safely and successfully implanted with the appropriate management.[23,25,100]

Radiographic Indicators and Clinical Management of Cerebrospinal Fluid Leak and Meningitis

Recurrent meningitis has been reported in patients with malformed cochleae. Among 33 patients in two larger series, three cases of recurrent pneumococcal meningitis were documented.[7,101] The most likely etiology is thought to be tympanogenic in association with congenital CSF fistula. The medial defect is thought to be most likely in the region of the modiolus, as has been found on histologic examination of malformed inner ears.[7,82] The lateral defect is thought to be most likely in the region of the stapes footplate, which has been described by Schuknecht histologically as partly or totally replaced by a thin membrane in selected ears with congenital cochlear malformation.[7,82]

Burton et al[82] in 1990 documented the flow of iohexol from the fundus of the internal auditory canal into the vestibule and cochlea after instillation into a lumbar subarachnoid drain in a patient with recurrent pneumococcal meningitis and a malformed inner ear. The malformation was described as consisting of a hypoplastic basal turn of the cochlea

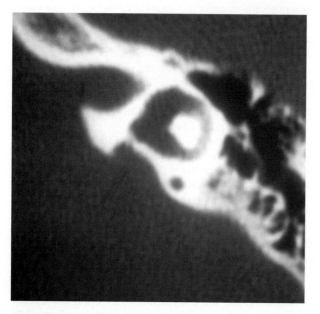

Figure 7–15 Axial CT image in a deaf child with an enlarged vestibular aqueduct.

and cochlear promontory, ectatic vestibule, and common vestibulocochlear chamber. It was further noted at surgical exploration that the stapes footplate was small and scalloped and did not completely fill the oval window, which was judged to be of normal size. The oval window was the site of the leak and was managed successfully with stapedectomy and obliterative grafting with fat and fascia.

Additional authors have described various management options ranging from isolated grafting of identifiable oval window defects without stapedectomy, to stapedectomy and fascia or muscle obliteration of the entire vestibule and middle ear space with or without spinal drainage, depending on the severity of the leak.[102,103] In cases of severe cochlea dysplasia with obvious radiologic absence of partitioning between the fundus and cochleovestibular cavity, there should be a high index of suspicion that there will be encountered CSF at intracranial pressure. This is true not only for the management of a postmeningitic patient with a cochlear anomaly but also during the cochlear implantation surgery of a patient in whom a CSF leak is encountered. In general, it has been found in our center that cases of severe deformity associated with profuse CSF egress required generous packing of fascia or harvested periosteum around the cochleostomy until egress has abated, as well as packing of the middle ear, eustachian tube, and spinal drainage in selected cases. Low-flow CSF egress is more commonly encountered in specific cases of enlarged vestibular aqueduct or incomplete partition, and it generally responds to generous packing of the cochleostomy without additional measures. Nonetheless, it would be prudent to anticipate and be prepared to handle CSF leakage in any patient with a cochlear malformation, as well as an obvious abnormality of either of the aqueducts or an abnormally dilated and bulbous internal auditory canal. Because we have successfully implanted and managed such cases, we do not consider the anticipation of an intraoperative CSF leak to be a contraindication to cochlear implantation. It may, however, play a factor in side selection in specific patients. Because the abnormal inner ear has the propensity to develop tympanogenic or meningogenic labyrinthitis, a given patient may possess varying degrees of both malformation and obstruction[82,101] (**Figs. 7–10** and **7–11**).

There have been three cases in the literature to date of postoperative meningitis in cochlear implant recipients; all patients had cochlear malformations.[103,104] One patient, a 5-year-old boy, developed meningitis following minor head trauma 2 years after cochlear implantation. His malformation was reported as being of the "Mondini type," without further characterization. At surgical exploration he was noted to be leaking CSF from the cochleostomy site. Treatment consisted of temporalis muscle and fascial packing into the vestibule and around the electrode array and into the middle ear, and a course of spinal drainage.[103]

Another patient had bilateral cochlear malformations characterized by cochleae consisting of approximately one turn with a hypoplastic modiolus with wide communication between the scala tympani and the internal auditory canal secondary to dehiscence in the cribrose area. At age 4 he underwent a left-sided cochlear implant with successful management of an intraoperative CSF leak. Two years later he had a fatal case of meningitis associated with a

right-sided acute otitis media. Histopathologic evaluation was consistent with a right-sided (contralateral) tympanogenic meningitis with a perforation of the round window and significant inflammatory infiltrate identified in the scala tympani, cochlear basal turn, and IAC. The side with the implant showed the cochleostomy sealed by fibrous tissue and bone consistent with minimal and typical implant-induced pathologic changes.[104]

The third reported case was in a patient implanted at age 5 who had bilateral common cavity deformities and developed meningitis 7 months postoperatively that was successfully treated with intravenous antibiotics.[23] The etiology of the meningitis was clinically determined to be from a contralateral acute otitis media. Fluorescein and radionuclide scanning demonstrated bilateral CSF leaks into the middle ear. Surgical exploration revealed CSF leakage bilaterally from oval window defects, which were managed with stapedectomy and packing of the vestibule with temporalis fascia. On the side of the implant, the device was temporarily removed and then reinserted after extension of the cochleostomy toward the oval window to allow for generous packing of the vestibule and cochleostomy opening around the reinserted device. Lumbar drainage was also utilized in this patient.

Retrocochlear Pathology

Appropriate evaluation of retrocochlear pathology with MRI must be considered in selected cases. This is especially true in adult patients who have lost hearing in a previously only hearing ear. Two such patients in our implant population underwent implantation in one side and a translabyrinthine resection of their acoustic neuroma in the other.

Summary

Preoperative sectional imaging is a vital tool for confirming the presence and nature of an implantable cochlear lumen. Imaging analysis should include the detection of malformations, luminal obstruction, and anatomic variants or middle ear pathology that could complicate the implantation process. Preimplant evaluation of these patients is often quite complex, taking into account a variety of clinical and electrophysiologic data. Appropriate preparedness and experience in handling the potential complications, especially an intraoperative CSF leak and facial nerve anomalies, are necessary for safe management. Numerous reports attest to the benefits received by these patients from cochlear implants.[18–25,37]

◆ Postoperative Imaging

Postoperative imaging goals for cochlear implant patients include imaging of the implant hardware itself as well as diagnostic imaging of either adjacent or distant structures. Plain film radiography can confirm proper initial surgical placement of the cochlear implant electrode array. Interval plain films may be obtained when there is suspicion of movement or malfunction that is often heralded by changes in program maps. Patients with cochlear implants may also require diagnostic sectional imaging for reasons unrelated to the implant itself. Because cochlear implants contain metallic components with varying ferromagnetic properties, their presence affects both the safety and the possibility of obtaining useful images of adjacent structures, depending on which sectional imaging technique is utilized. With the increased popularity of MRI as a diagnostic imaging modality, it is important to understand the issues surrounding its compatibility with the currently manufactured as well as previously implanted devices that may be encountered in patients today.

Determination and Monitoring of Electrode Position

Plain radiographs are currently the simplest, least expensive, and most reliable method of determining electrode position.[105] Many centers, including our own, routinely obtain an intraoperative portable plain radiograph to confirm final electrode position at the conclusion of surgery, prior to reversal of anesthesia. This image will confirm foremost that the implant has been placed intracochlearly in normal cochleae and in cases with severe malformation. These films also serve as a baseline for comparison with any future films. Further, it makes the implant team aware of malpositioning or damage to the electrode array, which would be extremely useful if there was undue difficulty during insertion or suspected device malfunction on intraoperative electrophysiologic monitoring. Additional information that can be gained from analysis of intraoperative and postoperative plain films includes detection of device extrusion as an etiology of malfunction, and electrode positioning relative to the labyrinthine portion of the facial nerve in cases of undesired postoperative facial nerve stimulation. It is our policy to compare a recently obtained postoperative plain film with an earlier film in the evaluation of suspected malfunction or significant changes in psychophysical measurements.

Intraoperative portable films are usually taken in an oblique anti-Stenver's view or a transorbital orientation. A three-view mastoid series (Stenver's, transorbital, base) may be obtained on postoperative day 1. Follow-up films are obtained in multiple views so that an appropriate film can be found to best match the intraoperative film orientation.

It is essential to be familiar with the characteristic appearances of electrode arrays in both normal and malformed cochleae and to utilize a consistent method of determination of electrode insertion depth. Trigonometric techniques of determining round window location on plain radiographs have been described.[106-108] Intracochlear electrode position is then discerned from this reference point. These techniques are dependent on good-quality radiographs with appropriate views so that the important landmarks are readily visible. Intraoperative films are often of poorer quality than postoperative films due to the nature of portable x-ray equipment and the inability to place the implanted side closer to the x-ray film. They are frequently of low contrast and do not allow the easy visualization of the fine structures of the labyrinth. In these situations, we have found it useful

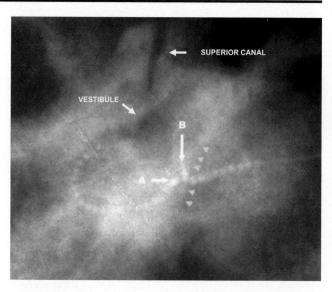

Figure 7–16 Plain radiograph of a cadaver head with an intracochlear electrode array in place. Barium markers were placed at the round window (A) and cochleostomy (B). The position of the cochleostomy can be approximated relative to the point at which the electrode array crosses the dense otic capsule bone, i.e., the inferior cochlear margin (arrowheads). The counted rings that lay posterior to this intersection are considered clearly outside the cochlea.

to utilize a computer enhancement method for determination of cochleostomy position. Our method of interpretation was developed through the analysis of cadaver temporal bones and confirmed using video analyses of several clinical cases. A description of the process is detailed in **Figs. 7–16** and **7–17**.

Plain Radiographs

Figures 7–18 through **7–27** illustrate the expected appearance of both properly and improperly placed electrode arrays as determined by plain radiographs. Several interesting clinical case examples are also provided.

Stability of the Implant Electrode Array

Electrode migration due to future skull growth was a concern that initially led to prohibiting implantation of children younger that 2 years of age. Recently, the high level of performance achieved by young implantees has led to a reevaluation of this lower age limit, requiring an assessment of the effects of skull growth over time. The reported electrode extrusion rate is 1% in all age groups.[109] The largest proportion of skull growth occurs during the first of life, which is below the age of all implanted children in the United States to date, after which there is a gradual increase to full adult size.[110,111] The distance from the cortically anchored receiver stimulator to the cochleostomy is influenced by head circumference changes and mastoid air cell development. Surgical fixation techniques and lead wire redundancy theoretically compensate for these skull growth concerns.

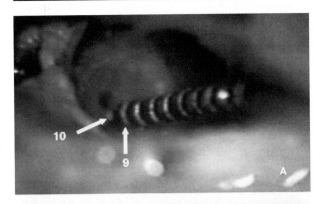

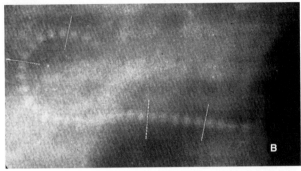

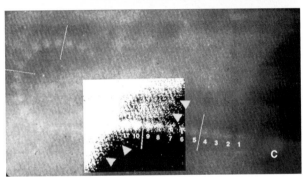

Figure 7–17 Confirmation of the validity of the landmark for electrode counts was evaluated with several clinical cases. The intraoperative video analysis is compared with the immediate postoperative radiograph. The films are digitally scanned into a graphics workstation. Image contrast filters enhance the visibility of the electrode array and surrounding osseous structures. The inferoposterior cochlear margin is readily visible, and determination of the point at which the electrode array enters the dense bony otic capsule is made. **(A)** Video-captured postinsertion image from a clinical case reveals that band 10 is intracochlear whereas band 9 is at the cochleostomy. **(B)** Image of digitally scanned x-ray with reference markers placed to facilitate counting. **(C)** Threshold adjustments demonstrate the inferoposterior cochlear margin (arrowheads) and the relative positions of the electrode bands. Note the positions of bands 9 and 10.

The factors influencing electrode array migration and extrusion are many and not solely quantifiable on the basis of skull circumference. These factors include intracochlear conditions such as ossification and fibrosis, which may force the electrodes out of the scala tympani. Mastoid factors, including adhesive bands and attachments, may influence the electrode lead wire position. During several revision operations performed on other implantees, a thick

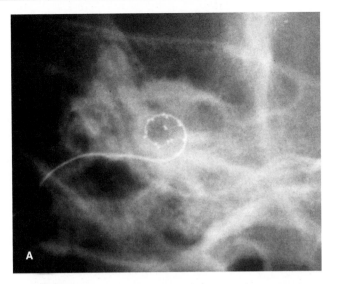

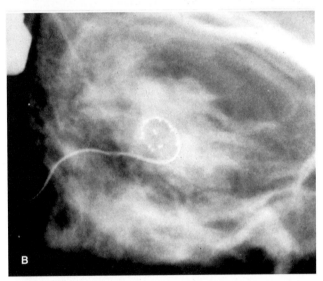

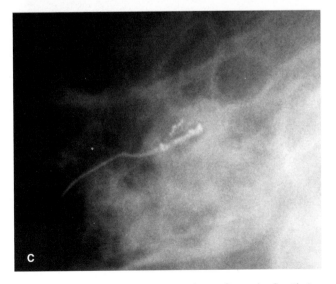

Figure 7–18 Normal postoperative plain radiograph of a Clarion multichannel cochlear implant electrode array implanted into the right cochlea. **(A)** Stenver's, **(B)** transorbital, and **(C)** base views.

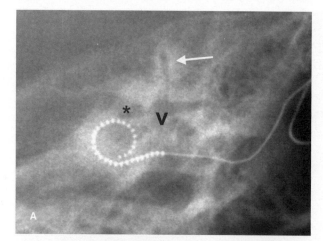

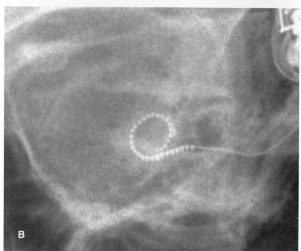

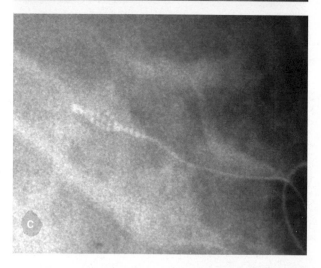

Figure 7–19 Normal postoperative plain radiograph of a Nucleus 24 multichannel cochlear implant electrode array implanted into the left cochlea. **(A)** Stenver's, **(B)** transorbital, and **(C)** base views. **(A)** The IAC (∗), vestibule (V), and superior semicircular canal (white arrow) are labeled.

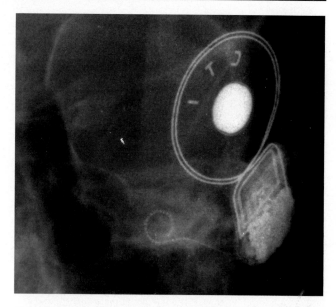

Figure 7–20 Intraoperative portable plain radiograph (transorbital projection) of the patient depicted in **Fig. 7–19**. Note that despite the diminished image resolution, the electrode array can clearly be identified within the density of the otic capsule and conforms appropriately to the shape of the cochlear lumen.

factors, such as trauma and infection, may also cause electrode migration. Electrode design may also affect electrode migration.

To address this concern, we studied a representative sample of our pediatric cochlear implant population, which confirmed the stability of the intracochlear electrode position over time.[112] A group of 151 children age 5 or younger were implanted at New York University (NYU) Medical Center between 1987 and 1997. Of these patients, 27 were followed with plain radiographs over an interval ranging from 1 to 75 months. The age range at the time of implantation was 14 months to 5 years 6 months. The study population encompassed the most common causes of deafness: congenital, 14; meningitis, three; genetic, three; cytomegalovirus (CMV), three; and mumps, Mondini malformation, Waardenburg syndrome, and kernicterus, one each. Twenty-three Nucleus (Cochlear Corporation, Englewood, CO) and four Clarion (Advanced Bionics; Valencia, CA) devices were evaluated. Fourteen of the patients had modified hemoclips placed.[109] In no case was there evidence of electrode migration in this study population. Although no case of extrusion has been radiographically or clinically identified in our pediatric implantees, one case of electrode extrusion in an adult patient from our center has been reported.[109] An incus bar modified hemoclip was not used with the Nucleus device in this case, and at reimplantation two hairpin turns in the proximal electrode were found. It was the operating surgeon's belief that these turns created uncoiling forces that resulted in electrode extrusion. No other cases of extrusion have been identified or suspected in our adult patients. This electrode may have in part been due to the strict adherence to surgical technique with regard to electrode and implant fixation utilized in our institution.

fibrous capsule was found attached to multiple adhesions encompassing the lead wire. Cortical factors including skull growth and receiver stimulator migration and other extrinsic

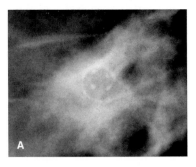
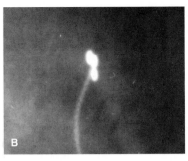

Figure 7–21 **(A)** Intraoperative portable plain radiograph of a Med-El multichannel cochlear implant electrode array. **(B)** Note the cloverleaf configuration of the free ground electrode.

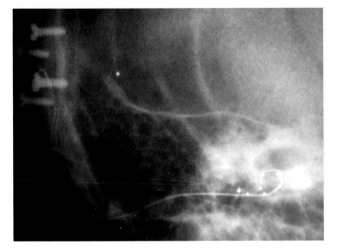

Figure 7–22 Normal plain radiograph of an Ineraid multichannel cochlear implant electrode array implanted into the right cochlea (Stenver's projection). Note the screws that fix the transcutaneous pedestal to the skull. Note that there are six ball electrodes as well as a two ground electrodes (promontory and free).

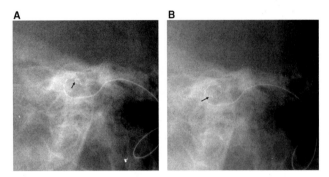

Figure 7–23 **(A)** Radiograph after insertion of a Clarion multichannel cochlear implant electrode array. Note that the tip has kinked and doubled over onto itself (arrow). **(B)** Radiograph after reinsertion of the same device. Note the proper position of the distal electrode pair (arrow).

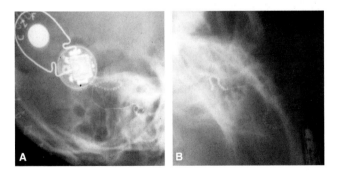

Figure 7–24 Postoperative plain radiographs of a multichannel electrode array inserted into a hypotympanic air cell tract. **(A)** The electrode has an unusual configuration and is located below the dense otic capsule bone. **(B)** A base view of the same implant.

In summary, implantation age should not be restricted by the concern for electrode migration with skull growth. The determination of implantation candidacy should be decided on other well-established and appropriate factors.

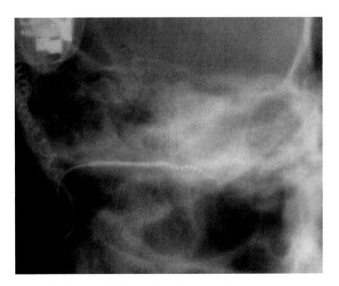

Figure 7–25 Transorbital plain radiograph after implantation of a multichannel electrode array into the drill-out of a straight tunnel into the basal turn of a patient with extensive bilateral labyrinthitis obliterans.

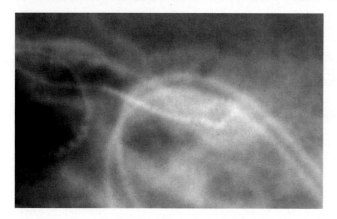

Figure 7–26 Intraoperative portable plain radiograph (lateral projection) of a multichannel cochlear implant electrode array implanted into the common cavity of the patient depicted in **Fig. 7–4**. Note how the electrode assumes a curved configuration and is located within the density of the otic capsule bone. In this image, there are superimposed electrode cables that are used for intraoperative electrophysiologic monitoring.

Magnetic Resonance Imaging Compatibility of Cochlear and Auditory Brainstem Implants

Magnetic resonance imaging is the diagnostic study of choice for many disease entities. Three electromagnetic fields are generated during acquisition of data for MR images. A constant, strong, static magnetic field aligns protons; a rapidly changing, small magnetic field gradient is developed for spatial localization; radiofrequency pulses produce proton energy state changes.[113] The strengths of the fields are proportional to the tesla rating of the MRI magnet. Imaging time, pulse sequences, and radiofrequency emissions also contribute to field strength. Although harmless to normal human tissue, these fields have the potential to generate torque and force on the ferromagnetic components of implanted devices. Additional concerns include the generation of heat or electrical currents in or around electronic devices that might damage surrounding tissues, damage the device, or cause unintentional device output. Internal magnets can become demagnetized, making them dysfunctional, and distortion of needed images may render the studies uninterpretable or inadequate.

It is a reasonable assumption that many people will need to have an MRI at some point during their lifetimes.[114] Issues of compatibility and potential human harm arise when the recipient of an implanted medical device needs to have an MRI study. The patient with a cochlear implant and the potential implant candidate requiring an MRI or serial MRIs present the physician with a unique clinical situation requiring a decision. Cochlear implants often contain ferromagnetic electronic parts and casings and an internal magnet that aligns an external antenna on the overlying scalp.

The Food and Drug Administration does not consider any currently available cochlear implant device MRI compatible. Although the 1995 National Institutes of Health (NIH) Cochlear Implant Consensus Development Conference Summary states that potential MRI risks should be part of the informed consent, a growing body of literature reports that patients with cochlear implants may safely undergo MRI evaluation when certain precautions are undertaken.[113]

Portnoy and Mattucci[113] examined the effects of MRI on the internal receiver/stimulator of several cochlear implants. They found that significant electrical currents were generated when the House/3M and 3M/Vienna cochlear implants were exposed to a 0.6-tesla (T) machine, and that these devices were magnetized and nonfunctional after exposure. The Nucleus 22 implant maintained its functionality but subjective "significant forces" were exerted on the device. The authors contend that these forces would potentially dislodge the implant and electrode array. Applebaum and Valvassori[115] discussed similar nonquantified forces exerted on the Nucleus Mini 22 device handheld within 1 m of a 1.5-T MRI. They noted that no movement of the electrode array occurred independent of the receiver/stimulator. Heller et al[116] evaluated the modified Nucleus Mini-22 and the auditory brainstem implant (ABI) (Cochlear Corporation, Englewood, CO) in a 1.5-T MRI machine. Both devices tested were magnetless and had nonferromagnetic casings around the internal electronics. The tests were conducted on a phantom body. No temperature elevations, negligible current inductions around the devices, and no output from the devices were found. A maximum force of 2818 dynes was exerted on the devices at the entrance to the bore of the machine. As expected, both devices caused a significant adjacent signal void of 2 to 6 cm on the MRI images. Chou et al,[117] in an extensive study using phantom head models, confirmed the absence of heating due to radiofrequency emissions from a 1.5-T machine on the ABI and modified Nucleus Mini-22 implant.

Studies performed on the Clarion 1.2 magnet-containing implant (Advanced Bionics Corp., Sylmar, CA) with a 1.5-T and 0.3-T magnet revealed no significant device output and no significant heating of the device or surrounding area.

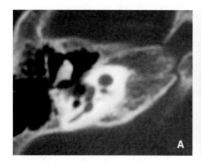
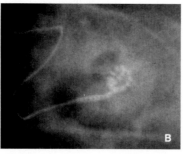

Figure 7–27 (A) Axial CT image of a patient with a severely hypoplastic cochlea. The cochlea is a small spherical cavity, which is seen in this image anterior to the vestibule and oval window. **(B)** A multichannel electrode array assumes a pigtail configuration as it coils inside the cochlear lumen.

Maximal torque and force production occurred when the implant magnet was aligned perpendicular to the axis of the MRI-generated magnetic field [0.19 Newton-meter (Nm)].[118] The magnetic field axis usually runs parallel to the long axis of the patient in a tunnel-design MRI machine. Torque production was much less with a 0.3-T magnet; however, force was approximately the same. These studies also reported no unintentional device output or heating. The authors did report as much as a 78.5% reduction in internal magnet strength after 20 minutes of exposure in the 1.5-T machine and only a maximal 10% reduction with the 0.3-T machine. It was recommended that MRI be performed, if absolutely necessary, with the internal magnet polarity aligned with the machine's magnet polarity to minimize induced forces.

The Digisonic magnet-containing cochlear implant (MXM Laboratories, Vallarius Cedex, France) was tested in a 1.0-T magnetic field where the device was anchored in a bony well in a human temporal bone and a pig's head.[119] No discernible change in position was observed in both specimens. No evoked stimulation, heating, magnetization, or device malfunction was incurred.

Teissel et al[120] performed in vitro experiments with the MED-ELCombi 40 cochlear implant (Innsbruck, Austria) in a 1.5-T head coil. The pulse sequences, radiofrequency (RF) settings, and image acquisition times were set to develop maximal detrimental effects. Similar forces were detected as with the other magnet containing devices (0.175 Nm). When anchored in a plastic cube with a binding around the implant, rotational movement was 2.7 degrees. The rotational forces decreased with distance from the MRI magnet isocenter. No significant heating, implant output, or device damage was observed. Demagnetization of the internal device magnet did occur (38%). Image signal voids were similar to other studies mentioned. The authors report that temperature change, voltage production, and heating could theoretically be reduced by choosing imaging sequences with low average RF power. It was also recommended that the patient's head be oriented parallel to the magnetic field of the MRI machine.

Tests on human cadaver skulls, volunteers with devices taped to their heads, and in two implantees requiring MRI for medical purposes were performed on the standard Med-El Combi 40 device with magnet strengths of up to 1.5 T.[121] Neither implantee patient reported abnormal sensations or impairments, and device function was not affected. Additionally, useful images were obtained of the anatomical areas of concern (pituitary and cervical spine).

In the event that an implantee requires an MRI, device compatibility must first be determined. The answers to the following three questions guide the clinical decision-making process: (1) Does the device contain an internal magnet? (2) Are the internal components and casing ferromagnetic? (3) Is the magnet removable?

Does the device contain an internal magnet? All major cochlear implant companies currently manufacture their standard devices containing internal magnets. These include the Nucleus Mini-22 and 24M, the Clarion 1.2, the Combi 40, and the Combi 40+. The companies also manufacture "special order" devices without internal magnets for implantation in patients with known MRI needs. These special devices require the use of an adhesive-backed external scalp magnet to position the external antenna over the receiver. If the status of a particular implant is unknown, the clinician should contact the company and provide the patient's identification number and device serial number.

Are the internal components and casing ferromagnetic and resistant to damage by the MRI's generated fields? Cochlear Corporation's Nucleus 22, 24M, and ABI (without the optionally installed magnet) contain titanium and other non-ferromagnetic materials and are resistant to damage by the strong magnetic fields generated by MRI scanning. The makeup of the internal components and casing of the Nucleus 22 device were eventually altered, making them MRI compatible in the absence of an internal magnet. Device construction can be determined by plain film analysis of radiopaque lettering or by contacting the company with device serial number and patient identification. The Ineraid (Cochlear Corporation, Englewood, CO) and House/3M devices are not MRI compatible, and MRI is not recommended in patients with these devices.[113,114] Clarion and Med-El both manufacture special-order, MRI-compatible devices that contain MRI-compatible components and no internal magnet.

Is the internal magnet removable? The internal magnet in the standard design Clarion and Med-El devices are housed within the ceramic casing and are therefore not removable. The standard-design Nucleus 24M and ABI have a magnet that is separately encased in Silastic and sits in a soft Silastic pouch and is therefore optionally removable at the time of initial implantation. Plain film analysis of radiopaque lettering around other Nucleus devices can determine magnet removability. The presence of a "J," "L," or "T" as the middle code letter near the magnet inside the antenna loop indicates that the device has a removable magnet (Cochlear Corporation, Englewood, CO; personal communication). The standard design Nucleus 22 has a magnet that is housed only in soft Silastic and may be "cut out" without damaging the integrity or function of the device electronics. If a device has a removable magnet, it can be removed under local anesthesia. An incision should be planned that will put the electrode lead wire at minimal risk and will avoid contact with the external antenna. It is wise to approach the device from posteriorly by raising a small flap and dissecting to the magnet housing. Ideally, the incision should avoid the external antenna's contact point with the skin.

If it is determined by the above three questions that a patient's device is MRI compatible, scanning can be undertaken. All external hardware must first be removed from the patient, as these components are not MRI compatible. Additionally, there will be a zone of susceptibility artifact with distortion of the local magnetic fields in the region of the implant regardless of its resistance to internal damage or local tissue injury. **Fig. 7–28** depicts a sequence of MR images obtained on a patient implanted with a modified Nucleus Mini-22 device who had an acoustic neuroma on the opposite side. Satisfactory serial images were obtained on a 1.5-T machine providing necessary information for patient management.

Susceptibility artifact is increased with the strength of the magnet in tesla and is related to the pulse sequence utilized. Consideration should be given to utilizing a lower tesla MRI system to obtain adequate imaging. Imaging time and

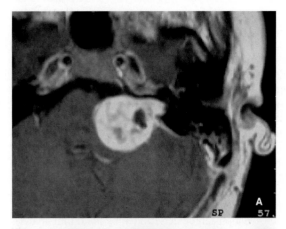

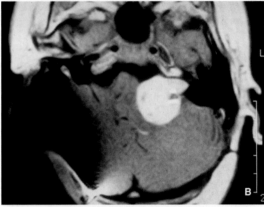

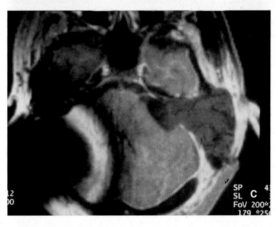

Figure 7–28 **(A)** T1-weighted, contrast-enhanced MRI of a large left-sided acoustic neuroma in a patient with contralateral auditory dyssynchrony long-term deafness. **(B)** MRI postimplantation of a modified Nucleus Mini-22 magnetless cochlear implant in the right ear. Note susceptibility artifact generated by magnetless device still allows for monitoring of contralateral disease process. **(C)** Baseline postoperative MRI following translabyrinthine total tumor removal delineates anatomy in tumor region despite susceptibility artifact from contralateral magnetless cochlear implant.

RF settings should also be optimized. The further away the anatomical area of concern for study is from the device, the less of an issue the tesla strength of the magnet becomes. When it is impossible to adequately study an anatomical region in proximity to an MRI compatible device, the adequacy of alternative imaging modalities (CT scan) must be weighed against the risks and benefits of explantation.

If it is determined that a patient's device is not MRI compatible, then several options may be entertained including the determination of the adequacy of alternative imaging modalities or temporary or permanent explantation with the possibility of reimplantation with an MRI-compatible device. Another possibility centers around a current area of controversy and recent investigation: There is a body of literature that suggests that standard-issue Clarion and Med-El devices may be safe with 1.5-T MRI machines when RF issues, imaging duration, and pulse sequencing are taken into consideration. The evidence suggests the possibility of mechanically binding a device with a nonremovable magnet whose other components will not be damaged by the MRI's generated fields. The patient's head must be aligned in the magnetic field so as to minimize the generated force. The typical tunnel MRI design generates a magnetic field in the long axis of the tunnel, which would generate the maximum torque on a magnet whose flat surface is perpendicular to this axis. Angulation of the head or utilization of an open MRI system may enable minimization of the torque to levels below those routinely applied to the skull and dura during surgical implantation and fixation. Firmly anchoring the receiver/stimulator in a deep bony well with tie-downs, at the time of implant surgery, may also prevent movement of a cochlear implant by the above-mentioned forces.

An additional concern is the demagnetization of the internal magnet after exposure to the MRI's magnetic field. Though this might result in the necessity of using alternative antenna fixation systems, such as with the magnetless custom designs, it does not necessarily preclude MRI scanning. A magnetless Clarion 1.2 device with an earmold-supported antenna was found to be stable and well tolerated by several patients.[122]

In the past, the presence of a cochlear implant was considered to be a major contraindication to MRI.[1] With advances in cochlear implant (CI) technology and an understanding of the RF, pulse sequences, and image time factors, it is now possible to obtain useful images. In current practice, the cochlear implant candidate with known future MRI needs should be implanted with a device considered MRI compatible by the above-mentioned criteria. Implantation of a device with a removable magnet would potentially provide the patient with the option of a magnet retrofit should future MRI no longer be required. Alternatively, a "special-order" magnetless device with non-ferromagnetic internal components can be obtained from all of the major implant manufacturers, and should be implanted until further studies demonstrate the safety of a magnet-containing device. An external scalp adhesive will be required for antenna attachment. Because a growing body of evidence suggests that MRI image acquisition with a 1.5-T magnet or less may be possible without incurring damage to the patient or to currently manufactured magnet-containing devices, these recommendations may change in the future. It is important to note, however, that currently in the United States an MRI is contraindicated in the presence of a magnet-containing cochlear implant. Consulting with CI and ABI manufacturers is highly recommended when issues of MRI compatibility arise. Because MRI machines now exist with magnet strengths up to 5 T, continued investigation will be necessary.

◆ Fluoroscopically Assisted Cochlear Implantation

Fluoroscopically assisted cochlear implantation allows visualization of electrode insertion in real time. This technique was initially developed for laboratory study of electrode prototypes, and to evaluate surgical technique.[123,124] Insertion angle, depth, and cochleostomy position were studied and optimized with fluoroscopic evaluation. Complication simulation provided useful information regarding the avoidance of cochlear and electrode damage. Cadaver temporal bones were implanted under fluoroscopic guidance to evaluate insertion dynamics and mechanisms of intracochlear trauma using conventionally implanted electrode arrays as well as a variety of perimodiolar prototypes. The information gleaned from these studies provided necessary feedback that eventually affected electrode design by the engineers. Real-time fluoroscopy provides a visual image that correlates with tactile sensations that a surgeon may experience during electrode insertion.[125]

Technique

Intraoperative fluoroscopy (IF) is performed using the C-arm unit utilized for conventional neurosurgical, orthopedic, and angiographic surgeries. The patient is placed on the table in a standard position for cochlear implantation—supine with the head turned away from the operating surgeon. The C-arm is placed with the beam generator beneath the table directed in an anti-Stenvers view (in contrast to traditional Stenvers where the ear of concern is placed against the image plate). Narrowing and centering the beam on the cochlea magnifies the image. Fluoroscopic assistance may be employed in the case of inner ear malformation at the time of cochleostomy for determination of proper placement, as well as during electrode insertion. Images are recorded on video in real time for future analysis. Care is taken to avoid placement of radiodense monitoring leads in the imaging path. Preset settings utilized for orthopedic procedures typically yield the best image quality. Adjustments of both position and beam characteristics are made so that the dense otic capsule is well visualized with minimal interference from adjacent skull structures and instrumentation. Surgery is performed as per routine.

Safety

Fluoroscopy is utilized as briefly as possible to keep exposure levels well below exposure tolerance of the human lens, the structure most vulnerable to exposure.[126] Narrowing the beam will minimize the radiation received by the patient. Direct penetration of the orbit should be avoided. Consultation with the radiation safety officer is recommended, at which time information regarding the fluoroscopy unit's calibrated skin entrance exposure level may be obtained. Most modern units produce a dose well below 10 rad per minute of use. The dose to the lens may be estimated by calculating 20% of this value. The total exposure should be kept below 200 rad. The typical exposure time should be no more than a total of 1 to 3 minutes of short multiple exposures for

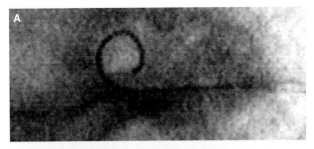

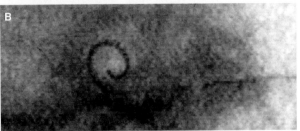

Figure 7–29 Intraoperative real-time fluoroscopic images taken from one of the five Contour preclinical trial insertions. Note the actively coiling properties are demonstrated after the stylet is removed. This can be seen by comparing **(A)** pre–stylet removal to **(B)** post–stylet removal). (From Fishman AJ, Roland Jr JT, Alexiades G, Mierzwinski J, Cohen NL. Fluoroscopically assisted cochlear implantation. Otol Neurotol 2003;24(6):882–886, with permission.)

cochlear implantation yielding a maximally calculated dose of 10 rad/min × 3 min × 0.2 = 6 rad for a 3-min exposure. Exposure can usually be limited to well under one minute. Lead aprons and thyroid shields are worn by the operating room staff. The patient is similarly protected.

Contour Preclinical Trials

During the Contour preclinical trial, five patients were implanted at NYU with the Nucleus 24 RCS Contour Cochlear Implant (Cochlear Corporation, Englewood, CO) under fluoroscopic assistance to verify and document the intracochlear performance of the newly designed electrode array, a precoiled design that assumes a perimodiolar position after removal of a straightening stylet. The device was easily implanted and a decreased diameter was observed after stylet removal (**Fig. 7–29**).

Case Studies of Inner Ear Malformations

Case 1

A 4-year-old congenitally deaf girl was recently implanted with a Nucleus CI24M (Cochlear Corporation, Englewood, CO) device in her right ear. Preoperative radiographical evaluation revealed that her right cochleovestibular apparatus is composed of a small common cavity measuring 7 mm in maximum diameter with hypoplastic semicircular canals and an absent endolymphatic duct (**Fig. 7–30**). Her left cochleovestibular was consistent with cochlear aplasia and was therefore not suitable for implantation.

Implantation surgery was performed via a transmastoid approach with facial recess. Intraoperative fluoroscopy

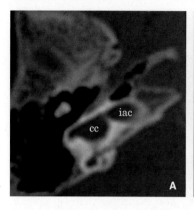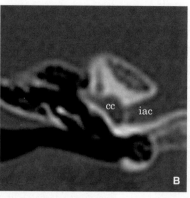

Figure 7–30 Axial **(A)** and coronal **(B)** images of a patient with a common cavity malformation who was implanted under fluoroscopic guidance. Note the common cavity (cc) and internal auditory canal (iac). (From Fishman AJ, Roland Jr JT, Alexiades G, Mierzwinski J, Cohen NL. Fluoroscopically assisted cochlear implantation. Otol Neurotol 2003;24(6):882–886, with permission.)

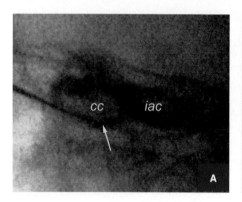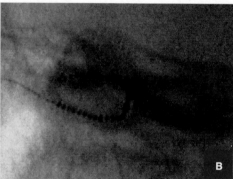

Figure 7–31 Intraoperative real-time fluoroscopic images taken from the same patient as in **Fig. 7–2**. **(A)** The cochleostomy position is verified by placement of a fine pick (arrow). cc, common cavity; iac, internal auditory canal. Note all 22 active electrodes are inserted in a C-shaped configuration within the common cavity. **(B)** The morphology on fluoroscopic image approximates the coronal CT image. (From Fishman AJ, Roland Jr JT, Alexiades G, Mierzwinski J, Cohen NL. Fluoroscopically assisted cochlear implantation. Otol Neurotol 2003;24(6):882–886, with permission.)

was utilized during cochleostomy localization and electrode insertion. The cochleostomy was performed on the promontory bulge inferior to the oval window. The patient had no round window. The position was determined by correlation of CT images with intraoperative surface landmarks as well as confirmed by intraoperative fluoroscopy (**Fig. 7–31A**). There was no egress of CSF. All 22 active electrodes were inserted in a C-shaped fashion (**Fig. 7–31B**). Intraoperative electrophysiologic monitoring revealed present stapedial reflexes and neural response telemetry in multiple electrodes tested throughout the array. Her postoperative course has been unremarkable.

Case 2

This patient is a congenitally deaf girl with a common cavity malformation who required reimplantation of a right common cavity malformation 3 years after the original surgery. She was originally implanted with a Nucleus CI24M. Her right cochleovestibular apparatus is the larger of her bilateral defects and is composed of a small common cavity measuring 6.5 mm in maximum diameter with hypoplastic semicircular canals and an absent endolymphatic duct (**Fig. 7–32A**). This is associated with an internal auditory canal measuring 2.5 mm in mid-diameter (**Fig. 7–32B**).

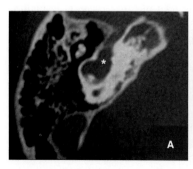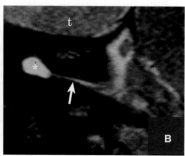

Figure 7–32 Axial CT **(A)** and coronal MRI **(B)** in a patient with common cavity malformation. Note the small common cavity (∗) with the narrow internal auditory canal (arrow). The temporal lobe (t) is labeled for orientation on coronal image. (From Fishman AJ, Roland Jr JT, Alexiades G, Mierzwinski J, Cohen NL. Fluoroscopically assisted cochlear implantation. Otol Neurotol 2003;24(6):882–886, with permission.)

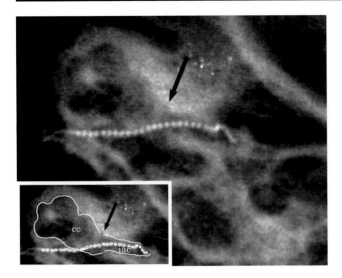

Intraoperative plain radiography revealed the electrode array had traversed the common cavity and passed into the internal auditory canal (**Fig. 7–33**). Because most of the electrodes were located within the common cavity, the decision was made not to reposition the array for fear of cochlear or facial nerve damage. Four electrode bands required deactivation secondary to facial nerve stimulation. Although the patient had not achieved open-set speech recognition, improvements have been noted.

She was performing well, mainstreamed in a regular class with an oral interpreter until 3 years postimplantation at which time she had increased channel interaction and decreased performance. A decision was made to reposition the array under fluoroscopic guidance so that intrameatal insertion could be avoided and the maximum number of available electrodes could be positioned into the common cavity. The same array was first removed and then reinserted with 17 electrode bands forming a C-shaped configuration inside the common cavity (**Fig. 7–34**). There was no CSF leak. The patient uses 17 electrodes postoperatively with performance currently improved over the preoperative one.

Figure 7–33 A transorbital intraoperative view taken during surgery of the patient in **Fig. 7–4**. Note that the array has passed into the internal auditory canal. The arrow denotes the junction between the common cavity and the internal auditory canal as seen in this orientation. The inset view outlines the lumen of the common cavity (cc) as well as the internal auditory canal (iac). (From Fishman AJ, Roland Jr JT, Alexiades G, Mierzwinski J, Cohen NL. Fluoroscopically assisted cochlear implantation. Otol Neurotol 2003;24(6):882–886, with permission of author.)

Case Studies of Cochlear Luminal Obstruction with Split Array

Case 3

A 44-year-old woman with labyrinthine ossification secondary to meningitis received an incomplete insertion of a CI24M electrode array on the left side (AS) at another institution. **Fig. 7–35A** demonstrates a kinked array on plain film. Due to a device failure, the patient underwent revision at our center and received a Nucleus (Cochlear Corporation, Englewood, CO) CI24 Double Array under fluoroscopic guidance. A basal turn drill-out allowed full insertion of all 11 electrodes of the lower array. Seven of the 11 available

At the time of initial implantation, the cochleostomy was performed anterior to a common window depression. There was no egress of CSF during cochleostomy. Seventeen electrode bands passed easily. With the introduction of three additional electrode bands, a copious egress of CSF was encountered. This could not be controlled with packing the cochleostomy alone, and the patient was managed with a course of continuous lumbar spinal drainage. The CSF leak resolved without consequence.

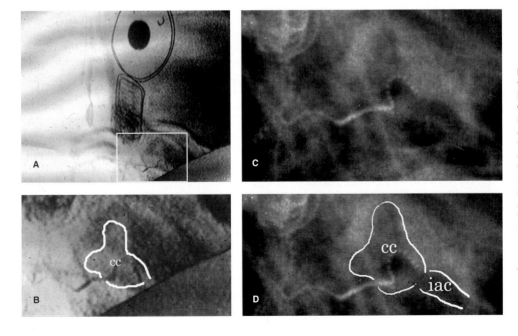

Figure 7–34 **(A)** Intraoperative fluoroscopy reveals the implant has been repositioned entirely within the common cavity. Inset (enlarged in **B**) displays outline of common cavity lumen (cc). Insertion was stopped at this point due to the visualization of cessation of advancement and kinking. **(C)** The postoperative plain film confirms proper placement. Arrows denote the cc–iac junction. **(D)** Detail reveals common cavity lumen (outline cc) and internal auditory canal (outline iac). (From Fishman AJ, Roland Jr JT, Alexiades G, Mierzwinski J, Cohen NL. Fluoroscopically assisted cochlear implantation. Otol Neurotol 2003;24(6):882–886, with permission of author.)

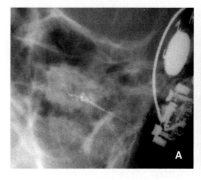 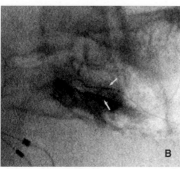

Figure 7–35 (A) Plain x-ray reveals kinked array and partial insertion in a patient with history meningitis. Patient was referred for reimplantation for a device failure. **(B)** Intraoperative fluoroscopy was utilized to confirm proper placement during revision surgery of same patient. A Nucleus 24 Double Array was utilized. Arrows denote the upper and lower electrode arrays in proper position without kinking or bending. (From Fishman AJ, Roland Jr JT, Alexiades G, Mierzwinski J, Cohen NL. Fluoroscopically assisted cochlear implantation. Otol Neurotol 2003;24(6):882–886, with permission of author.)

upper electrodes were inserted through the apical cochleostomy. **Fig. 7–35B** demonstrates the split array in good position, without kinks or bends as visualized fluoroscopically. Seventeen electrodes are active in the program map.

Case 4

An 11-year-old girl with deafness secondary to meningitis was originally implanted at another center with a Nucleus CI22 at age 4 with four intracochlear electrodes. The patient was receiving some benefit from the device until 5 years postoperatively, when the device failed electronically. At revision surgery a CI24 Double Array was placed under fluoroscopic guidance. An 8-mm basal turn drill-out was performed with insertion of 10 lower electrodes and five upper electrodes through an apical cochleostomy. She currently uses 13 electrodes in the program map.

Use of Imaging for Evaluation and Pre-, Intra-, and Postoperatively

Imaging plays an essential role in evaluating the cochlear implant candidate, intraoperative monitoring, postoperative examination, as well as in research and experimental studies. Currently CT and MRI technology are routinely used in preoperative radiologic examination for the cochlear implant patient. For intraoperative and postoperative evaluation of implanted electrodes, plain film radiography is regarded as being the simplest, least expensive, and most reliable modality.[105,125,127] To improve the accuracy of these techniques some enhancement methods have been developed.[105,128,129] However, none of these allow visualization of electrode insertion in real time during surgery.

In routine cases of normal anatomy and luminal patency, proper insertion can usually be ascertained by visual inspection of cochleostomy position and proprioception at the time of insertion. In these cases an intraoperative postinsertion plain film radiograph is sufficient to confirm the ultimate electrode position.

Fluoroscopic assistance is utilized when the intracochlear behavior of the electrode array cannot be predicted. New electrode prototypes have been routinely studied in both cadaver and animal models so that their safety and reliability may be assessed.[123,124] We utilized fluoroscopic assistance during the Nucleus Contour preclinical trials to monitor the electrode behavior in the live human cochleae.

In the case of severely malformed inner ears, there is an increased chance of complications such as extracochlear array placement, intrameatal array insertion, or kinking or bending of the electrodes.[21,25] Histologic evaluation of severe cochlear deformities reveals scattered malformed neuroepithelial elements with adjacent neuronal elements along the outer wall of the common cavity.[129] Insertional trauma to these delicate structures can be minimized by avoiding the application of pressure to the electrode after significant resistance to advancement occurs. Insertion end-point determination can be precisely defined using fluoroscopy, thereby avoiding both electrode and structural damage. Pushing more electrodes into a common cavity is not necessarily better if excessive damage will occur to the outer wall of the cavity. We currently implant a straight array with concentric bands so that outer wall electrode contact may be achieved in these small spherical and ovoid cavities.

The other group of difficult insertions includes cases of severe intraluminal obstruction, which may require a drill-out procedure or double array insertion.[50] With the aid of intraoperative fluoroscopy, the entire electrode array can be continually visualized so that bending and kinking can be avoided.

For electrode placement imaging, fluoroscopy has been reported by Yang et al[130] in laboratory study and by Lawson et al[131] in postoperative electrode evaluation with good results. Now, direct observation of the electrode behavior in real time during live surgery has been reported as well.[132] Recorded on video, these implantations have been reviewed and have helped to localize intracochlear positions where smooth array excursion may be most likely to be compromised even in normal inner ears. In combination with fluoroscopically assisted cadaver implantation, these live recordings have provided an important contribution for the design of both the current and future implants.

Summary

In summary, intraoperative fluoroscopy is a useful adjunct to cochlear implantation that can be performed with minimum risk to the patient and operating room staff if the above-mentioned precautions are taken. Intraoperative fluoroscopy is indicated in cases where the intracochlear behavior of the electrode array cannot be predicted, a condition encountered when implanting new electrode designs; in cases with severely malformed inner ears; or in cases of severe intra-luminal obstruction requiring a double array insertion. We currently implant a straight array with concentric bands so that outer wall electrode contact may be achieved in these small spherical or ovoid cavities.

◆ Conclusion

Preoperative imaging, appropriately selected and performed, provides useful information for the cochlear implant candidacy evaluation and surgical procedure, and assists in the avoidance of abnormal electrode placement and complications. Both high-resolution CT scan and MRI with the proper sequencing are important and useful modalities and are often complementary. Intraoperative imaging, including plain film radiographs and real-time fluoroscopic guidance, provides very useful information that can maximize the outcome in cochlear implantation, especially when implanting the malformed or obstructed cochlea. Additionally, the intraoperative radiograph serves as a baseline to which any future images can be compared. The cochlear implant professional must consider the principles outlined in this chapter to provide the benefits of cochlear implantation.

References

1. Abrams HL. Cochlear implants are a contraindication to MRI. Letter to the editor. JAMA 1989;261:46
2. Jensen J. Malformations of the inner ear in deaf children. Acta Radiol Diagn (Stockh) 1968;286:1–97
3. Jackler RK, Luxford WM, House WF. Congenital malformations of the inner ear: a classification based on embryogenesis. Laryngoscope 1987;97(suppl 40):2–14
4. Schuknecht HF, Gulya AJ. Anatomy of the Temporal Bone with Surgical Implications. Philadelphia: Lea & Febiger, 1986
5. Mondini C. Minor works of Carlo Mondini: the anatomical section of a boy born deaf. Am J Otol 1997;18:288–293
6. Swartz JD, Harnsberger HR. Imaging of the Temporal Bone, 2nd ed. New York: Thieme, 1992
7. Schuknecht HF. Mondini dysplasia: a clinical and pathological study. Ann Otol Rhinol Laryngol Suppl 1980;89(1 pt 2):1–23
8. Phelps PD. Cochlear dysplasias and meningitis. Am J Otol 1994;15:551–557
9. Shelton C, Luxford WM, Tonokawa LL, Lo WW, House WF. The narrow internal auditory canal in children: a contraindication to cochlear implants. Otolaryngol Head Neck Surg 1989;100: 227–231
10. Phelps PD. Cochlear implants for congenital deformities. J Laryngol Otol 1992;106:967–970
11. Phelps PD, Lloyd GAS, Sheldon PW. Deformity of the labyrinth and internal auditory meatus in congenital deafness. Br J Radiol 1975;48:973–978
12. Naunton RF, Valvassori GE. Inner ear anomalies: their association with atresia. Laryngoscope 1968;78:1041–1049
13. Lo WM. Imaging of cochlear and auditory brain stem implantation. AJNR Am J Neuroradiol 1998;19:1147–1154
14. Phelps PD, Reardon W, Pembry ME, Bellman S, Luxon L. X-linked deafness, stapes gushers and a distinctive defect of the inner ear. Neuroradiology 1991;33:326–330
15. Reardon W, Middelton-Price HR, Sandkuijl L, et al. A multipedigree linkage study of X-linked deafness: linkage to Xq13-q12 and evidence for genetic heterogeneity. Genomics 1991;11:885–894
16. Casselman JW, Kuhweide R, Deimling M, Ampe W, Dehaene I, Meeus L. Constructive interference in steady state-3DFT MR imaging of the inner ear and cerebellopontine angle. AJNR Am J Neuroradiol 1993;14:47–57
17. Casselman JW, Kuhweide R, Ampe W, Meeus L, Steyaert L. Pathology of the membranous labyrinth: comparison of T1 and T2-weighted and gadolinium-enhanced spin-echo and 3DFT-CISS imaging. AJNR Am J Neuroradiol 1993;14:59–69
18. Molter DW, Pate BR, McElveen JT. Cochlear implantation in the congenitally malformed ear. Otolaryngol Head Neck Surg 1993;108:174–177
19. Jackler RK, Luxford WM, House WF. Sound detection with the cochlear implant in five ears of four children with congenital malformations of the cochlea. Laryngoscope 1987;97(suppl 40):2–14
20. Silverstein H, Smouha E, Morgan N. Multichannel cochlear implantation in a patient with bilateral Mondini deformities. Am J Otol 1988;9:451–455
21. Tucci DL, Telian SA, Zimmerman-Philips MS, Zwolen TA, Ceylon PR. Cochlear implantation in patients with cochlear malformations. Arch Otolaryngol Head Neck Surg 1995;121:833–838
22. Slattery WH III, Luxford WM. Cochlear implantation in the congenital malformed cochlea. Laryngoscope 1995;105:1184–1187
23. Woolley AL, Jenison V, Stroer BS, Lusk RP, Bahadori RS, Wippold FJ II. Cochlear implantation in children with inner ear malformations. Ann Otol Rhinol Laryngol 1998;107:492–500
24. Weber BP, Lenarz T, Dillo W, Manke I, Bertran B. Malformations in cochlear implant patients. Am J Otol 1997;18:S64–S65
25. Hoffman RA, Downey LL, Waltzman SB, Cohen NL. Cochlear implantation in children with cochlear malformations. Am J Otol 1997;18:184–187
26. Kotzias SA, Linthicum FH. Labyrinthine ossification: differences between two types of ectopic bone. Am J Otol 1985;6:490–494
27. Suga F, Lindsay JR. Labyrinthitis ossificans. Ann Otol Rhinol Laryngol 1977;86:17–29
28. Rarey KE, Bicknell JM, Davis LE. Intralabyrinthine osteogenesis in Cogan's syndrome. Am J Otolaryngol 1986;7:387–390
29. Green JD Jr, Marion MS, Hinojosa R. Labyrinthitis ossificans: histo-pathologic considerations for cochlear implantation. Otolaryngol Head Neck Surg 1991;104:320–326
30. Becker TS, Eisenberg LS, Luxford WM, House WF. Labyrinthine ossification secondary to childhood bacterial meningitis: Implications for cochlear implant surgery. AJNR Am J Neuroradiol 1984;5:739–741
31. Johnson MH, Hasenstab MS, Seicshnaydre MA, Williams GH. CT of postmeningitic deafness: observations and predictive value for cochlear implants in children. AJNR Am J Neuroradiol 1995;16:103–109
32. Kaplan SL, Catlin FL, Weaver T, Feigin RD. Onset of hearing loss in children with bacterial meningitis. Pediatrics 1984;73:575–578
33. Silberman B, Garabedian EN, Denoyelle F, Moatti L, Roger G. Role of modern imaging technology in the implementation of pediatric cochlear implants. Ann Otol Rhinol Laryngol 1995;104:42–46
34. Dodge PR, Davis H, Feigin RD, et al. Prospective evaluation of hearing impairment as a sequela of acute bacterial meningitis. N Engl J Med 1984;311:869–874
35. Berlow SJ, Calderelli DD, Matz FJ, Meyer DH, Harsch GG. Bacterial meningitis and sensorineural hearing loss: a prospective investigation. Laryngoscope 1980;90:1445–1452
36. Seidman DA, Chute PM, Parisier S. Temporal bone imaging for cochlear implantation. Laryngoscope 1994;104:562–565
37. Balkany T, Gantz B, Nadol JB Jr. Multichannel cochlear implants in partially ossified cochleas. Ann Otol Rhinol Laryngol Suppl 1988;135:3–7
38. Harnsberger HR, Dart DJ, Parkin JL, Smoker WR, Osborn AG. Cochlear implant candidates: assessment with CT and MR imaging. Radiology 1987;164:53–57
39. Luxford WM, House WF. House 3M cochlear implant: surgical considerations. International Cochlear Implant Symposium and Workshop, Melbourne, 1985, Clark GM, Busby PA, eds. Ann Otol Rhinol Laryngol 1987;96(suppl 128):12–14
40. Schuknecht HF. Pathophysiology. In: Schuknecht HF, ed. Pathology of the Ear, 2nd ed. Philadelphia: Lea & Febiger, 1993:77–113

41. Igarashi M, Shuknecht HF. Pneumococcic otitis media, meningitis and labyrinthitis. Arch Otolaryngol 1962;76:126–130

42. Igarashi M, Saito R, Alford BR, Filippone MV, Smith JA. Temporal bone findings in pneumococcal meningitis. Arch Otolaryngol 1974;99:79–83

43. Balkany T, Dreisbach J, Cohen N, Martinez S, Valvassori G. Workshop: surgical anatomy and radiologic imaging of cochlear implant surgery. Am J Otol 1987;8:195–200

44. Ketten D. The role of temporal bone imaging in cochlear implants. Curr Opin Otolaryngol Head Neck Surg 1994;2:401–408

45. Otte J, Shucknecht HF, Kerr AG. Ganglion cell populations in normal and pathological human cochlea. Implications for cochlear implantation. Laryngoscope 1978;88:1231–1245

46. Saunders M, Fortnum HM, O'Donoghue GM, Gibbon KP. Retrospective analysis of children profoundly deafened by bacterial meningitis [abstract No. 34]. In: Lutman ME, Archbold SM, O'Donaghue GM, eds. First European Symposium on Paediatric Cochlear Implantation. Nottingham, England: Nottingham Paediatric Implant Programme, 1992

47. Hinojosa R, Green JD Jr, Marion MS. Ganglion cell populations in labyrinthitis ossificans. Am J Otol 1991(suppl);12:3–7, 18–21

48. Schuknecht HF. Anatomy. In: Schuknecht HF, ed. Pathology of the Ear, 2nd ed. Philadelphia: Lea & Febiger, 1993:31–75

49. Linthicum FH Jr, Fayad J, Otto S, et al. Inner ear morphologic changes resulting from cochlear implantation. Am J Otol 1991;12(suppl):8–10

50. Balkany T, Gantz BJ, Steenerson RL, Cohen NL. Systematic approach to electrode insertion in the ossified cochlea. Otolaryngol Head Neck Surg 1996;114:4–11

51. Druss JG. Labyrinthitis secondary to meningococcic meningitis: a clinical and histopathologic study. Arch Otolaryngol 1936;24:19–28

52. Sugiura S, Paparella MM. The pathology of labyrinthine ossification. Laryngoscope 1967;77:1974–1989

53. Novak MA, Fifer RC, Barkmeier JC, Firszt JB. Labyrinthine ossification after meningitis: its implications for cochlear implantation. Otolaryngol Head Neck Surg 1990;103:351–356

54. Paparella MM, Sugiura S. The pathology of suppurative labyrinthitis. Ann Otol Rhinol Laryngol 1967;76:554–586

55. Kimura R, Perlman HB. Arterial obstruction of the labyrinth. Part I: Cochlear changes. Part II: Vestibular changes. Ann Otol Rhinol Laryngol 1958;67:5–40

56. Belal A. Pathology as it relates to ear surgery. III: Surgery of the cerebello-pontine angle tumors. J Laryngol Otol 1983;97:101–115

57. Belal A, Ylikoski J. Pathology as it relates to ear surgery. II: Labyrinthectomy. J Laryngol Otol 1983;97:1–10

58. Belal A, Linthicum FH Jr, House WF. Middle fossa vestibular nerve section. A histopathological report. Am J Otol 1979;1:72–79

59. Belal A. The effects of vascular occlusion on the human inner ear. J Laryngol Otol 1979;93:955–968

60. Gorham LW, Test WT. Circulatory changes in osteolytic and osteoblastic reaction. Arch Pathol 1964;78:673–680

61. Harnsberger HR, Dart DJ, Parkin JL, Smoker WR, Osborn AG. Cochlear implant candidates: assessment with CT and MR imaging. Radiology 1987;164:53–57

62. Frau GN, Luxford WM, Lo WM, Berliner KI, Telishi FF. High resolution computed tomography in evaluation of cochlear patency in implant candidates: a comparison with surgical findings. J Laryngol Otol 1994;108:743–748

63. Jackler RK, Luxford WM, Schindler RA, McKerrow WS. Cochlear patency problems in cochlear implantation. Laryngoscope 1987;97:801–805

64. Seicshnaydre MA, Johnson MH, Hasenstab MS, Williams GH. Cochlear implants in children: reliability of computed tomography. Otolaryngol Head Neck Surg 1992;107:410–417

65. Langman AW, Quigley SM. Accuracy of high resolution computed tomography in cochlear implantation. Otolaryngol Head Neck Surg 1996;114:38–43

66. Laszig R, Terwey B, Battmer RD, Hesse G. Magnetic resonance imaging (MRI) and high resolution computer tomography (HRCT) in cochlear implant candidates. Scand Audiol Suppl 1988;30:197–200

67. Yune HY, Miyamoto RT, Yune ME. Medical imaging in cochlear implant candidates. Am J Otol 1991;12(suppl):11–17

68. Phelps PD. Fast spin echo MRI in otology. J Laryngol Otol 1994;108:383–394

69. Tomura N, Sashi R, Kobayashi M, et al. Normal variations of the temporal bone on high-resolution CT: their incidence and clinical significance. Clin Radiol 1995;50:144–148

70. Curtin HD, Vignaud J, Bar D. Anomaly of the facial canal in a Mondini malformation with recurrent meningitis. Radiology 1982;144:335–341

71. House JR III, Luxford WN. Facial nerve injury in cochlear implantation. Otolaryngol Head Neck Surg 1993;109:1078–1082

72. Kelsall DC, Shallop JK, Brammeier TG, Prenger EC. Facial nerve stimulation after Nucleus 22-channel cochlear implantation. Am J Otol 1997;18:336–341

73. Valvassori GE, Naunton RF, Lindsay JR. Inner ear anomalies: clinical and histopathological considerations. Ann Otol Rhinol Laryngol 1969;78:929–938

74. Phelps PD. Congenital lesions of the inner ear demonstrated by polytomography. Arch Otolaryngol 1974;100:11–18

75. Jackler RK, Hwang PH. Enlargement of the cochlear aqueduct: fact of fiction? Otolaryngol Head Neck Surg 1993;109:14–25

76. Mukherji SK, Baggett HC, Alley J, Carrasco VH. Enlarged cochlear aqueduct. AJNR Am J Neuroradiol 1998;19:330–332

77. Anson BJ, Donaldson JA, Warpeha RL, Winch TR. Surgical anatomy of the endolymphatic sac and perilymphatic duct. Laryngo scope 1964;74:480–497

78. Palva T, Dammert K. Human cochlear aqueduct. Acta Otolaryngol 1969;suppl 246:1–58

79. Allen G. Fluid flow in the cochlear aqueduct and cochlear hydrodynamic considerations in perilymph fistula, stapes gusher, and secondary endolymphatic hydrops. Am J Otol 1987;8:319–322

80. Schuknecht HF, Reisser C. The morphologic basis for perilymphatic gushers and oozers. Adv Otorhinolaryngol 1988;39:1–12

81. Park TS, Hoffman HJ, Humphreys RP, Chuang SH. Spontaneous cerebrospinal fluid otorrhea in association with a congenital defect of the cochlear aqueduct and Mondini dysplasia. Neurosurgery 1982;11:356–362

82. Burton EM, Keith JW, Linden BE, Lazar RH. CSF fistula in a patient with Mondini deformity: demonstration by CT cisternography. AJNR Am J Neuroradiol 1990;11:205–207

83. Beal DD, Davey PR, Lindsay JR. Inner ear pathology of congenital deafness. Arch Otolaryngol 1967;85:134–142

84. Valvassori GE, Clemis JD. The large vestibular aqueduct syndrome. Laryngoscope 1978;88:723–728

85. Valvassori GE. The large vestibular aqueduct and associated anomalies of the inner ear. Otolaryngol Clin North Am 1983;16:95–101

86. Jackler RK, de la Cruz A. The large vestibular aqueduct syndrome. Laryngoscope 1989;99:1238–1243

87. Levenson MJ, Parisier SC, Jacobs M, Edelstein DR. The large vestibular aqueduct in children. Arch Otolaryngol. 1989;115:54–58

88. Hirsch BE, Weissman JL, Curtin HD, Kamerer DB. Magnetic resonance imaging of the large vestibular aqueduct. Arch Otolaryngol Head Neck Surg 1992;118:1124–1127

89. Dahlen RT, Harnsberger HR, Gray SD, et al. Overlapping thin-section fast spin-echo MR of the large vestibular aqueduct syndrome. AJNR Am J Neuroradiol 1997;18:67–75

90. Okamoto K, Ito J, Furusawa T, Sakai K, Tokiguchi S. Large vestibular aqueduct syndrome with high CT density and high MR signal intensity. AJNR Am J Neuroradiol 1997;18:482–484

91. Phelps PD, Mahoney CF, Luxon LM. Large endolymphatic sac. A congenital deformity of the inner ear shown by magnetic resonance imaging. J Laryngol Otol 1997;111:754–756

92. Okamoto K, Ito J, Furusawa T, Sakai K, Horikawa S, Tokiguchi S. MRI of enlarged endolymphatic sacs in the large vestibular aqueduct syndrome. Neuroradiology 1998;40:167–172

93. Welling DB, Martyn MD, Miles BA, Oehler M, Schmalbrock P. Endolymphatic sac occlusion for the enlarged vestibular aqueduct syndrome. Am J Otol 1998;19:145–151

94. Tong KA, Harnsberger HR, Dahlen RT, Carey JC, Ward K. Large vestibular aqueduct syndrome: a genetic disease? AJR Am J Roentgenol 1997;168:1097–1101

95. Antonelli PJ, Agnes NV, Lemmerling MM, Mancuso AA, Kublis PS. Hearing loss with cochlear modiolar defects and large vestibular aqueducts. Am J Otol 1998;19:306–312

96. Lemmerling MM, Mancuso AA, Antonelli PJ, Kublis PS. Normal modiolus: CT appearance in patients with a large vestibular aqueduct. Radiology 1997;204:213–219

97. Abe S, Usami S, Shinkawa H. Three familial cases of hearing loss associated with enlargement of the vestibular aqueduct. Ann Otol Rhinol Laryngol 1997;106:1063–1069

98. Phelps PD, Coffey RA, Trembath RC, et al. Radiological malformations of the ear in Pendred syndrome. Clin Radiol 1998;53:268–273

99. Wilson DF, Hodgson RS, Talbot JM. Endolymphatic sac obliteration for large vestibular aqueduct syndrome. Am J Otol 1997;18:101–106 discussion 106–7

100. Aschendorff A, Marangos N, Laszig R. Large vestibular aqueduct syndrome and its implication for cochlear implant surgery. Am J Otol 1997;18(6 suppl):S57

101. Mafee MF, Selis JE, Yannias DA, et al. Congenital sensorineural hearing loss. Radiology 1984;150:427–434

102. Stevenson DS, Proops DW, Phelps PD. Severe cochlear dysplasia causing recurrent meningitis: a surgical lesson. J Laryngol Otol 1993;107:726–729

103. Page EL, Eby TL. Meningitis after cochlear implantation in Mondini malformation. Otolaryngol Head Neck Surg 1997;116:104–106

104. Suzuki C, Sando I, Fagan JJ, Kamerer DB, Knisely AS. Histopathoogical features of a cochlear implant and otogenic meningitis in Mondini dysplasia. Arch Otolaryngol Head Neck Surg 1998;124:462–466

105. Shpizner BA, Holliday RA, Roland JT, Cohen NL, Waltzman SB, Shapiro WH. Postoperative imaging of the multichannel cochlear implant. AJNR Am J Neuroradiol 1995;16:1517–1524

106. Cohen LT, Xu J, Xu SA, Clark GM. Improved and simplified methods for specifying positions of the electrode bands of a cochlear implant array. Am J Otol 1996;17:859–865

107. Marsh MA, Jin XU, Blamey PJ, et al. Radiological evaluation of multiple-channel intracochlear implant insertion depth. Am J Otol 1993;14:386–391

108. Skinner MW, Ketten DR, Vannier MW, et al. Determination of the position of Nucleus cochlear implant insertion depth. Am J Otol 1994;15:644–651

109. Cohen NL, Kuzma J. Titanium clip for cochlear implant electrode fixation. Ann Otol Rhinol Laryngol Suppl 1995;166:402–403

110. Barone MA. The Harriet Lane Handbook. St. Louis: Mosby Publishers, 1996:272

111. Hamill PVV, Drizd TA, Johnson CL, et al. Physical growth: National Center for Health Statistic Percentiles. Am J Clin Nutr 1979;32:607–629

112. Roland JT Jr, Fishman AJ, Waltzman SB, Alexiades G, Hoffman RA, Cohen NL. Stability of the cochlear implant array in children. Laryngoscope 1998;108:1119–1123

113. Portnoy WM, Mattucci K. Cochlear implants as a contraindication to magnetic resonance imaging. Ann Otol Rhinol Laryngol 1991;100:195–197

114. NIH Consensus Conference. Cochlear implants in adults and children. JAMA 1995;274:1955–1961

115. Applebaum EL, Valvassori GE. Further studies on the effects of magnetic resonance imaging fields on middle ear implants. Ann Otol Rhinol Laryngol 1990;99:801–804

116. Heller JW, Brackman DE, Tucci DL, et al. Evaluation of MRI compatibility of the modified nucleus multichannel auditory brainstem and cochlear implants. Am J Otol 1996;17:724–729

117. Chou CK, McDougall JA, Chan KW. Absence of radiofrequency heating from auditory implants during magnetic resonance imaging. Bioelectromagnetics 1995;16:307–316

118. Weber BP, Goldring JE, Santogrossi T, et al. Magnetic resonance imaging compatibility testing of the Clarion 1.2 cochlear implant. Am J Otol 1998;19:584–590

119. Ouayoun M, Dupuch K, Aitbenamou C, Chouard CH. Resonance magnetique nucleaire et implant cochleaire. Ann Otolaryngol Chir Cervicofac 1997;114:65–70

120. Teissel C, Kremser C, Hochmair ES, Hochmair-Desoyer IJ. Magnetic resonance imaging compatibility of a cochlear implant. Presented at the Vth International Cochlear Implant Conference, May 1–3, 1997, New York

121. Baumgartner WD, Youssefzadeh S, Franz P, Gstoettner W. First results of magnetic resonance imaging in the Combi 40 cochlear implanted patients. Presented at the Vth International Cochlear Implant Conference, May 1–3, 1997, New York

122. Weber B, Neuberger J, Pillo W, et al. Clinical results of the Clarion magnetless cochlear implant. Presented at the Vth International Cochlear Implant Conference, New York, NY, May 1–3, 1997.

123. Roland JT Jr, Fishman AJ, Alexiades G, Cohen NL. Electrode to modiolus proximity: a fluoroscopic and histologic analysis. Am J Otol 2000;21:218–225

124. Roland JT Jr, Fishman AJ, Alexiades G, Cohen NL. Modiolar hugging cochlear implant electrodes. Presented at the Combined Otologic Society Meeting, Palm Springs, CA, Spring 1999

125. Fishman AJ, Roland JT Jr, Alexiades G, Waltzman SB, Shapiro WS, Cohen NL. Implantation of the Severely Malformed Cochlea. Presented at the American Otologic Society Annual Meeting, May 14, 2000, Orlando FL

126. Brown NP. The lens is more sensitive to radiation than we had believed. Br J Ophthalmol 1997;81:257

127. Rosenberg RA, Cohen NL, Reede DL. Radiographic imaging for the cochlear implant. Ann Otol Rhinol Laryngol 1987;96(3 pt 1):300–304

128. Xu J, Xu SA, Cohen LT, Clark GM. Cochlear view: postoperative radiography for cochlear implantation. Am J Otol 2000;21:49–56

129. Fishman AJ, Holliday RA. Principles of cochlear implant imaging. In: Waltzman SB, Cohen NL, eds. Cochlear Implants. New York: Thieme, 2000

130. Yang NW, Hodges AV, Balkany TJ. Novel intracochlear positioner: effects on electrode position. Ann Otol Rhinol Laryngol Suppl 2000;185:18–20

131. Lawson JT, Cranley K, Toner JG. Digital imaging: a valuable technique for the postoperative assessment of cochlear implantation. Eur Radiol 1998;8:951–954

132. Fishman AJ, Roland JT Jr, Alexiades G, Mierzwinski J, Cohen NL. Fluoroscopically assisted cochlear implantation. Otol Neurotol 2003;24:882–886

8

Electrophysiology and Device Telemetry

Paul J. Abbas,

Carolyn J. Brown, and

Christine P. Etler

The performance of individuals receiving cochlear implants has improved significantly over the course of the past two decades. This improvement is likely the result of several factors including advances in cochlear implant technology, changes in patient criteria (both age and degree of hearing loss), and advances in fitting procedures. However, despite these advances, the range of postimplant outcomes is still quite large. The variability in performance among cochlear implant users undoubtedly reflects several factors including the status of the auditory nerve and central auditory system, electrode placement, and the integrity of the implanted electronics. Although imaging techniques have improved significantly in the past decade and can be used to assess electrode placement, such techniques have not proven to be effective in determining neural survival, assessing device function, or predicting postimplant performance (Skinner et al, 2002; Wang et al, 1996, 2005). It is possible, however, to use the telemetry systems available with present-day cochlear implants to assess the function of the implanted components of the cochlear implant. Additionally, both the Nucleus (Cochlear Corporation; Sydney, Australia) and Advanced Bionics (Valencia, CA) devices have neural telemetry systems that allow the user to record the response of the auditory nerve to electrical stimulation. This chapter reviews the information about how both devices function as well as the status of the peripheral auditory nervous system that can be obtained using these telemetry systems. Specifically, this chapter discusses how telemetry systems can be used to assess device function, the specific methodology used to measure electrically evoked compound action potentials (ECAPs), and the application of these measures both in terms of direct clinical applications and as a research tool.

96

◆ Techniques to Assess Device Function

Cochlear implants are designed to last for the life of the recipient. Unfortunately, the internal components of the cochlear implant can and do fail. Consequently, clinicians need to assess and monitor the function of the implanted electronics on a regular basis. Today, all three of the major cochlear implant manufacturers (Cochlear Corporation; Advanced Bionics Corporation; and Med-El Corporation, Innsbruck, Austria) have incorporated telemetry systems that can be used to measure the impedance of the intracochlear electrodes. Additionally, surface electrodes and standard evoked potential recording techniques can be used to evaluate the function of the internal electronics for a range of different stimulation conditions. The following sections discuss the information about device function that can be obtained and how that information can be used in clinical practice.

Telemetry Systems

All of the cochlear implants that are available today have built-in telemetry systems that allow limited information about the function of the internal device to be assessed directly. In general, these telemetry systems work by sampling and digitizing the voltage generated on the internal electrodes during stimulation. This information is then transmitted back through the computer interface to the programming software. No external recording electrodes are needed and the stimulation levels used to assess device function are typically low enough that the patient does not hear the stimulus.

One of the most important applications for this technology is that it allows clinicians to measure the impedance of the intracochlear electrodes directly. It is not unusual to find that an individual patient has an electrode or two that are either shorted together or open. Most cochlear implant recipients either are unable to detect stimulation or experience very abnormal growth of loudness with increases in stimulation level when an open circuit electrode is stimulated. Consequently, these electrodes should not be used in these recipients' regular program for their speech processor. Stimulation of electrode pairs that are shorted together can result in an auditory percept. However, these electrodes also are generally programmed out because they can significantly distort the place-frequency relationship that is critical for speech coding.

It is possible, using the standard programming software, to measure the impedance of the implanted electrodes in the Nucleus, Advanced Bionics, and Med-El implants in a monopolar stimulation mode, that is, in each intracochlear electrode relative to an external reference. Monopolar impedance measures can be used to identify open circuit electrodes but do not allow identification of a malfunction where two intracochlear electrodes are shorted. To identify electrodes that are shorted to each other, either the impedance must be measured in a common ground stimulation mode, or testing must be conducted for all possible bipolar electrode pairs. The clinical programming software used with both the Nucleus and Med-El devices does flag short-circuited electrodes. Identifying shorts between intracochlear electrodes for the Advanced Bionics implant, however, requires access to specialized electrical field imaging (EFI) software that allows the user to sample the electrical field across the length of the cochlea during stimulation.

It is also possible to use the telemetry systems of the cochlear implant to assess whether or not compliance voltage has been reached. Every current source has some limitation in maximum output that is dependent, in part, on the impedance of the electrodes and, in part, on battery capacity. That maximum level is called the compliance voltage. In order for the cochlear implant user to have adequate loudness growth, it is important that all stimulation provided by the speech processor stays below this compliance voltage. The software used to program the Nucleus, Advanced Bionics, and Med-El speech processors includes flags that can alert the user that compliance voltage has been reached so appropriate adjustments in the stimulation parameters (e.g., increasing pulse duration) can be made for the individual patient.

Average Electrode Voltages

A second technique that can be used to assess function of the internal components of the cochlear implant is to use surface electrodes to record the voltages generated when one of the intracochlear electrodes is stimulated. These potentials have been referred to in the literature as averaged electrode voltages (AEVs). When the intracochlear electrodes are activated, the voltages associated with stimulation that are measured at the scalp are large and can be recorded relatively easily and quickly using standard evoked potential recording systems. These are not physiologic potentials; rather, they are far-field recordings of the stimulus artifact that accompanies stimulation.

AEVs can be measured with any of the available cochlear implant systems but have proven to be particularly useful with older implants, like the Nucleus CI22 device, where it is not possible to measure intracochlear electrode impedance directly. The primary clinical application for AEVs is to monitor device function in cochlear implant users (Heller et al, 1991; Kileny et al, 1995; Mens et al, 1994, 1995). Several investigators have published reports demonstrating how abnormal electrode impedance or function can be inferred from examination of AEV recordings (Kileny et al, 1995; Mahoney & Proctor, 1994; Mens et al, 1994). A recent study by Hughes et al (2004) demonstrated that AEVs recorded in response to stimulation in a common ground electrode configuration could consistently detect both open circuits and short circuits among electrodes. At a simple level, these results suggest that AEVs could serve as an efficient test of electrode integrity for implants without impedance telemetry systems.

It should be understood, however, that the morphology of the AEV recording is affected by more than simply the impedance of the stimulated electrode. The size and general shape of the recording that is made from surface electrodes is affected by many different factors including current level, mode of stimulation, spatial orientation of the stimulating and recording electrodes, the current path within the tissue, as well as changes in position and tissue growth over time. It is precisely because the AEV is a reflection of more than simply the electrode impedance that recording this potential may be useful even in patients who use implants that are equipped with impedance telemetry systems. Although electrode impedance may be normal for a given electrode, other factors, such as unusual tissue growth or electrode position, may influence the ability of an implant to effectively stimulate the neural population. Malfunction of the internal components of the device can also result in a broad range of percepts ranging from complete lack of stimulation to intermittent overstimulation or a subtle change in the level or quality of stimulation provided by the implant. Such failures may not be common but are certainly not insignificant. Two recent studies (Franck and Shah, 2004; Hughes et al, 2004) also demonstrated that abnormally functioning electrodes can be missed with clinical impedance measures, but correctly identified with AEVs. Such data suggest that in addition to monitoring electrode impedance using the standard telemetry systems available with the clinical software, baseline AEV measures should be obtained some time during the first few months following implantation. For pediatric patients or other cochlear implant recipients who may not be reliable reporters of changes in sound quality over time, it might be advisable to measure AEVs on a routine basis to monitor electrode function over time.

◆ Techniques to Assess the Response of the Auditory System

Over the course of the past several decades, several electrophysiologic tools have been developed and used with acoustic stimulation to assess the response of the auditory system at various levels of neural processing. These include the whole nerve action potential, the auditory brainstem response, middle and long latency responses, as well as more cognitively related brain potentials, such as the mismatch negativity (MMN) response and event-related cortical responses such as the P-300 response. Counterparts to each of these potentials have been recorded in response to electrical stimulation. Studies using the electrically evoked compound action potential (ECAP) (Brown et al, 1990), the electrically evoked auditory brainstem response, (EABR) (van den Honert & Stypulkowski, 1986), the electrically evoked middle latency response (EMLR) (Kileny & Kemink, 1987), MMN (Kraus et al, 1993), the N1-P2 complex (Sharma et al, 2002), and the P-300 (Kaga et al, 1991) have been reported. In addition, there have been several studies published describing techniques for using electrical stimulation to evoke the stapedius reflex (Battmer et al, 1990).

In general, all of these electrically evoked potentials have characteristics that are very similar to their acoustically evoked counterparts. On a global level this suggests that the basic organization of the auditory system in implant users is intact. Electrical stimulation, however, bypasses the normal cochlear processes including the compressive effects of the basilar membrane mechanics and the hair cell and synaptic process. The resulting excitation of the auditory nerve is known to have shorter latency, greater synchrony, and steeper response growth in response to electrical stimulation as compared with acoustic stimulation (Kiang & Moxon, 1972). The characteristics of evoked potentials measured with implant patients reflect these differences in the mode of stimulation. Response latencies of early potentials (ECAP and EABR) tend to be shorter, response amplitudes tend to be greater, and the growth of response with the level tends to be faster than is observed with acoustic stimulation (Brown et al, 1990; van den Honert & Stypulkowski, 1986).

Initially, most of the research that was published exploring ways in which electrophysiologic techniques could be adapted for use with patients with cochlear implants focused on the EABR and the EMLR. Recording either of these potentials requires the application of surface recording electrodes, the use of sophisticated recording instrumentation, and a quiet subject. Although several investigators described clinical applications for these electrically evoked responses, many clinical settings did not routinely record these responses because of these practical limitations. In the mid-1990s, Cochlear Corporation introduced a telemetry system that allows the user to record a response from the auditory nerve by using one of the electrodes in the intracochlear array. The telemetry system used to record the response of the auditory nerve that was introduced with the Nucleus 24M and 24R implants has been termed neural response telemetry (NRT). A similar system was later introduced by Advanced Bionics Corporation with the Clarion CII and HiResolution 90k implants and is referred to as neural response imaging (NRI). Although the current generation of Med-El cochlear implants (the Combi 40+) are not equipped with neural response telemetry systems, the next generation Med-El implant (the PULSARci) will have a comparable recording system that they refer to as auditory nerve response telemetry (ART). All of these telemetry systems include software to control the stimulation and recording parameters as well as methods for averaging, filtering, and analyzing the recorded waveforms. The response that is recorded by each of these systems has been called the electrically evoked compound action potential (ECAP or EAP) and compared with the electrically evoked auditory responses recorded previously (the EABR or EMLR), the ECAP is a very peripheral measure of the response of the auditory system to electrical stimulation.

It is often difficult and time-consuming to program the speech processor for very young cochlear implant recipients, and it is for these patients in particular that having the ability to measure the response of the auditory nerve to electrical stimulation has proven useful. There are several reasons that this response has gained popularity during the past decade. First, recording the response does not require the application of external recording electrodes. Also, because the internal electrodes are placed close to the neural elements (in contrast to surface electrodes), the amplitude of the response is relatively large compared with other biologic activity, such as that originating in superficial muscle. As a result, subjects can move around without negatively affecting the quality of the recording. It is not necessary for the child to sleep during the recording procedure. Finally, because of this favorable signal-to-noise ratio, fewer sweeps are needed per average and data collection time is reduced considerably relative to that typically required to record the EABR.

It is largely because of these advantages that there has been a great increase in experimental studies related to ECAP measures made through telemetry systems, and those studies are the focus of the rest of this chapter. Although we are convinced that the ECAP can prove to be a powerful tool in the management of patients with cochlear implants, we also recognize that that there are several very important issues that *cannot* be addressed with the ECAP. For example, there are changes that are known to take place in the central nervous system as a result of peripheral hearing loss (Miller et al, 1996) and as the result of subsequent electrical stimulation. The ECAP is a measure of the response of the auditory nerve and as such clearly is not sensitive to changes in structures central to the auditory nerve. Studies involving both EABR and late potentials (Gordon et al, 2003; Ponton and Eggermont, 2001; Sharma et al, 2002) have demonstrated plastic changes in the central auditory system in young children receiving cochlear implants. Such measures show considerable promise in characterizing the ability of the central auditory system to adapt to a relatively novel input provided by the cochlear implant. Degenerative changes in structures central to the auditory nerve are likely to affect the amplitude, sensitivity, tuning, and temporal response properties of the auditory system to electrical stimulation. The EABR and/or other more centrally evoked auditory potentials could potentially be used as comparative measures to assess such affects. Because the ECAP and EABR are related and share many of the same properties, the following sections describe experimental methods that can be used to record these responses and provide the reader with an overview of their potential clinical applications. This chapter does not discuss how electrically evoked potentials might be used to assess higher level processes such as learning, adaptation, and cortical plasticity.

◆ Experimental Methods

Electrically Evoked Auditory Brainstem Response

The EABR is typically recorded by stimulating the auditory nerve with a series of pulses applied to a single electrode at a relatively slow rate (i.e., under 50 Hz). The response of the auditory system to this electrical stimulation is then recorded using a differential amplifier and standard averaging techniques. Stimulation is typically achieved using software that is provided by the manufacturer. This software allows for discrete stimulation of individual electrodes with single pulses or trains of pulses and provides an external trigger pulse that can be used to initiate sampling on a separate evoked potential system. Any one of several commercially available evoked potential recording systems that has the capability of being externally triggered can be used to record the EABR. Because stimulus artifact can be problematic, radiofrequency (RF) shielding at the electrode interface and contralateral rather than ipsilateral recording electrode montages are typically used. Despite the use of both RF shielding and a contralateral recording electrode montage, the stimulus artifact associated with the electrical stimulus provided by the cochlear implant can be large enough to saturate the recording amplifier and significantly distort the recordings that are made. Generally, this problem can be managed by using very short duration pulsatile stimuli, by decreasing the gain in the recording amplifier, by increasing the width of the analog filter pass-band that is used to record the EABR (e.g., using 1–3000 Hz rather than 100–3000 Hz), or by alternating the polarity of stimulation in the recording. Some investigators have also used blanking circuits to minimize the effects of stimulus artifact on the EABR (Black et al, 1983). Finding a way to successfully manage stimulus artifact is the key to recording EABRs successfully, and most of the major implant companies and evoked potential manufacturers can provide information to the clinician about how to achieve this goal.

Electrically Evoked Compound Action Potential

The first direct recordings of the ECAP in humans were made in Ineraid cochlear implant users (Brown et al, 1990). With the Ineraid cochlear implant system (Symbion Inc., Utah), all of the implanted electrodes were accessible via a percutaneous plug that could be directly connected to external stimulation and recording equipment (with appropriate ground isolation). The relative simplicity of this design allowed us to experiment with techniques for using one of the intracochlear electrodes to record a response directly from the auditory nerve. Although the proximity of the recording electrode to the auditory nerve was advantageous, the use of an intracochlear electrode to record the ECAP also results in extremely large stimulus artifact recordings. Typically, the electrical stimulus artifact that is recorded from an intracochlear electrode is several orders of magnitude larger than the associated neural response. Additionally, the relatively short latency of the ECAP also made separation of the stimulus artifact from the neural response problematic. Most investigators have used either a two-pulse subtraction technique (Brown et al, 1990) or a polarity alternation technique (Wilson et al, 1997) to reduce the effects of stimulus artifact. Additionally, use of low gain, fast sampling rates (50–100 kHz) and good sampling resolution ($\geq$16 bits) allowed for minimization of stimulus artifact and amplifier saturation effects.

Although much was learned about how to record the ECAP from Ineraid cochlear implant users, the development of telemetry systems such as NRT for the Nucleus implant and NRI for Advanced Bionic implants has provided the means to record the ECAP in patients with cochlear implants that used transcutaneous transmission. With these systems, special software is used to control both stimulation and recording parameters. A stimulus pulse or series of pulses is applied to a specific intracochlear electrode, and the voltages on a nearby electrode are measured for a period of time following the presentation of that stimulus pulse. These voltages are then transmitted to an external receiver through the reverse telemetry system. The neural response telemetry system that was first introduced by Cochlear Corporation in 1995 was not perfect. In fact, it has several important limitations, many of which are directly related to how the recording amplifier responds to large levels of stimulus artifact. We have developed a procedure for adjusting stimulus parameters to minimize the effects of these complications and to assist with recording of responses that are not excessively contaminated by artifact (Abbas et al, 1999). Many of these same techniques for minimizing the impact of excessive stimulus artifact are also useful when the NRI system is used to record the ECAP from Advanced Bionics cochlear implant recipients.

Fig. 8–1 shows examples of the ECAP waveforms that can be recorded using the NRI software. These recordings were obtained from the same individual using the same stimulation levels. The waveforms on the left were obtained using a subtraction procedure to minimize stimulus artifact contamination. The subtraction method takes advantage of neural refractory properties to extract a template of the artifact with no response (masker + probe), which can then be subtracted from the recorded response to the probe alone. Details regarding how this technique works have been published previously (Abbas et al, 1999). The waveforms on the right were collected using alternating polarity stimuli. With both methods, there is some residual stimulus artifact that is followed by a negative peak (N1) and, in many cases, a positive peak (P2). As illustrated in this example, our experience with both telemetry systems has been that the subtraction method is more reliable in reducing stimulus artifact and has typically been our method of choice.

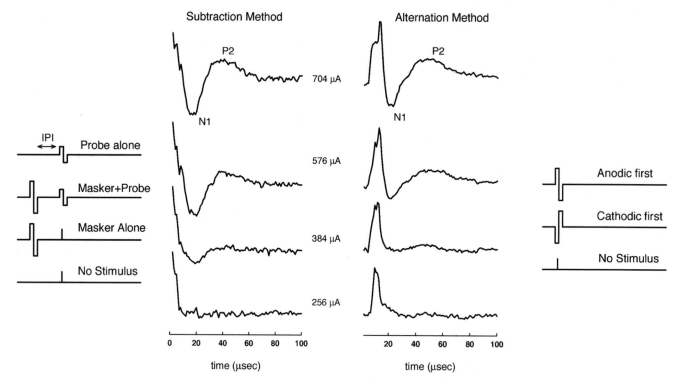

Figure 8–1 Schematic of stimulus paradigms used to measure evoked compound action potential (ECAP) responses and examples of response waveforms at several stimulus levels recorded from an Advanced Bionics CII implant user. Left column illustrates the stimuli used for the "subtraction" method. The second column illustrates resulting responses at four stimulus levels. The typical response morphology of a negative peak followed by a positive peak is indicated by N1, P2 labels. The fourth and third columns illustrate the stimulus used for the "alternation" method of reducing stimulus artifact, and shows examples of responses from the same individual at the same stimulus using the alternation method.

The waveforms illustrated in **Fig. 8–1** show responses to four levels of probe. Unlike acoustically evoked auditory potentials, electrically evoked responses change very little in latency as stimulus level is changed. Consequently response amplitude (measured between the negative trough and the following positive peak) rather than latency is commonly used to quantify the response. To measure an ECAP growth function using the subtraction method,

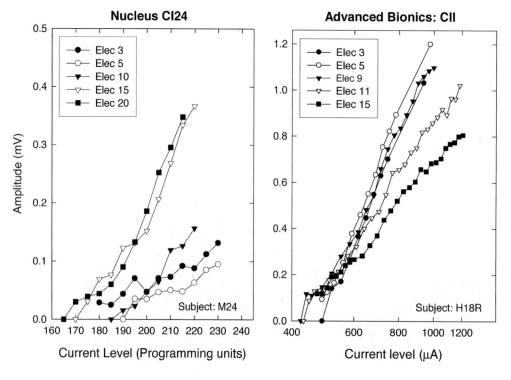

Figure 8–2 Amplitude of the ECAP (P2–N1) is plotted as a function of stimulus level. Measurements from a Nucleus CI24 implant user are plotted at left and those from an Advanced Bionics CII user are plotted at the right. In each case responses to stimulation of five different electrodes are shown as indicated in the key (*top*). Stimulus level for Nucleus implant is indicated in clinical programming units. The abscissa for the Advanced Bionics implant is shown in current level on a logarithmic scale.

the interpulse interval (IPI) is fixed (typically at 500 μs), the masker pulse is fixed at a relatively high level [near the uncomfortable loudness level (UCL)], and the level of the probe is varied. A high-level masker pulse is used because the sole purpose of the masker is to put all of the neurons that may respond to the probe into a refractory state. Probe levels are then chosen that do not exceed the level of the masker. Although we cannot be certain that all of the stimulable fibers are refractory at the time the probe is presented, we would argue that the best way to ensure this is true is to use of the highest level of masker possible. Alternatively, the level of the masker pulse can be varied, keeping it at a fixed level relative to the level of the probe (typically 5 to 10 current units above the probe). Comparisons of growth functions using the two methods have yielded no significant differences (Hughes et al, 2001).

Fig. 8–2 shows examples of ECAP growth functions. The panel on the left shows data recorded using the Nucleus NRT system. The panel on the right shows data obtained using the NRI system available with the Advanced Bionics device. One important difference between these two systems is that the stimulation levels used to control output of the implant are roughly proportional to current for the Advanced Bionics device but are logarithmically related to current in the Nucleus device. In **Fig. 8–2**, a logarithmic scale is on the abscissa for data obtained from the Advanced Bionics device, whereas a linear scale is used to show results obtained using the Nucleus device. In general, ECAP growth functions recorded from the two implant types are similar and tend to show little evidence of saturation as stimulus amplitude is increased. For both implant types we have observed differences across subjects and across electrodes within a subject not only in sensitivity (threshold), but also in the rate of growth in response amplitude with increases in stimulus level (i.e., slope).

◆ Application of Electrophysiological Measures to Device Programming

Using Electrically Evoked Compared Action Potential Thresholds to Predict Programming Levels

Implanting children 12 months of age or younger not only presents problems in candidate identification but also in postoperative, speech processor programming. For very young cochlear implant recipients, simply establishing threshold and upper levels of stimulation can be a difficult task. Because electrophysiologic measures of auditory function do not require behavioral responses from the subject, these measures have the potential to be particularly useful in the clinical management of pediatric cochlear implant recipients. Central to this issue is the extent to which electrophysiologic thresholds correlate with behavioral threshold measures.

In general, when the stimuli used for both physiologic and behavioral measures are similar, the correlation between the two measures of threshold has been shown to be strong. This finding applies to both acoustically evoked responses as well as to their electrical counterparts, the ECAP and the EABR (Abbas & Brown, 1991; Brown et al, 1994; Coats & Martin, 1977; Gorga et al, 1985; Hodges et al, 1994; Miller et al, 1995; Shallop et al, 1991; Smith et al, 1994). Typically, however, the stimuli used to measure ECAP or EABR thresholds are very different from the stimuli used to program the speech processor. Pulse trains at rates of 30 to 80 Hz are generally used to measure the ECAP and EABR thresholds. Pulse trains of 250 Hz or greater are generally used to program the speech processor. Because behavioral measures of threshold and maximum comfort reflect temporal integration whereas ECAP or EABR thresholds do not, it is not surprising that the correlation between ECAP and EABR thresholds and behavioral programming levels to be only moderate and to include significant cross-subject variability (Brown et al, 1994, 2000; Chen et al, 2002; Cullington, 2000; DiNardo et al, 2003; Gordon et al 2002; Hughes et al, 2000; Mason et al, 1993, 2001; Shallop et al, 1990, 1991; Thai-Van et al, 2001). **Fig. 8–3** shows examples of our data obtained from both subjects who use the Nucleus cochlear implant as well as those who use the Advanced Bionics device. Scatter plots of threshold levels used in speech processor programming versus ECAP threshold demonstrate that ECAP thresholds are consistently higher than behavioral thresholds but that, for these particular stimuli, the correlation is relatively weak. That variability is due, at least in part, to differences in temporal integration among cochlear implant users (Brown et al, 1999).

Much of the literature that has been published to date comparing ECAP thresholds with programming levels has shown cross-subject correlations such as those shown in **Fig. 8–3**. These studies have shown that while there can be large differences between behavioral and electrophysiologic thresholds, the ECAP threshold is generally recorded within the implant users' electrical dynamic range and in many cases the pattern or "profile" of ECAP across electrodes within an individual subject can be similar to the profile of programming T-level, M-level, or C-levels across electrodes. The plots in column A of **Fig. 8–4** illustrate this trend for two individual Nucleus implant users. In one case the ECAP thresholds lie approximately halfway between the T and C levels; in the other case the ECAP thresholds approximate the C level but in both cases, the general shape of the ECAP profile matches that of the "MAP" used in programming the speech processor. This trend has led several investigators to propose combining NRT/NRI/EABR thresholds with a limited amount of behavioral data to predict speech processor programming levels (Brown et al, 2000; Franck and Norton, 2001; Hughes et al, 2000; Smoorenburg et al, 2002). Although the techniques suggested by each group differ somewhat, they were all able to show improved correlations between ECAP thresholds and MAP C- or T-levels by adjusting threshold levels using either a behavioral threshold on a particular electrode or a detection threshold for speech stimuli presented through the processor.

The procedure recommended for programming the Advanced Bionics CII and HiResolution 90k implants in the high-resolution mode is somewhat different from that used

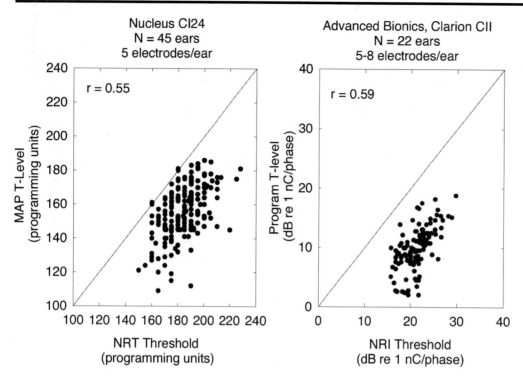

Figure 8–3 Scatter plots show the relationship between the behavioral determined T-level used for programming the implant and ECAP threshold. Data from a group of Nucleus CI24 implant users are plotted at left; data from Advanced Bionics CII implant users are shown at right.

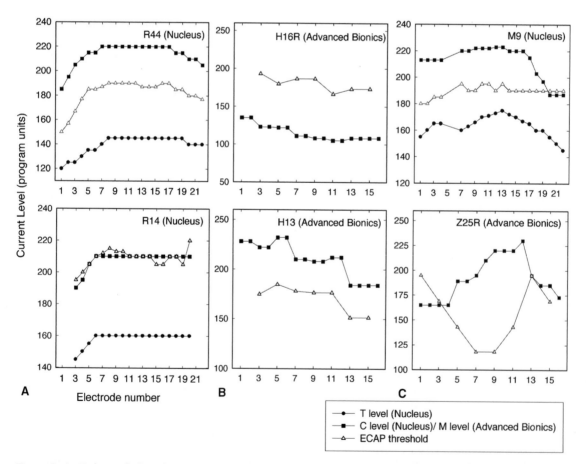

Figure 8–4 Each panel plots the programming levels determined behaviorally as well as ECAP thresholds as a function of electrode number (position) for an individual subject. Data from six subjects are illustrated with the type of implant indicated in each panel. For the Advance Bionics implant, the behavioral M-levels are plotted; for the Nucleus implant users, both T and C levels are plotted (see text).

with the Nucleus implant. That procedure requires determining a most comfortable level (M level) for the electrodes, typically at a relatively high pulse rate. Measures of threshold are not used to program the processor. The two plots shown in column B of **Fig. 8–4** were obtained from subjects who used the Advanced Bionics CII device. In these subjects, ECAP thresholds can be used with reasonable accuracy to estimate the program profile. However, as we have previously observed with the Nucleus implant, the absolute level at which the ECAP falls relative to M-level can vary greatly across individuals. In one subject (H16R), ECAP thresholds significantly exceeded the M-levels. In the other subject (H13), ECAP thresholds were recorded well below the M-levels.

Despite these positive results there are clear limitations in using ECAP measures to program implant speech processors. The two plots in column C of **Fig. 8–4** illustrate cases where the profile of ECAP thresholds across electrodes does not correspond with the behaviorally determined T-, M- or C-levels. We recently conducted a study in Nucleus implant users where we applied the combined ECAP and behavioral threshold method of predicting the T- and C-levels (Brown et al, 2000) to a large group of adult Nucleus 24 implant users. That method calls for using the behavioral threshold on one electrode (electrode 10) to adjust the ECAP threshold profile up or down to match the T- and C-levels. We used these predictions in comparison with behavioral MAPs determined according to normal clinical procedure. For each subject we calculated a prediction error, that is, the deviation of the predicted MAP from the behaviorally determined MAP across all electrodes. We also determined an error for a "flat" MAP, that is, one where the T and C levels were the same across electrodes, based on the values for electrode 10. We observed that although some subjects clearly benefited from using the ECAP profile, the overall results with the flat MAP showed similar error. Because many behavioral MAPs are relatively flat, the additional data provided by the ECAP measures did not improve the ability to predict MAP levels and in fact degraded the prediction in many cases.

To summarize, several studies have examined possible roles for ECAP measures in programming the implant in young children. There is a clear need and potential for such measures. However, no study has demonstrated a clear prescriptive procedure to reliably determine the most appropriate levels for programming the speech processor. Nevertheless, it is important to note that much of the research to date has used behaviorally determined programming levels as a "gold standard" to which electrophysiologically based paradigms are compared. Several studies have compared performance with electrophysiologically based MAPs compared with clinically determined MAPs (Seyle and Brown, 2002; Smoorenburg et al, 2002). In both cases performance was similar with both MAPs, suggesting that programming of an implant using ECAP is at least a reasonable MAP.

Consequently, there are several ways in which we presently use the ECAP in clinical practice. First, because NRT/NRI thresholds always indicate a point where programming stimulus is audible, those values can provide a place to start behavioral conditioning for young children. These initial values can be particularly useful for a clinician who works with very young children. In addition, as speech processor programs are refined, NRT/NRI thresholds can reveal errors in behavioral measures allowing faster approximation of a final program. For instance, ECAP thresholds lower than the behavioral determined T-level are an indication that behavioral responses may not accurately indicate true sensitivity. Finally, some children are unable to respond consistently to electrical stimulation at initial stimulation and in some cases for several months thereafter. NRT/NRI and/ or EABR can provide reassurance to the family and to the medical professionals that the device is, in fact, effectively stimulating the auditory system. In such children, ECAP thresholds can be used to guide device programming until the child is able to participate in behavioral testing. We have used ECAP thresholds (plus or minus some predetermined value) for estimating the T- and C-levels, typically choosing relatively conservative values initially and adjusting levels up gradually as the individual gains experience with the device.

Documenting Changes Over Time

A second application for the ECAP is in documenting changes in stimulability over time. Although there are some initial changes in sensitivity during the first few weeks after implantation, NRT/NRI measures have also been shown to be quite stable over time (Hughes et al, 2001; Lai et al, 2004), suggesting that long-term electrical stimulation provided with this implant likely has no negative consequences in terms of sensitivity to electrical stimulation. Therefore, these neural responses coupled with AEV and electrode impedance measures can be used to assist in determining whether an apparent change in response to stimulation is due to a change in device function or a change in neural responsiveness. Obtaining baseline NRT/NRI measures on all cochlear implant recipients at some time during the first few months of stimulation and annually or even biannually thereafter can be useful as a baseline of comparison for future measurements. Such information can be invaluable in trying to determine why a child might be failing to progress with his/her implant.

Role for Evoked Auditory Brainstem Response

As noted earlier, much of the recent literature on evoked neural responses in cochlear implant users has focused on the ECAP due to the ease of measurement, peripheral response measure, and the advantageous signal-to-noise ratio. Nevertheless, the EABR shares many of the same response characteristics, and the sensitivity of the two measures is similar (Brown et al, 2000). Consequently, the EABR may be used interchangeably with the ECAP for many applications. We have observed several instances where the EABR can be recorded at slightly lower stimulation levels than the ECAP. Additionally, in some instances, it is not possible to record an ECAP in a patient for whom the internal device is apparently functioning appropriately. This occurs in patients with cochlear malformations and those with either high thresholds or small dynamic ranges. In many cases, these individuals require relatively wide pulse durations to perceive the stimulus. At high stimulation levels and long pulse durations, stimulus artifact is problematic and often causes saturation of the amplifier used to record the ECAP. In these cases, the EABR can be used in much the same way as the ECAP to assist with programming. In cases where a child is not exhibiting any overt response to electrical stimulation despite indications that the internal device is functional, the presence of an EABR is a good indication that the auditory system is intact at the level of the brainstem and that the stimulus generated by the speech processor should be audible.

◆ Future Research Directions

An outstanding need in cochlear implant research is to develop methods of improving speech perception in low-performing individuals. Because the interface between the electrode and the remaining neurons in the auditory nerve is a likely source of variability among implant users, there have been several studies that have attempted to use the ECAP as a means of characterizing the responses of the auditory nerve with an eye toward modifying the electrical stimulation to improve neural response. Two general areas have been the focus of that research. The first area of research has been to explore how the auditory nerve codes rapid and continuous trains of pulses such as those generated by the speech processor. We know that auditory neurons can vary both in terms of their relative refractory properties as well as in terms of how much adaptation they exhibit to continuous stimulation (Zhou et al, 1995). Both of these factors are likely to affect the response of the nervous system to speech as well as to other environmentally relevant stimuli. The second general area of research has been to explore how the response of the auditory nerve is affected by channel interaction. It is clear that individual electrodes in a multichannel cochlear implant are not likely to stimulate completely separate populations of neurons. It is probable that the degree of overlap, or interaction, between these electrodes will be a factor in determining the ability of the implant to transmit information to the auditory nervous system. ECAP measures provide the ability to assess both the temporal and spatial patterns of the auditory nerve response in individual users. The following sections describe the methods for measuring these responses and review the general results that have been reported to date in these two general areas.

Temporal Response Properties

Individual, electrically stimulated, auditory nerve fibers demonstrate refractory behavior (Hartmann et al, 1984). This means that there is a time of reduced stimulability (increased threshold) following generation of an action potential. With two-pulse stimuli, recovery from the refractory state is relatively fast, on the order of 4 to 5 milliseconds. For sustained stimulation, as with pulse trains, recovery

is slower (Javel, 1990; Matsuoka et al, 2000; Schmidt-Clay, 2003; Vischer et al, 1997). Other studies have demonstrated an enhanced sensitivity following a subthreshold "conditioning" pulse (Cartee et al, 2000; Dynes, 1995), presumably due to a favorable biasing of residual charge on the neural membranes. As a result, in modern implants with speech processors using relatively high stimulation rates, refractoriness, adaptation, and temporal integration can all affect the response to a given stimulus pulse depending on the recent history of stimulation through the implant.

Refractory properties of the auditory nerve have been assessed using two current pulses presented in a forward-masking paradigm and recording either single-unit responses or the compound action potential (Brown et al, 1990; Hartmann et al, 1984; Miller et al, 2001). The normal subtraction method used to reduce stimulus artifact can be easily adapted to demonstrate refractory properties. As noted previously, ECAP growth functions are measured by fixing the IPI and systematically varying the level of the probe stimulus. ECAP refractory recovery functions can be measured by fixing the level of the masker and probe stimuli and systematically varying the length of the interval between the masker and the probe (IPI). **Fig. 8–5** shows ECAP recovery functions from two subjects recorded using a range of IPIs. In each case the amplitude of the response (normalized to the amplitude at IPI = 500 milliseconds) is plotted as a function of IPI. As IPI is increased, there is more time after the masker pulse for neurons to recover from refractoriness and therefore be able to respond to the probe in the two-pulse sequence. With the subtraction method, when short IPIs are used, the neural response to the probe in the probe-alone condition is large while the neural response to the probe in the masker-plus-probe condition is quite small. As a result, in the subtraction method, a relatively large amplitude ECAP is recorded. As IPI is increased and the response to the probe in the masker-plus-probe condition recovers, the neural response to the probe in the masker-plus-probe condition becomes increasingly similar to the neural response to the probe

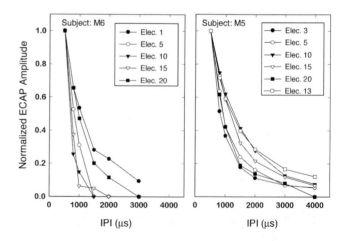

Figure 8–5 ECAP refractory recovery functions for two Nucleus CI24 implant users are plotted. ECAP amplitude (normalized to the amplitude at IPI of 500 μs) is plotted as function of the interpulse interval (IPI). The parameter is stimulation electrode as indicated in the legend.

that is recorded in the probe-alone condition. Thus, the amplitude of the subtracted response decreases with increasing IPI.

The results in **Fig. 8–5** suggest that the rate of recovery from the refractory state can vary both across electrodes within a subject as well as across subjects. Such differences may be due to several factors including effects of nerve fiber degeneration and demyelination (Stypulkowski & van den Honert, 1984; Zhou et al, 1995). An important caveat in making comparisons of this type is that measured ECAP refractory functions are highly dependent on stimulus level (Finley et al, 1997). The extent to which these differences in physiologic refractory recovery functions are reflected in perceptual differences was addressed by Brown et al. (1996), who measured psychophysical recovery functions with a similar two-pulse stimulus. Psychophysical recovery generally showed a time course similar to ECAP recovery functions, demonstrating similar variation across electrodes within the implant.

The responses to continuous stimulation through a cochlear implant may be characterized to some extent by refractory properties as measured with two-pulse stimuli. The extent to which other factors, such as cumulative adaptation and stochastic nerve discharge, may have an effect on the responses can be evaluated in a more comprehensive way by using trains of pulses. The NRT software does not allow for direct averaging of the response to each pulse in a train. By using a modification of a technique used by Wilson et al. (1997), we have been able to evaluate responses to individual pulses in a train. To measure the response to the nth pulse in a train, we set the number of masker pulses to $n − 1$ and set the IPI between masker and probe to be equal to that between masker pulses. The "masker + probe" stimulus in the normal NRT subtraction paradigm is then a series of n pulses. The "masker alone" stimulus is a train of $n − 1$ pulses of the same amplitude. Subtracting the responses to these two stimuli is therefore the response to the last pulse in the train. To measure the response to the first 15 pulses of the train, n is varied and 15 different averaged responses must be collected.

Fig. 8–6 shows examples of responses recorded using NRT as a function of the number of pulses within a continuous pulse train. In the graph at the top, waveforms in response to each pulse are arranged according to pulse number. Each trace is 1.5 millisecond in duration. The response to the first pulse is largest, because fibers are presumably nonrefractory. The response to the second pulse in the train is typically small because many fibers, which have responded to the first pulse, are still refractory. The response to the third pulse, in this case, is relatively large because many of those fibers responding to the first pulse are now recovered. Across the rest of the pulse train, a clear alternating pattern of response is observed in response to the constant level

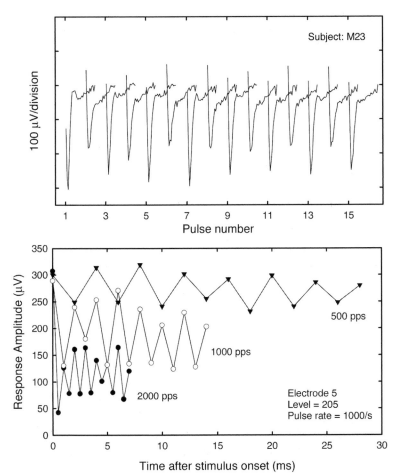

Figure 8–6 *Top*: The waveforms of the response to a series of pulses with fixed current level presented at 1000/s. The response to each successive pulse in the train is plotted as a function of pulse number. *Bottom*: The measured amplitude of the response is plotted as a function of time after stimulus onset three different pulse rates, illustrating both the adaptation and response amplitude alternation that is typically observed.

pulses. We interpret this alternating pattern to be at least partially the result of refractory recovery properties, for example, many fibers alternating between a refractory and a recovered state.

The lower graph in **Fig. 8–6** illustrates response amplitudes, demonstrating a clear alternating pattern in response amplitude. The degree of alternation varies somewhat across subjects and across electrodes within a subject, possibly related to the variations in refractory properties. We observe a decrease in average response amplitude to subsequent pulses within the train. This decrease is likely due to, in part, two-pulse refractory effects as shown in **Fig. 8–5** but also, in part, due to cumulative effects across several pulse presentations.

Responses to pulse trains in humans with cochlear implants generally demonstrate an alternating pattern of ECAP amplitude in response to a constant-amplitude pulse train (Hay-McCutcheon, 2004; Wilson et al, 1997). Measures in animal subjects with acute hearing loss have demonstrated a smaller alternation effect but also a decrease in amplitude across the duration of the electrical pulse train (Javel, 1990; Matsuoka et al, 2000; Vischer et al, 1997). More recent data with electrical pulse trains suggest that cumulative effects of electrical stimulation may be evident for even longer periods. Data with both animal and human subjects have shown long-term decreases in responsiveness over the course of several minutes (Abkes et al, 2003; Schmidt-Clay, 2003).

Refractoriness and adaptation may also have a significant effect on stimuli, such as high-rate amplitude-modulated pulses used in cochlear implant speech processors. Temporal information is encoded as a series of amplitude modulated pulses where the IPI is typically less than ECAP recovery time. Consequently, the response to each pulse in a sequence of amplitude-modulated pulses is affected by the previous sequence of stimulation. Experiments with ECAP have been extended to include more complex or realistic stimuli. Amplitude modulated pulse trains simulate the type of stimulus that is typically used with a continuous interleaved sampling (CIS)-type speech processor (Lawson et al, 1997; Wilson et al, 1997). The degree to which the response amplitude of the ECAP distorts the pattern of stimulus pulse amplitudes is of interest in that the response of the nerve is clearly the medium through which information is transferred. The ability of the neural response to accurately follow stimulus modulations may depend on pulse rate, modulation rate, and on individual subjects. In addition, responses occurring more centrally may place further constraints on the ability of the nervous system to encode modulations in the stimulus waveforms. The extent to which such variations determine performance with the implant are important questions for further research.

Channel Interaction

An important feature of multichannel implants is the ability of each electrode or each channel to stimulate a different population of neurons. If each channel stimulated the same neurons, then there would be no inherent benefit to multiple- versus single-channel implants. Clearly there can be significant overlap in the neurons stimulated among the channels. Electrophysiologic studies (Kral et al, 1998; Liang et al, 1991; Miller et al, 1993; Shepherd et al, 1993) and computer-modeling efforts (Finley et al, 1990; Frijns et al, 1996; Kral et al, 1998) have clearly demonstrated the influence of electrode position, configuration, and stimulus level on the pattern of fiber recruitment and consequently the degree of overlap among stimulated channels. One may also expect that the number and spatial pattern of surviving neurons in an individual may have a significant effect on the degree of channel interaction. For instance, if all surviving neurons were remote to two monopolar stimulating electrodes, then significant overlap in the stimulated populations would be expected.

Consequently there has been interest in electrophysiologic assessment tools to measure spread of excitation and channel interaction in individual cochlear implant users. Here we make a distinction between spread of excitation, how the population of neurons excited by an electrical stimulus is distributed along the length of the cochlea, and channel interaction, the degree to which stimulation through one electrode affects the responses to another electrode at a different longitudinal location in the cochlea. Although these measures are clearly related, the methodology to measure each is quite different.

One method of assessing spread of excitation or spatial selectivity assumes that the recording electrode primarily measures response from neurons near that electrode so that if one measures the amplitude of response as a function of recording electrode position for a fixed level and position of stimulating electrode, then the pattern of response across electrode number reflects the spread of excitation across the population (Cohen et al, 2004). Consequently, if one measures the amplitude of response as a function of recording electrode position for a fixed level and position of stimulating electrode, then the pattern of response across electrode number reflects both the spread of excitation across the population and the spread of the response field from active neuron populations to the recording electrode. The interpretation of such measures therefore should be tempered somewhat in that they do not directly represent simply the spread of excitation.

Alternatively, it is also possible to measure channel interaction among stimulating electrodes directly, by modifying the subtraction technique so that different electrodes are used for the masker and probe pulses (Abbas et al, 2004b; Cohen et al, 2003). If the masker and probe pulses are on different electrodes, the response to the probe will be dependent on the extent of overlap in the stimulated neural population. Measures of probe response as a function of probe position would then reflect the degree of overlap between the population of neurons responding to the masker and the population that is stimulated by the probe.

Examples of measures of spatial selectivity and channel interaction using these two methods are illustrated in **Fig. 8–7**. They demonstrate a general trend that measures of spatial selectivity (measured by varying the recording

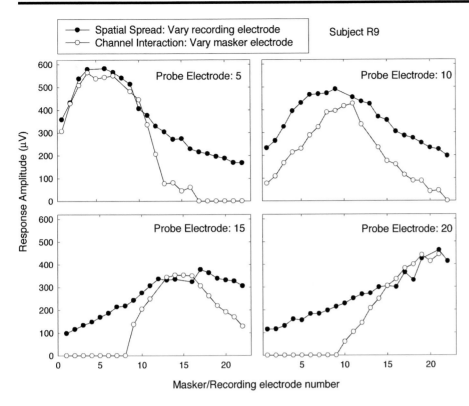

Figure 8–7 Comparison of spatial spread of responses as measured by varying the recording electrode and channel interaction as measures by varying masker electrode. Probe electrode is indicated on each panel. In each case the response amplitude is plotted as a function of recording electrode using a fixed masker, indicated as spatial spread. The second plot in each panel utilized a fixed recording electrode position and responses are plotted as a function of masker electrode position, indicated as channel interaction.

electrode and shown with filled symbols in **Fig. 8–7**) generally show a broader function than those of channel interaction (measured by varying the masker electrode and shown with open symbols in **Fig. 8–7**). We expect that the difference is due to the methodology; that is, as noted above, the basic assumption that a recording electrode reflects neural activity from only that place in the cochlea is likely not true. Consequently, channel interaction measures likely more accurately reflect the spatial selectivity of the peripheral auditory nerve stimulation.

◆ Conclusion

Because of the availability of telemetry systems in modern cochlear implants, there have been many reports in the literature of experiments aimed at exploring the utility of electrophysiologic potentials to provide information about the electrically stimulated auditory nervous system. The primary clinical application for such measures is generally seen to be young children and difficult-to-test populations. Although recent data suggest that programming the implant based solely on electrophysiologic measures such as the ECAP may not result in an optimal program, there is clearly a role for such measures in providing complementary information relative to stimulability of the auditory nerve. We also note that as recording systems are improved, there is the potential for more sensitive measures and possibly more accurate predictions of behavioral sensitivity. For instance, recent recordings with a new system from Nucleus (Research Platform 8/Nucleus

System 4) demonstrated lower noise floor and nonlinear growth functions, suggesting a more sensitive recording system that can detect with slow growth at low stimulus level (Abbas et al, 2004a).

In addition to assistance with programming the implant, there are several other immediate applications of physiologic recording methods and telemetry. These include impedance testing and the assessment of current generation within an implant with external electrodes (AEVs).

Finally, there are several applications for ECAP and other evoked potentials that are currently under investigation. In general they can be useful in gaining a better understanding of the underlying differences in performances among individual implant users. The variety of measures that can be recorded from an individual, including growth, temporal response patterns, and spatial spread, may potentially allow us to better understand their specific abilities and deficits. With such an understanding, a next step could be a modification of the stimulus parameters to overcome these deficits in processing.

Acknowledgments

This work is supported by research grant DC00242 from the National Institutes of Health–National Institute on Deafness and Other Communication Disorders (NIH/NIDCD); grant RR59 from the General Clinical Research Centers Program, NIH; and the Iowa Lions Sight and Hearing Foundation.

References

Abbas PJ, Brown CJ. (1991). Electrically evoked auditory brainstem response: growth of response with current level. Hear Res 51:123–138

Abbas PJ, Brown CJ, Shallop JK, et al. (1999). Summary of results using the Nucleus CI24M implant to record electrically evoked compound action potential. Ear Hear 20:45–49

Abbas PJ, Etler CP, Brown CJ, Van Voorst TL, Zubrod LJ, Dunn SM. (2004a). Electrically evoked compound action potential using Nucleus RP8. International Congress Series 1273:80–83

Abbas PJ, Hughes ML, Brown CJ, Miller CA, South H. (2004b). Channel interaction in cochlear implant users evaluated using the electrically evoked compound action potential. Audiol Neurootol 2004;9:203–213

Abkes BA, Miller CA, Nu N, Abbas PJ. (2003). Adaptation in the auditory nerve in response to a continuous electric pulse train. 26th Midwinter Meeting of the Association for Research in Otolaryngology, Daytona Beach, FL

Battmer RD, Laszig R, Lehnhardt E. (1990). Electrically elicited stapedius reflex in cochlear implant patients. Ear Hear 11:370–374

Black RC, Clark GM, O'Leary SJ, Walters C. (1983). Intracochlear electrical stimulation: brainstem response audiometric and Histopathological studies. Acta Otolaryngol Suppl 399:5–17

Brown CJ, Abbas PJ, Borland J, Bertschy MR. (1996). Electrically evoked whole nerve action potentials in Ineraid cochlear implant users: Responses to different stimulating electrode configurations and comparison to psychophysical responses. J Speech Hear Res 39:453–467

Brown CJ, Abbas PJ, Fryauf-Bertschy H, Kelsey D, Gantz BJ. (1994). Intraoperative and postoperative electrically evoked auditory brainstem responses in Nucleus cochlear implant users: Implications for the fitting process. Ear Hear 15:168–176

Brown CJ, Abbas PJ, Gantz BJ. (1990). Electrically evoked whole-nerve action potentials: data from human cochlear implant users. J Acoust Soc Am 88:1385–1391

Brown CJ, Hughes ML, Lopez SM, Abbas PJ. (1999). Relationship between EABR thresholds and levels used to program the CLARION Speech Processor. Ann Otol Rhinol Laryngol Suppl. 177(Suppl):50–57

Brown CJ, Hughes ML, Luk B, Abbas PJ, Wolaver A, Gervais J. (2000). The relationship between EAP and EABR thresholds and levels used to program the Nucleus CI24M speech processor: data from adults. Ear Hear 21:151–163

Cartee LA, van den Honert C, Finley CC, Miller RL. (2000). Evaluation of a model of the cochlear neural membrane. I. Physiological measurement of membrane characteristics in response to intrameatal electrical stimulation. Hear Res 146:143–152

Chen X, Han D, Zhao X, et al. (2002). [Comparison of neural response telemetry thresholds with behavioral T/C levels.] Zhonghua Er Bi Yan Hou Ke Za Zhi 37:435–439 (in Chinese)

Coats AC, Martin JL. (1977). Human auditory nerve action potentials and brainstem evoked responses: effect of audiogram shape and lesion location. Arch Otolaryngol 103:605–622

Cohen LT, Richardson LM, Cowan RS. (2003). Spatial spread of neural excitation in cochlear implant recipients: comparison of improved ECAP method and psychophysical forward masking. Hear Res 179:72–87

Cohen LT, Saunders E, Richardson LM. (2004). Spatial spread of neural excitation: comparison of compound action potential and forward-masking data in cochlear implant recipients. Int J Audiol 43:346–355

Cullington H. (2000). Preliminary neural response telemetry results. Br J Audiol 34:131–140

Di Nardo W, Ippolito S, Quaranta N, Cadoni G, Galli J. (2003). Correlation between NRT measurement and behavioral levels in patients with the Nucleus 24 cochlear implant. Acta Otorhinolaryngol Ital 23:352–355

Dynes S. (1995). Discharge characteristics of auditory nerve fibers for pulsatile electrical stimuli. Ph.D. Thesis, Massachusetts Institute of Technology, Cambridge, MA

Finley CC, Wilson B, van den Honert C, Lawson D. (1997). Sixth quarterly progress report, speech processors for auditory prostheses, NIH project NO1-DC-5-2103</unknown

Finley CC, Wilson BS, White MW. (1990). Models of neural responsiveness to electrical stimulation. In: Miller JM, Spellman FA, eds. Cochlear Implants. Models of the Electrically Stimulated Ear (pp. 55–96). New York: Springer-Verlag

Franck KH, Norton SJ. (2001). Estimation of psychophysical levels using the electrically evoked compound action potential measured with the neural response telemetry capabilities of Cochlear Corporation's CI24M device. Ear Hear 22:289–299

Franck KH, Shah UK. (2004). Averaged electrode voltage testing to diagnose an unusual cochlear implant internal device failure. J Am Acad Audiol 15:643–648

Frijns JH, de Snoo SL, ten Kate JH. (1996). Spatial selectivity in a rotationally symmetric model of the electrically stimulated cochlea. Hear Res 95:33–48

Gordon KA, Ebinger KA, Gilden JE, Shapiro WH. (2002). Neural response telemetry in 12- to 24-month old children. Ann Otol Rhinol Laryngol Suppl 189:42–48

Gordon KA, Papsin BC, Harrison RV. (2003). Activity-dependent developmental plasticity of the auditory brain stem in children who use cochlear implants. Ear Hear 24:485–500

Gorga MP, Worthington DW, Reiland JK, Beauchaine KA, Goldgar DE. (1985). Some comparisons between auditory brainstem response threshold, latencies, and the pure-tone audiogram. Ear Hear 6:105–112

Hartmann R, Topp G, Klinke R. (1984). Discharge patterns of cat primary auditory fibers with electrical stimulation of the cochlea. Hear Res 13:47–62

Hay-McCutcheon MJ. (2004). The impact of peripheral auditory nerve adaptation upon central measures of temporal integration in nucleus 24 cochlear implant recipients. PhD Dissertation, University of Iowa, Iowa City, IA

Heller JW, Sinopoli T, Fowler-Brehm N, Shallop JK. (1991). Characterization of averaged electrode voltages from the Nucleus cochelar implant. Proceedings of the Annual International Conference of the IEEE Engineering in Medicine and Biology Society 13:1907–1908

Hodges AV, Ruth RA, Lambert PR, Balkany TJ. (1994). Electrical auditory brain-stem responses in Nucleus multichannel cochlear implant users. Arch Otolaryngol Head Neck Surg 120:1093–1099

Hughes ML, Brown CJ, Abbas PJ. (2004). Sensitivity and specificity of averaged electrode voltage (AEV) measures in cochlear implant recipients. Ear Hear 25:431–446

Hughes ML, Brown CJ, Abbas PJ, Wolaver A, Gervais J. (2000). The relationship between EAP and EABR thresholds and levels used to program the Nucleus CI24M speech processor: data from children. Ear Hear 21:164–174

Hughes ML, Vander Werff KR, Brown CJ, et al. (2001). A longitudinal study of electrode impedance, the electrically evoked compound action potential, and behavioral measures in Nucleus 24 cochlear implant users. Ear Hear 22:471–486

Javel E. (1990). Acoustic and electrical encoding of temporal information. In: Miller JM, Spellman FA, eds. Cochlear Implants. Models of the Electrically Stimulated Ear. New York: Springer-Verlag

Kaga K, Kodera K, Hirota E, Tsuzuku T. (1991). P300 responses to tones and speech sounds after cochlear implant: a case report. Laryngoscope 101:905–907

Kiang NY, Moxon EC. (1972). Physiological considerations in artificial stimulation of the inner ear. Ann Otol Rhinol Laryngol 81:714–730

Kileny PR, Kemink JL. (1987). Electrically evoked middle-latency auditory potentials in cochlear implant candidates. Arch Otolaryngol Head Neck Surg 113:1072–1077

Kileny PR, Meiteles LZ, Zwolan TA, Telian SA. (1995). Cochlear implant device failure: diagnosis and management. Am J Otol 16:164–171

Kral A, Hartmann R, Mortazavi D, Klinke R. (1998). Spatial resolution of cochlear implants: the electrical field and excitation of auditory afferents. Hear Res 121:11–28

Kraus N, Micco AG, Koch DB, et al. (1993). The mismatch negativity cortical potential elicited by speech stimuli in cochlear implant patients. Hear Res 65:118–124

Lai WK, Aksit M, Akdas F, Dillier N. (2004). Longitudinal behaviour of neural response telemetry (NRT) data and clinical implications. Int J Audiol 43:252–263

Lawson DT, Wilson BS, Finley CC, et al. (1997). Cochlear implant studies at Research Triangle Institute and Duke University Medical Center. Scand Audiol Suppl 46:50–64

Liang DH, Kovacs GT, Storment CW, White RL. (1991). A method for evaluating the selectivity of electrodes implanted for nrve simulation. IEEE Trans Biomed Eng 38:443–449

Mahoney MJ, Proctor LA. (1994). The use of averaged electrode voltages to assess the function of Nucleus internal cochlear implant devices in children. Ear Hear 15:177–183

Mason SM, Cope Y, Garnham J, O'Donoghue GM, Gibbin KP. (2001). Intra-operative recordings of electrically evoked auditory nerve action potentials in young children by use of neural response telemetry with the Nucleus CI24M cochlear implant. Br J Audiol 35:225–235

Mason SM, Sheppard S, Garnham CW, Lutman ME, O'Donoghue GM, Gibbin KP. (1993). Improving the relationship of intraoperative EABR thresholds to T-level in young children receiving the Nucleus cochlear implant. In Hochmair-Desoyer IJ, Hochmair ES, eds. Advances in Cochlear Implants (pp. 44–49). Vienna: Manz

Matsuoka AJ, Abbas PJ, Rubinstein JT, Miller CA. (2000). The neuronal response to electrical constant-amplitude pulse train stimulation: evoked compound action potential recordings. Hear Res 149:115–128

Mens LH, Brokx JP, van den Broek P. (1995). Averaged electrode voltages: management of electrode failures in children, fluctuating threshold and comfort levels, and otosclerosis. Ann Otol Rhinol Laryngol Suppl 166:169–172

Mens LHM, Oostendorp T, van den Broek P. (1994). Identifying electrode failures with cochlear implant generated surface potentials. Ear Hear 15:330–338

Miller CA, Abbas PJ, Brown CJ. (1993). Electrically evoked auditory brainstem response to stimulation of different sites in the cochlea. Hear Res 66:130–142

Miller CA, Abbas PJ, Robinson BK. (2001). Response properties of the refractory auditory nerve fiber. J Assoc Res Otolaryngol 2:216–232

Miller CA, Woodruff KE, Pfingst BE. (1995). Functional responses from guinea pigs with cochlear implants. I. Electrophysiological and psychophysical measures. Hear Res 92:85–99

Miller JM, Altschuler RA, Dupont J, Lesperance M, Tucci D. (1996). Consequences of deafness and electrical stimulation in the auditory system. In Salvi RJ, Henderson D, Fiorino F, Colletti V, eds. Auditory System Plasticity and Regeneration, (pp. 378–391). New York: Thieme

Ponton CW, Eggermont JJ. (2001). Of kittens and kids: Altered cortical maturation following profound deafness and cochlear implant use. Audiol Neurootol 6:363–380

Schmidt-Clay KM. (2003). Variations in neural adaptation across nucleus C124 cochlear implant users and the relationship to behavioral dynamic range and word recognition performance. PhD Dissertation, University of Iowa, Iowa City, IA

Seyle K, Brown CJ. (2002). Speech perception using maps based on neural response telemetry measures. Ear Hear 23(1 suppl):72S–79S

Shallop JK, Beiter AL, Goin DW, Mischke RE. (1990). Electrically evoked auditory brainstem responses (EABR) and middle latency responses (EMLR) obtained from patients with the Nucleus multichannel cochlear implant. Ear Hear 11:5–15

Shallop JK, VanDyke L, Goin DW, Mischke RE. (1991). Prediction of behavioral threshold and comfort values for Nucleus 22-channel implant patients from electrical auditory brain stem response test results. Ann Otol Rhinol Laryngol 100:896–898

Sharma A, Dorman MF, Spahr AJ. (2002). A sensitive period for the development of the central auditory system in children with cochlear implants: implications of age of implantation. Ear Hear 23:532–539

Shepherd RK, Hatsushika S, Clark GM. (1993). Electrical stimulation of the auditory nerve: the effect of electrode position on neural excitation. Hear Res 66:108–120

Skinner MW, Ketten DR, Holden LK, et al. (2002). CT-derived estimation of cochlear morphology and electrode array position in relation to word recognition in Nucleus-22 recipients. J Assoc Res Otolaryngol 3:332–350

Smith DW, Finley CC, van den Honert C, Olszyk VB, Konrad KEM. (1994). Behavioral and electrophysiological responses to electrical stimulation in the cat absolute threshold. Hear Res 81:1–10

Smoorenburg GF, Willeboer C, van Dijk JE. (2002). Speech perception in Nucleus CI24M cochlear implant users with processor settings based on electrically evoked compound action potential thresholds. Audiol Neurootol 7:335–347

Stypulkowski PH, van den Honert C. (1984). Physiological properties of the electrically stimulated auditory nerve. I. Compound action potential recordings. Hear Res 14:205–223

Thai-Van H, Chanal JM, Coudert C, Veuillet E, Truy E, Collet L. (2001). Relationship between NRT measurements and behavioral levels in children with the Nucleus 24 cochlear implant may change over time: Preliminary report. Int J Pediatr Otorhinolaryngol 58:153–162

van den Honert C, Stypulkowski PH. (1986). Characterization of the electrically evoked auditory brainstem response in cats and humans. Hear Res 21:109–126

Vischer M, Haenggeli A, Zhang J, Pelizzone M, Hausler R, Rouiller EM. (1997). Effect of high frequency electrical stimulation of the auditory nerve in an animal model of cochlear implants. Am J Otol 18:S27–S29

Wang G, Vannier MW, Skinner MW, Kalender WA, Polacin A, Ketten DR. (1996). Unwrapping cochlear implants by spiral CT. IEEE Trans Biomed Eng 43:891–900

Wang G, Zhao S, Yu H, et al. Design, analysis and simulation for development of the first clinical micro-CT scanner. Acad Radiol 2005;12:511–525

Wilson BS, Finley CC, Lawson DT, Zerbi M. (1997). Temporal representations with cochlear implants. Am J Otol 18(6 suppl):S30–S34

Zhou R, Assouline JG, Abbas PJ, Messing A, Gantz BJ. (1995). Anatomical and physiological measures of auditory system in mice with peripheral myelin deficiency. Hear Res 88:87–97

9

Cochlear Implant Electrode History, Choices, and Insertion Techniques

J. Thomas Roland Jr.,

Tina C. Huang, and

Andrew J. Fishman

◆ History of Cochlear Implantation

The history of cochlear implantation begins with the use of electricity to stimulate the ear in an attempt to produce a sensation of sound. Volta, in 1790, was the first to publish his results. Using his recently invented voltaic cell, he connected 30 or 40 cells, the equivalent of ~50 V, to two metal rods, which he then inserted into his ears. When he closed the circuit, he received a sensation akin to being hit in the head and then described a sound like thickly boiling paste. Luckily, he chose not to repeat his experiment. Ritter reported his attempt to repeat Volta's experiment using a battery with 100 to 200 cells in 1801. He also experienced disagreeable cerebral effects. Not until 1855 did another experimenter stimulate the ear with electricity. Duchenne used alternating current to produce a crackling sound. Brenner, in the 1860s, was able to use short current pulses to produce a sensation of sound, and in the 1930s several other researchers were able to use alternating currents in the ear to produce sound.[1,2]

Stevens at Harvard described the effect of auditory sensation due to alternating current passed through the head as the electrophonic phenomenon. He did several experiments using subjects with normal hearing and intact tympanic membranes and middle ears as well as patients who had prior surgery and no tympanic membranes. His first published report in 1937 showed that, in people with normal hearing and intact tympanic membranes, alternating current passed through the ears could produce sound of different frequencies. In addition, the subjects could recognize speech and music, but the quality was extremely poor and no word discrimination was possible. This led him to propose three different mechanisms for the production of sound: (1) direct stimulation of the auditory nerve, (2) cochlear receptors electrically tuned to different frequencies, and (3) mechanical vibrations produced by the alternating currents that stimulate the auditory organs in the same manner as sound vibrations. Further experiments led him to refine his three hypotheses. He proposed that in patients with normal ears, alternating current displaces the tympanic membrane, leading to mechanical vibration. Patients lacking a tympanic membrane either had the hair cells of the organ of Corti set into motion by the electrical current or had direct stimulation of the auditory nerve.[3] Some subjects also experienced vertigo with stimulation, presumably from stimulation of the vestibular nerves.

The year 1957 ushered in the modern era of cochlear implants with the implantation of an electrode into a human patient by Djourno and Eyriès. A patient with large bilateral cholesteatomas had undergone bilateral temporal resections and was left with bilateral facial nerve paralysis and deafness. During the surgery for facial nerve grafting, an electrode was implanted into the stump of the remaining cochlear nerve. The patient was able to hear sound and differentiate frequency and intensity, but not speech. Unfortunately, the electrode broke twice and was not replaced a third time. Interestingly, Djourno is also the first person to describe using promontory stimulation with a transtympanic needle to verify a functioning cochlear nerve.[4] Chouard, who had worked in Eyriès laboratory, carried on the work and developed one of the early multichannel implants.[5,6]

In the 1960s, Simmons at Stanford, Michelson at University of California–San Francisco, and House in Los Angeles all began implanting human subjects with various types of implants. Simmons, in 1964 and 1966, placed multiple electrodes into human subjects with no adverse effects. Both patients had direct auditory nerve stimulation and both patients were able to distinguish different frequencies, but no speech.[7] He also performed several histologic studies in cats that did not show significant damage to auditory structures from prolonged electrical stimulation and damage limited to the most distal portions of the basal turn of the cochlear from electrode insertion.[8] He, too, encountered what continues to plague implant makers today: the fragility of the electrical wires leading to the electrodes.[9] In 1977, two patients were implanted with a four-electrode system into the auditory nerve. Their initial results showed that the patients were able to differentiate various frequencies and loudness levels.[10]

Michelson had also published experiments on cats in the late 1960s that showed no adverse effects from long-term stimulation with multiple electrodes placed within the cochlea. He then published his results on four patients with a bipolar electrode placed through the round window into the cochlea. Two patients perceived only noise with activation, but the other two patients were able to identify pure tones and had limited speech recognition.[7] Again, technical failures due to breakage of the wires were a major impediment. This was corrected using methyl methacrylate cement to fix the receiver and wires to the temporal bone.[11]

House first implanted two patients with a single electrode system into the scala tympani in 1961. However, one was quickly explanted secondary to an increase in current requirements. The second patient had the single electrode replaced with a five-wire electrode system several months after his first implantation. This system, too, was explanted secondary to an inflammatory reaction.[12] He teamed up with Urban and, in 1969, implanted another patient with their five-electrode system. Two more were then implanted in 1970. The third patient moved away from the area and the second patient had a device failure, but their first patient was able not only to differentiate sounds but also to carry on simple telephone conversations.[12,13]

Clark developed an early multichannel implant using biphasic current stimulation. He also began using a banded electrode array, instead of a two-dimensional electrode array, placed within the cochlea and driven with a transcutaneous data and power link. This was the precursor of the Nucleus cochlear implant.[5,14] In Austria, Hochmair and Hochmair-Desoyer were also experimenting with multichannel bipolar electrode arrays.[5,14]

Once clinical trials began, cochlear implantation advanced rapidly in terms of device design as well as device placement. Clark's first patient, implanted in 1978, was able to perceive pitch and gained some open set speech discrimination. Several other patients were implanted in 1979 and this experience led to the formation of Cochlear Ltd. by a collaboration between the University of Melbourne, Nucleus Ltd., and the Australian Government. The Nucleus 22 device (Cochlear Corporation, Sydney, Australia) was developed in 1981 and clinical trials began in 1982. The Nucleus 22 then evolved into the Mini 22 receiver/stimulator (Cochlear Corporation, Sydney, Australia). The Mini 22 improved on the original Nucleus 22 in terms of its smaller size as well as the incorporation of a magnet to hold the transmitting coil against the device instead of the previously used headset. The electrode array contained 22 evenly spaced platinum band electrodes

supported within a straight silicone rubber molding and an additional 10 platinum bands to provide extra stiffness to facilitate insertion. The array had a maximal insertion depth of 25 mm into the scala tympani.[15] The Mini 22 was then replaced with the Nucleus CI24M/SP5 cochlear implant system (Cochlear Corporation, Sydney, Australia). The Nucleus 24 device consisted of a titanium-encapsulated receiver-stimulator connected to 22 intracochlear electrodes and two extracochlear electrodes with the ability to deliver biphasic pulses in either bipolar or monopolar configuration.[16]

In 1987, the Clarion multichannel cochlear implant was developed by MiniMed Technologies, now the Advanced Bionics Corporation (Valencia, CA), in collaboration with the Department of Otolaryngology of the University of California–San Francisco and the Neuroscience Program Office of the Research Triangle Institute (Research Triangle Park, NC). The Clarion used 16 platinum-iridium (90:10) wire contacts encased within a curved silicone rubber carrier. Each wire ends in a 0.3-mm-diameter ball with the balls arranged in eight near-radial pairs with 2 mm between pairs. The 16 wires are stacked in a double-rib configuration and the total length of the electrode array was 25 mm. The external antenna connected to the internal components via a magnet.[17] Because the electrode was precurved, the device required a special insertion tool to straighten the electrode prior to insertion.[18] The electrode was inserted into a Teflon tube, which is then mated to the insertion tool, which contained a retractable slide. The tube containing the electrode was then placed into the cochleostomy and the slide advanced. As the slide advanced, the electrode was advanced into the cochlea. The original device, version 1.0, was introduced in 1991. Version 1.2, with a smaller case, was introduced in 1995.[19] The Clarion was approved for use in adults in 1996 and for children in 1997.

The last company currently manufacturing cochlear implants is Med-El (Innsbruck, Austria). Its original device, the Med-El Combi 40, was a multichannel fast-stimulator device with eight intracochlear electrodes housed in a straight soft silicone carrier. The 16 electrode contacts, two interconnected contacts per electrode, were arranged in diametrically opposite pairs. The electrodes were driven in monopolar mode. The electrodes were spaced over 20.6 mm and had an average insertion depth of 30 mm. The device became available in the mid-1990s and, at the time, was the fastest implant available.[20,21] The company's next device, the Combi 40+ implant, was a 12-channel system with a thinner receiver/stimulator housing.[22] The newest device is the Pulsar CI[100], which continues to use the same design for the electrode array, but has improved processing capability.

As research into device design progressed, the potential advantages of perimodiolar placement of the electrode array came to light. With this goal in mind, several implant companies produced implants that brought the electrodes closer to the modiolus. Though the original Clarion array was already precurved, the array assumed an intermediate position within the scala tympani. The Advanced Bionics Corp. developed an intracochlear Silastic positioner that was inserted adjacent to the electrode to bring the array even closer to the medial wall. The positioner was a curved piece of Silastic thinner at the distal tip and thicker at the proximal end. The positioner was inserted using the insertion tool after the electrode was in position.[23] In addition, the company developed a new electrode, the HiFocus electrode, to be used specifically with the electrode positioning system. It still contained 16 electrode contacts, but these contacts were arranged longitudinally along the carrier and had a large rectangular surface area. Dielectric partitions were located between each contact to reduce the spread of current. The HiFocus device was approved for use in adults in 2000.[24] Unfortunately, the positioner was associated with an increased risk of meningitis and was taken off the market. The company's current device, the HiResolution 90K, uses the "J" electrode, which maintains the precurved shape of the carrier and has a thinner case housed in Silastic for the receiver/stimulator. A perimodiolar Helix electrode is also currently under development and refinement.

Cochlear Ltd. developed the perimodiolar Contour electrode. The Nucleus CI-22 and CI-24 systems were both straight electrodes and assumed a position along the lateral wall of the scala tympani. The Contour electrode was precurved and tapered from 0.8 mm at the proximal end to 0.5 mm at the tip to minimize its volume. A platinum stylet within the lumen of the array holds the electrode straight before insertion. Removal of the stylet either after or during insertion allows the array to assume its perimodiolar shape and position. The array contains 22 platinum half-band electrodes positioned on the modiolar side of the array along the proximal 15.5 mm of the carrier. The array also has a silicone marker rib at 22 mm measured from the tip to guide the depth of insertion.[25] It was approved for use in adults in 2000.[26] The Contour electrode has recently been replaced with the Contour Advance electrode, which continues to utilize the perimodiolar design with 22 electrodes, but a softer tip to guide insertion and minimize insertion trauma. This device is deployed with the Advance Off Stylet (AOS) technique.

The initial debate between single versus multiple electrode systems has produced modern devices that all utilize multichannel systems. The most current challenge for cochlear implant manufacturers is to design an electrode that assumes the closest position to the modiolus without causing excessive insertional trauma and perhaps preserve residual cochlear elements and hearing.

◆ Intracochlear Trauma Due to Cochlear Implantation

Intracochlear trauma caused by cochlear implantation has been extensively reported in the literature. The short- and long-term structural and functional detrimental effects of trauma have been documented in animals but not in humans. The long-term functional effects of trauma are unknown in humans. In 1981 Leake-Jones et al[27] showed that basilar membrane perforation caused focal spiral ganglion cell degeneration in animals. In a later report, Leake-Jones and Rebscher[28] comment that neuronal elements can withstand chronic implantation if two prerequisites are met. The shape and mechanical properties of the array must be precisely controlled such that insertional trauma is minimized and that the materials and fabrication

must be highly biocompatible. Miller et al[29,30] in 1983 showed that fracture of the osseous spiral lamina in monkeys was associated with a significant decrease in spiral ganglion cell population and that degeneration might continue along the auditory neural pathways to the inferior colliculus. In a large postmortem human study, four separate studies reported no correlation between spiral ganglion cell counts and speech perception performance.[31–34] Significant medial osseous trauma and neo-ossification was reported. Spiral ganglion cell counts, however, are not the only variable related to performance with a cochlear implant. Nadol[35] suggests that there is no firm evidence that intracochlear trauma, found in several human postmortem temporal bones, caused further spiral ganglion cell degeneration. In 1999, Ketten[36] performed computed tomographic (CT) radiographic analysis of living postimplantation patients showing cochlear trauma and ossification related to electrode trajectory and final position. Animal studies, human temporal bone studies, and radiologic studies document intracochlear trauma following cochlear implantation. Despite the discrepancy between findings in animal studies and human clinical results and postmortem temporal bone histopathology, few would argue against preservation of cochlear structures during cochlear implantation. Perhaps the subtle detrimental outcomes from cochlear trauma will become more apparent as patients with better hearing are implanted and more complicated signal processing and neuronal stimulation strategies are utilized. One might also argue that, within a single subject, performance would certainly be better with more surviving neurons to stimulate.

Currently, there are three cochlear implant electrode array designs: straight, precurved, and perimodiolar. As mentioned earlier, the recent designs have attempted to position the electrode array closer to the modiolus in an effort to decrease power consumption and prolong battery life as well as provide more specific neuronal subpopulation stimulation. Among the perimodiolar devices, there are three conceptual models: straight electrode design with a lateral tension band; precurved electrode with a straightening stylet; and space-occupying positioner lateral to the electrode array. The nature of observed intracochlear trauma differs with each of these designs.[37–39]

Other than the design characteristics of the aforementioned electrodes, surgical technique is a variable in cochlear trauma during cochlear implantation. Cochleostomy position, electrode insertion angle in two dimensions, insertional forces, kinking of electrodes, and the use of various tools and lubricants all affect the potential degree of trauma resulting from cochlear implantation.

Observations and conclusions in this chapter are based on the cumulative experience of more than 10 years of work developing and refining a cadaver temporal bone model for the study of cochlear implant electrode insertion dynamics, position analysis, and trauma reporting.[40]

The Model for Electrode Evaluation

Temporal bones are harvested from human cadavers, and the otic capsule is removed with limited surrounding bone to minimize bone density and allow optimal fluoroscopic

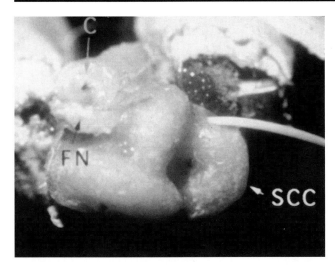

Figure 9–1 Thinned otic capsule with catheter placed in superior semicircular canal (SCC) ampulla. FN, facial nerve; C, cochleostomy. Fluoroscopic measurement evaluation, histologic sections, and hydraulic pressure measurements are obtainable from these specimens.

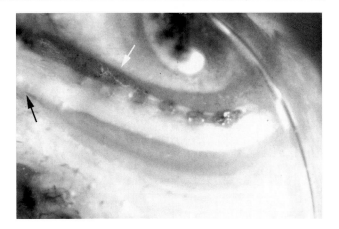

Figure 9–2 Longitudinal section through the basal turn of the cochlea. Black arrow cochleostomy; white arrow modiolar wall. Note the tip of the electrode in the second turn of the cochlea.

imaging. A basal cochleostomy is performed and a lubricant (surgical grade glycerin diluted to 50% with saline) is infused into the cochlea to facilitate insertion and for bone dust removal, as is performed in all our live patient implantations. Under real-time fluoroscopic guidance, using standard microsurgical instrumentation and technique, electrodes are inserted through the cochleostomy. Multiplanar real-time images are captured to videotape, so that detailed analyses may be performed. Additionally, hydraulic pressure measurements can be performed by inserting a catheter into the superior semicircular canal ampulla and connecting to a pressure transducer and monitor (**Fig. 9–1**). Pressure fluctuations can be detected during lubricant infusion, and during electrode insertion and withdrawal.

The temporal bones are next dehydrated and fixed in resin. Radial sections allow observation and imaging of the pars inferior, pars ascendens, and pars descendens in a plane perpendicular to the scalar lumen. This technique, which has been previously described, facilitates measurements of electrode position relative to cochlear structures and the evaluation of trauma.[40,41] Additional sections at the cochleostomy and the cochlear apex can also be made (**Fig. 9–2**). Alternatively, serial sections can be performed as with standard thick section temporal bone histologic techniques.

Anatomic Regions of Potential Trauma

The anatomic sites and the potential mechanisms of cochlear implant–related trauma are categorized in **Table 9–1**. Damage to the *spiral ligament* and the *outer scalar wall endosteum* undoubtedly occurs with every cochlear implantation. Straight electrodes strike the outer wall at the mid pars ascendens in most cases.[40–42] This outer wall contact is well seen on both fluoroscopic evaluations and in histologic preparations, and the trauma has been shown to cause neo-ossification and fibrosis that may affect electrode impedance characteristics and will also affect cochlear

reimplantation. No evidence exists in human studies that injuries to the outer scalar wall and the spiral ligament affect spiral ganglion cell survival.

Damage to the *basilar membrane* also occurs in many cochlear implantations. Tears and disruptions have the potential to destroy the organ of Corti and the terminal dendritic processes that may result in spiral ganglion cell degeneration in humans.

Osseous spiral lamina fractures are a rare occurrence, but trauma to this structure disrupts the dendrites of the spiral ganglion cells, which might lead to further spiral ganglion cell degeneration.

Modiolar wall trauma and fracture represents the most severe form of cochlear implant injury. The immediately adjacent spiral ganglion cells would be directly injured or exposed to ongoing inflammatory and fibrotic processes.

Cochlear and vestibular *neuroepithelial* damage may occur secondary to perilymphatic and endolymphatic flow and composition alterations as well as by hydraulic forces.

Table 9–1 Anatomic Sites and Mechanisms of Cochlear Implant–Related Trauma

Anatomic Region of Injury	Mechanism
Lateral wall/spiral ligament	High cochleostomy
	Inappropriate angle of insertion
	Electrode friction/design
	Outer wall forces
Basilar membrane	High cochleostomy
	Inappropriate angle of insertion
	Outer wall forces
	Electrode size
Osseous spiral lamina	Electrode pressure on medial wall
	Medial movement after basilar membrane perforation
Modiolar wall	Electrode pressure of perimodiolar designs
	Direct insertion trauma
	Chronic electrode pressure
Neuroepithelium	Hydraulic forces
	Adjacent structural violations

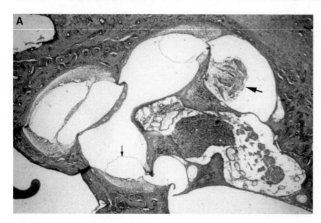

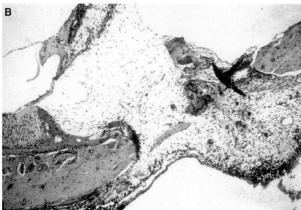

Figure 9–3 **(A)** A section through guinea pig cochlea harvested 8 weeks after cochleostomy. Note island of neo-ossification in basal turn (large black arrow). Small black arrow shows endolymphatic hydrops. **(B)** Magnified view of healed cochleostomy demonstrating advancing fibrosis.

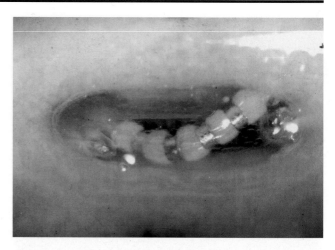

Figure 9–4 Focal basilar membrane perforation in pars ascendens by perimodiolar prototype electrode array.

basilar membrane trauma. All electrode designs have been found to potentially disturb or penetrate the basilar membrane to varying degrees.

All electrode designs, with the exception of the Contour Advance deployed with the AOS technique, produce outer wall contact and forces during insertion, some more than others. The outer wall of the scala tympani is upwardly sloping. Any outward force applied against a rigid wall will be met with a force of equal magnitude, less frictional forces, perpendicular to the wall at the point of contact. The sum of the two force vectors is an upward force toward the spiral ligament and the basilar membrane (**Fig. 9–5**). This upward force drives the electrode into, and sometimes through, the spiral ligament and lateral

Mechanisms of Trauma

The surgical cochleostomy represents the first step in the traumatic process of cochlear implantation. Direct injury to the spiral ligament, basilar membrane, and the osseous spiral lamina may occur with a cochleostomy that is made in a superior position closer to the oval window. Blood and bone dust created by the drilling process might enter the cochlea, initiating an irritative or inflammatory process leading to fibrosis and ossification. Fibrosis and neo-ossification were found in nearly every control and test guinea pig cochlea, adjacent to the cochleostomy and more distally in the scala tympani, during a lubricant safety study[43] (**Fig. 9–3**). Bone dust introduced during cochleostomy can be pushed further into the scala by the electrode insertion.

Electrode introduction and insertion occurs after cochleostomy. An electrode will directly elevate or penetrate the basilar membrane if inserted at an inappropriate angle. Damage from this type of trauma is seen as either focal or diffuse elevation, focal penetration, or diffuse disruption (**Fig. 9–4**). An electrode that penetrates focally will occupy the scala vestibuli or scala media in the upper cochlea. Diffuse disruption represents the most severe form of

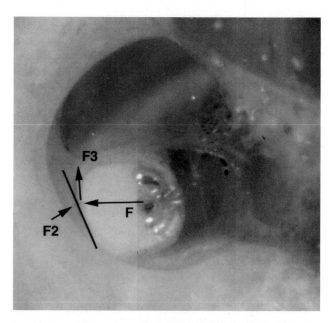

Figure 9–5 Surface view of an electrode lying along the outer wall of the scala tympani. Note the electrode exerts a force (F), which is met with a resistant force perpendicular to the point of outer wall contact (F2). The resultant force vector (F3) is directed superiorly.

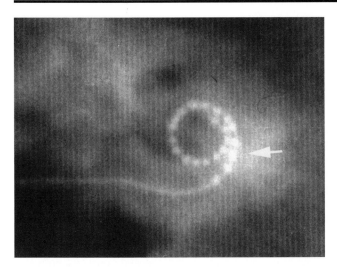

Figure 9–6 A fluoroscopic view of a deeply inserted perimodiolar electrode. White arrow denotes the initial point of contact during insertion at the level of the proximal pars ascendens.

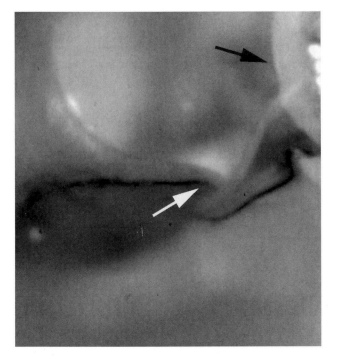

Figure 9–7 An osseous spiral lamina fracture (white arrow) caused by a perimodiolar electrode (black arrow) that penetrated the basilar membrane.

basilar membrane. The outer wall trauma is well documented in cadaver temporal bone studies and postmortem studies. Fluoroscopically, the first point of contact between the electrode and the outer wall is the lower mid-pars ascendens, the same region that is often shown to have the most neo-ossification on postmortem studies[41] (**Fig. 9–6**).

Medial osseous fractures, either of the osseus spiral lamina or the modiolar wall, occur from direct trauma to these bony structures by the electrode or by pressure against the modiolus caused by the active process of medialization of the perimodiolar electrodes. If an electrode penetrates the basilar membrane and lies proximally in the scala tympani and distally in the scala vestibuli, direct pressure will be exerted on the osseus spiral lamina during the coiling process. A space-occupying electrode that has penetrated the basilar membrane will also cause osseus spiral lamina fractures as the electrode is inserted and forced medially by the bulk of the more lateral positioning band (**Fig. 9–7**). Chronic modiolar pressure may cause a process of bony resorption and erosion over time, jeopardizing the integrity of the spiral ganglion cells. This potential mechanism of trauma cannot be evaluated by our model, as long-term animal studies are necessary to evaluate the effects of chronic modiolar wall pressure. Cervera-Paz and Linthicum[44] recently described an outer wall osseous erosive process in a human temporal bone in a patient who had a straight electrode placed prior to death. This defect was most likely from destructive outer wall pressure over time.

Intrascalar hydraulic forces are created during the insertion process. Because fluid is not a compressible substance, forces generated by intrascalar infusions of lubricant and electrode insertion are evenly distributed throughout the fluids of the cochlea and labyrinth (**Fig. 9–8**). Local cellular damage as well as more distal vestibular neuroepithelial damage may occur as a result of these hydraulic forces. This phenomenon may explain dizziness and balance disturbance in some patients immediately postimplantation. Larger, space-occupying electrodes may generate more fluid pressures, acting like a piston in a cylinder. Fluid egress around the advancing electrode is essential to avoid the potential for high hydraulic pressure generation. Further studies need to be conducted to evaluate the effects of hydraulic forces on intracochlear tissues.

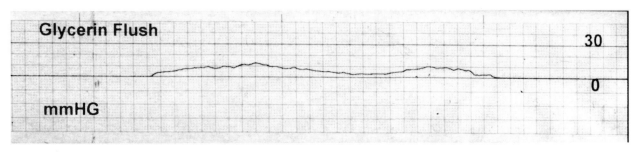

Figure 9–8 A hydraulic pressure tracing of a vigorous infusion of glycerin lubricant measured from the superior canal ampulla. Note pressures of up to 12 mmHg are generated.

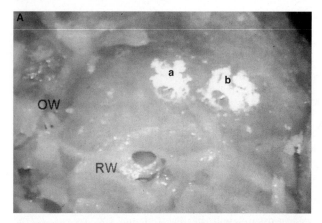

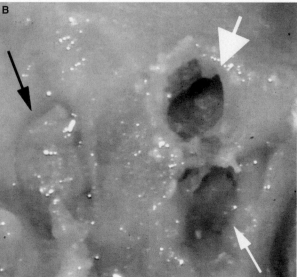

Figure 9–9 **(A)** A cadaver temporal bone depicting center point for cochleostomies 2 mm (a) and 2.5 mm (b) inferior to the oval window (OW) lip. RW, round window. **(B)** Completed cochleostomy (large white arrow) allowing visualization of the modiolar wall, outer cochlear wall, and the undersurface of the basilar membrane. Black arrow, oval window; small white arrow, round window niche.

Prevention of Cochlear Implant Trauma

The cochleostomy should be located inferior and anterior to the round window membrane, allowing entry into the scala tympani without causing direct injury to the spiral ligament, basilar membrane, or the medial osseous structures. Direct round window insertion is receiving renewed interest. Temporal bone insertions with various cochleostomy positions have shown that a cochleostomy centered ~2.5 mm from the lower edge of the oval window, anterior and inferior to the round window, always decreases the incidence of damage to the aforementioned structures (**Fig. 9–9**). Cochleostomy size is somewhat dependent on the electrode to be used; however, at a minimum it is advisable to visualize the outer wall of the scala tympani. Enlarging the cochleostomy in a more inferior, anterior, or superior direction might be necessary for larger electrodes. Care should be taken to avoid the introduction of blood and bone dust into the scalar lumen. This can be accomplished by burring down the cochlear bone until the endosteum is visualized, and then irrigating the field and suctioning away particulate matter before opening the endosteum. Next the endosteum is entered and a lubricating solution is gently infused over the cochleostomy. The solution should have a specific gravity that is denser than blood and bone particulate. Blood and bone dust will float out of the cochlea and not be driven deeper into the scalar lumen. The solution will also act as a lubricant, reducing frictional forces between the electrode and the cochlear walls. Sterile surgical grade glycerin is a safe, inexpensive option with all the favorable properties mentioned above.[43] The use of lubricants might be avoided when hearing preservation is attempted.

The angle of electrode insertion in both the superior-inferior and the medial-lateral direction is a controllable trauma variable. Care should be taken to direct the electrode carefully around the first turn without contacting the medial modiolar wall or the basilar membrane (**Fig. 9–10**). Tip rollover, electrode bending, modiolar injuries, and basal membrane injuries can be prevented to a large degree. Insertion tools may also assist in directing the electrode appropriately in the early insertion phase. A properly initiated cochlear implant electrode insertion reduces the chances of untoward events later in the insertion process.

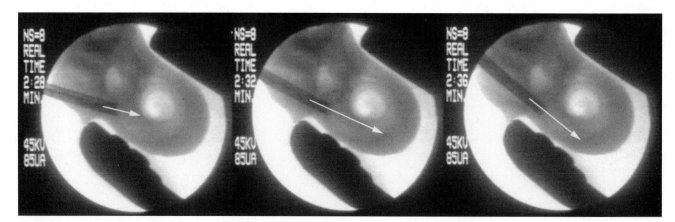

Figure 9–10   Fluoroscopic analysis of potential insertion angles showing initial point of electrode contact.

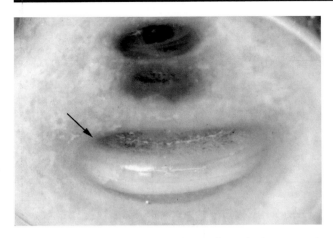

Figure 9–11 Smooth outer wall of new electrode design seen in pars ascendens under basilar membrane (arrow).

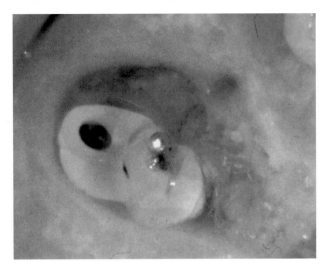

Figure 9–12 Early space filling perimodiolar design pushing electrode against modiolar wall.

Newer electrode designs have the raised or recessed electrical contacts directed medially with a smooth outer electrode wall. This design feature combined with a lubricant reduces frictional forces and insertional trauma (**Fig. 9–11**). The manufacturers should continue to refine electrodes with coiling and positioning properties that minimize outer wall forces during insertion. Appropriately sized space-occupying positioning electrodes will reduce hydraulic forces and basilar membrane trauma as well as limit osseous spiral lamina and modiolar wall pressure (**Fig. 9–12**). Calibrated insertional stop points and insertion tools that allow tactile feedback will prevent unnecessary overinsertion that might bend or damage the electrode or cause electrode displacement into the upper scala. With straight electrode designs, the surgeon is required to weigh the risks of electrode damage with the benefits of deeper insertion at every cochlear implantation. A well-placed, more shallow electrode insertion is undoubtedly of more benefit

to a patient than an overinserted, multiply bent and kinked electrode. Caution must be taken to avoid excessive insertional forces. Although cochlear implants are intended to survive 10 years or longer, failures and reimplantation are inevitable. Any electrode design must allow explantation without causing undue trauma and permit reimplantation in the same cochlea. Postimplantation cochlear fibrosis and neo-ossification affects the diameter of the cochlear lumen and replacement electrode, which argues for smaller diameter electrodes in the future.

Force Reduction with Advance Off-Stylet Technique and a Perimodiolar Electrode

In a recently published study, basal-turn intracochlear forces were quantified using a calibrated Instron 5543 Universal Force Measurement System (Instron, Canton, MA) utilizing

Insertion Force Analysis

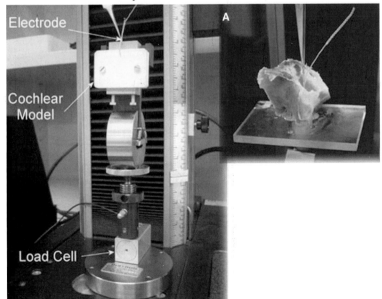

Figure 9–13 Instron System with cochlear Teflon model and load cell underneath (left image). Inset **(A)** is a close-up of electrode insertion in a temporal bone. (From Roland JT. A model for cochlear implant electrode insertion and force evaluation: results with a new electrode design and insertion technique. Laryngoscope 2005;115:1325–1339, with permission.)

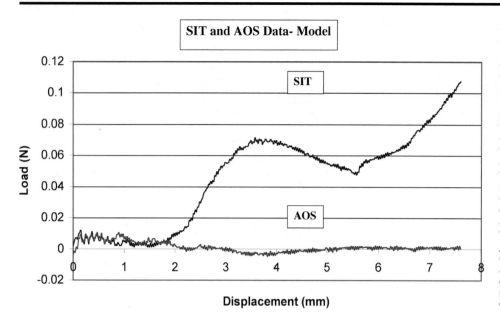

Figure 9–14 Cumulative mean force curves as measured with the Instron system with the Contour electrode and standard insertion technique (SIT) and the Advance electrode and the Advance Off Stylet (AOS) technique in the cochlear model. Note the two-peak force curve (SIT). The first peak occurs at the point where the electrode contacts the pars ascendens and forces rise as the electrode travels along the outer wall. The lower tracing shows the AOS curve where minimal force is exerted on the outer wall except when the tip first contacts the outer wall of the pars ascendens, prior to advancing off the stylet. N, newtons. (From Roland JT. A model for cochlear implant electrode insertion and force evaluation: results with a new electrode design and insertion technique. Laryngoscope 2005;115:1325–1339, with permission.)

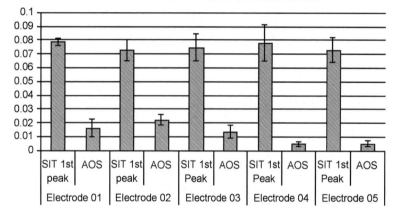

Figure 9–15 Insertion force results for all five trials with the Contour SIT and the Advance electrode with the AOS in the Teflon model. The SIT value is the first peak. (From Roland JT. A model for cochlear implant electrode insertion and force evaluation: results with a new electrode design and insertion technique. Laryngoscope 2005;115:1325–1339, with permission.)

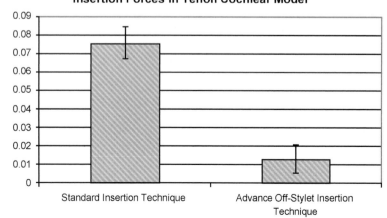

Figure 9–16 Mean insertion force results for all five trials with the Contour SIT and the Advance electrode with the AOS in the Teflon model. The SIT value is for the first peak. (From Roland JT. A model for cochlear implant electrode insertion and force evaluation: results with a new electrode design and insertion technique. Laryngoscope 2005;115:1325–1339, with permission.)

A

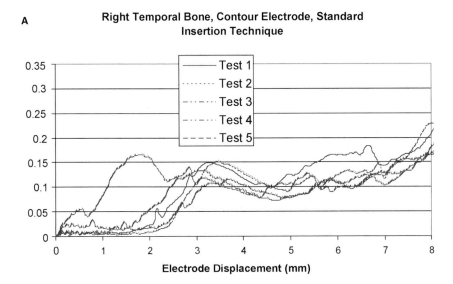

Right Temporal Bone, Contour Electrode, Standard Insertion Technique

Electrode Displacement (mm)

B

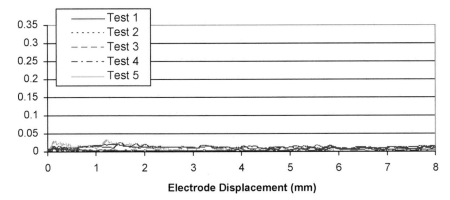

Right Temporal bone, Contour Electrode with Softip, Advance Off-Stylet Insertion Technique

Electrode Displacement (mm)

Figure 9–17 Insertion force results for all five trials with the Contour SIT **(A)** and the Advance electrode with the AOS **(B)** in the right temporal bone. These results reveal the same pattern as seen in the cochlear model. (From Roland JT. A model for cochlear implant electrode insertion and force evaluation: results with a new electrode design and insertion technique. Laryngoscope 2005;115:1325–1339, with permission.)

a static 50 N load cell. A personal computer running Instron Merlin Test Control Software version 5.11 (Instron) captured force and displacement data every 10 milliseconds. The direction of force is in the opposite direction from the direction of electrode insertion, and the force was first applied at approximately the midpoint of the ascending limb of the basal turn of the cochlea. This is the same region of the cochlea that sustains first contact and trauma with all existing cochlear implant electrodes. Electrode insertions are performed at a rate of 120 mm/min into a standard polytetrafluoroethylene (PTFE) cochlea model and in the temporal bones (**Fig. 9–13**). A 10% solution of Bathox Body Wash with cocoa butter (Bathox P/L, Cipping Norton, NSW, Australia) in deionized water was used as a lubricant to approximate the intracochlear environment and to reduce frictional forces between the Teflon walls and the Silastic electrode. The insertion rate and direction of insertion approximated the actual surgical experience in live humans.

Five Contour electrodes with the standard insertion technique (SIT) were evaluated in the plastic model and in a right and left temporal bone. The Contour electrode behaves as a straight electrode on initial insertion. Five Contour

Advance electrodes were inserted with the AOS technique in the plastic model and in a right and left temporal bone.

Results of force studies of the cochlear model with Contour electrode–SIT: A consistent and characteristic force curve was observed with each insertion (**Fig. 9–14**). The force began to rise after the electrode tip made contact with the back wall of the cochlea (145 to 180 degrees). The force rose to a first peak and then fell slightly as the electrode bent and rounded the first turn and then rose to a maximum nearing complete insertion.

Cochlear model with Advance electrode–AOS: Minimal force against the back wall of the cochlear was observed (**Fig. 9–14**). There was a minimal negative force observed at the same depth of insertion where the first peak was noted above. This most likely represents the tip touching the modiolar wall as it advances off the stylet and moves from the outer to the inner wall. **Fig. 9–15** presents the data, with standard deviations, for each insertion trial in the model, and **Fig. 9–16** presents the mean for all the trials. The SIT value represents the maximum value of the first peak. These data have statistical significance ($p = .001$).

A

Left Temporal Bone, Contour Electrode, Standard Insertion Technique

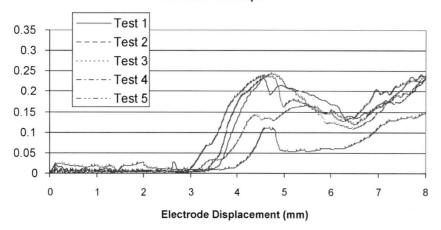

B

Left Temporal Bone, Contour Electrode with Softip, Advance Off-Stylet Insertion Technique

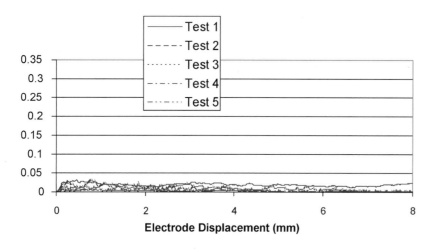

Figure 9–18 Insertion force results for all five trials with the Contour SIT **(A)** and the Advance electrode with the AOS **(B)** in the left temporal bone. These results reveal the same pattern as seen in the cochlear model. (From Roland JT. A model for cochlear implant electrode insertion and force evaluation: results with a new electrode design and insertion technique. Laryngoscope 2005;115:1325–1339, with permission.)

Right temporal bone with Contour electrode–SIT: A two-peak-force curve configuration was observed in the right temporal bone for all five trials (**Fig. 9–17A**). The forces measured in the right human temporal bone were higher than the forces measured in the cochlear Teflon model.

Right temporal bone with Advance electrode–AOS: Only slight forces were noted with the AOS technique using the Advance electrode in all five trials (**Fig. 9–17B**).

Left temporal bone with Contour electrode–SIT: A two-peak-force curve configuration was found in the left temporal bone for all five trials (**Fig. 9–18A**). The first force peak was observed at a deeper electrode insertion depth than in the right temporal bone. This appeared to be due to either a different insertion force measurement start point with the equipment or to variance in cochlear anatomy.

Left temporal bone with Advance electrode–AOS: Only slight forces were noted with the AOS technique using the Advance electrode in all five trials (**Fig. 9–18B**).

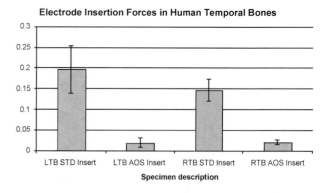

Figure 9–19 Summary mean insertion force results for all five trials with the Contour SIT and the Advance electrode with the AOS in both temporal bones. These results reveal the same pattern as seen in the cochlear model. (From Roland JT. A model for cochlear implant electrode insertion and force evaluation: results with a new electrode design and insertion technique. Laryngoscope 2005;115:1325–1339, with permission.)

Fig. 9–19 represents the mean summary data for the right and left temporal bone for the Contour with SIT and the Advance with AOS. The SIT data represent the maximum value of the first peak. These data have statistical significance ($p = .001$).

This study and data are from a recently published article by the first author (J.T.R.).[40] It is the feeling of the author that an appropriately sized (thin) perimodiolar electrode that is properly designed and inserted with an AOS technique (the electrode coils on insertion and avoids outer wall contact) is currently the best way to diminish intracochlear forces, avoid intracochlear trauma, and ensure reliable electrode positioning in normal cochleae.

◆ Current Surgical Technique and Electrode Choice

Full atraumatic scala tympani electrode placement is the goal of every cochlear implantation (CI) operation. This can be achieved in most CI surgeries except in patients with obstructed or malformed cochleae. Although there are many modifications and variations to the CI procedure, the electrode insertion is the vital step. Optimum CI results depend first on optimal electrode placement. Improperly or suboptimally placed electrodes and kinked or damaged electrodes result in poor cochlear implant functioning and poorer outcomes.

◆ The Normal Cochlea

CI electrode insertion requires access to the cochlea through the facial recess approach. Thinning the posterior external auditory canal is the first step in visualizing and performing the facial recess. After mastoidectomy the descending facial nerve is skeletonized so that it can be seen through a thin layer of bone. The short process of the incus is also visualized but a thin incus bar remains intact. (The incus bar can be taken down and the incus removed if more visualization is needed.) Preoperative imaging (CT scan) would reveal, and alert the surgeon to, an abnormal course of the facial nerve and pneumatization of the facial recess. The chorda tympani nerve is visualized through its course from the facial nerve to the chorda iter posterior, where it enters the middle ear. Bone between the facial nerve and the chorda tympani nerve is slowly removed with serially smaller diamond burrs.

An adequate facial recess facilitates good visualization of the stapedial tendon, the round window, and the cochlear promontory. To properly visualize and gain access to the cochlear promontory for the cochleostomy, the facial recess must be enlarged inferiorly and the bone inferior to the stapedial tendon must be removed, anterior to the facial nerve. The chorda tympani nerve can be spared in nearly all cases. Care should be taken not to injure the annular ligament of the tympanic membrane. Copious irrigation should be used to avoid thermal damage to the nerve when skeletonizing the facial nerve and removing the bone anterior to the facial nerve. An adequate facial recess approach to the middle ear allows full access to the round window niche and the inferior cochlea.

The cochleostomy is made, using a 1.5- or 1.0-mm diamond burr, inferior and anterior to the round window membrane (**Fig. 9–20**). Drilling off the round window niche may be required in some cases to properly visualize the membrane. The electrode choice and the insertion tool used for that electrode determine the cochleostomy size. Round window insertions can also be performed. Care should be taken not to drill into a hypotympanic air cell that might look just like the round window. The ideal cochleostomy position is inferior and slightly anterior to the round window membrane. A

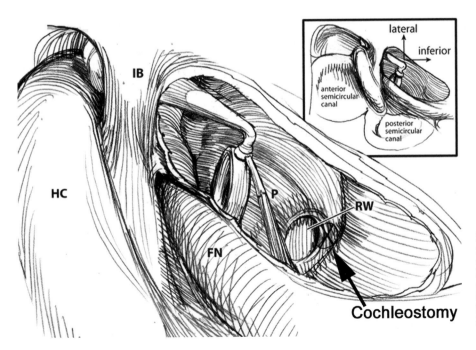

Figure 9–20 Representation of dissected mastoid and adequate facial recess and cochleostomy position. FN, facial nerve; HC, horizontal canal; IB, incus bar; P, promontory; RW, round window. (From Roland JT. Cochlear implant electrode insertion. Oper Tech Otolaryngol 2005;16:86–92, with permission from Elsevier.)

more superior cochleostomy placement would result in injury to the spiral ligament or the basilar membrane or even result in direct entry to the scala vestibuli.

The bone is slowly removed over the cochlea, by saucerizing the rounded dome, until the endosteum of the scala tympani is seen. After removal of bone dust and blood, the endosteum is carefully opened with a small pick or a rasp revealing the lumen of the scala tympani. Sharp edges of the cochleostomy should also be removed with the rasp. Healon or 50% glycerin can be used over the cochleostomy to prevent the ingress of blood or bone dust and to act as a lubricant. The egress of cerebrospinal fluid (CSF) might be encountered when operating on a cochlear malformation and is managed by slight head elevation and tight packing with strips of mastoid periosteum around the inserted electrode. Lumbar subarachnoid spinal fluid diversion is rarely necessary to seal a leak.

General Electrode Insertion Principles

In general, receiver/stimulator fixation is desirable prior to electrode array insertion. Manipulation of the device after electrode insertion may result in the extrusion of a perfectly placed electrode and require reinsertion. In some circumstances, however, rotating a straight electrode in a clockwise or counterclockwise direction may facilitate further insertion when the electrode appears to be hung up and significant resistance is encountered. To do this the receiver stimulator must be held in the noninserting hand.

Proper cochlear implant electrode insertion requires an understanding of the orientation of the cochlea when inserting through the facial recess. The lumen of the basal turn is oriented in a plane nearly parallel to the external auditory canal wall. Therefore, the direction of electrode insertion should be down the midportion of the proximal basal turn with care taken not to push the electrode through the basilar membrane or firmly against the medial modiolar wall or the outer wall. This will create potentially damaging forces on the cochlea or potentially lead to electrode misplacement or kinking and bending, which will complicate a smooth electrode insertion and potentially damage the electrode array. Likewise, the surgeon should avoid excessive force when inserting an electrode. The tactile perception of resistance to insertion indicates a problem with insertion, and reassessment and evaluation is prudent. Lubricants such as Healon and glycerin are used at many centers to facilitate electrode insertion but are not necessary. Various inserting tools are available from the manufacturers, and some centers have modified currently available inserting tools. Electrode insertion should proceed until the entire array is inside the cochleostomy or until significant resistance to insertion is felt. It is highly recommended that practice in a temporal bone laboratory be undertaken prior to inserting a new electrode design for the first time. Several different device-specific inserting tools including claws and forceps exist, and familiarity with these instruments makes the electrode insertion process easier.

Every cochleostomy should be packed with periosteum around the electrode array. This maneuver enhances the creation of scar tissue that seals the cochleostomy, thus preventing dizziness due to perilymph leak, infectious complications, and electrode extrusion.

◆ Electrodes for the Normal Cochlea

Straight Electrode Arrays

Cochlear Corporation K Electrode

The K electrode is available on the Nucleus receiver stimulators. It is a straight electrode array with 22 active banded contacts and 10 stiffening rings and occupies an antimodiolar or outer wall position when fully inserted. The cochleostomy can be as small as 1 mm in diameter when inserting this device. The receiver stimulator is held in the nondominant hand, and the electrode is introduced into the cochlea with a claw instrument provided by the Cochlear Corporation. Jeweler's forceps and alligator forceps are also useful instruments to have available. The receiver stimulator can be slightly rotated in a counterclockwise manner on the right ear and clockwise on the left ear if resistance to smooth insertion is encountered. Attempts at full electrode insertion should be made; however, the avoidance of kinking and damaging the electrode is essential. The insertion of all active electrodes and at least five stiffening rings is desirable for access to the speech frequency areas of the cochlea.

Med-El Combi 40+ Electrode

This 31-mm straight electrode is inserted with a claw or modified alligator forceps. The active contacts are on opposite sides of this oval-shaped array. The manufacturer recommends modifications to the aforementioned cochleostomy technique. Rather than saucerize the promontory, it is advantageous to make the cochleostomy with the 1-mm diamond burr straight through the cochlear wall creating a tunnel with a 1.2-mm diameter. The walls of the tunnel support the electrode during insertion. Additionally, the manufacturers recommend securing the receiver stimulator prior to electrode insertion. This electrode is the longest of the currently available electrodes, and Med-El recommends full insertion to the hub if possible.

Advanced Bionics J Electrode (Slightly Curved)

This slightly curved electrode is most commonly inserted with an inserting tool provided by the manufacturer. The cochleostomy should be drilled to a 1.2- to 1.4-mm diameter. The contacts are on the modiolar (inner) surface only, and therefore orientation of the electrodes toward the modiolus is essential. The J electrode can be inserted manually without the tool using a claw or forceps if needed in the case of a very narrow facial recess. A thinner metal insertion tube is available, which allows better visualization of the cochleostomy through the facial recess. The electrode should be expelled from the plastic tube that it is packaged with and reloaded in the metal tube prior.

Perimodiolar Electrodes

In the past 5 years, perimodiolar electrodes have been introduced to the market. These electrodes are designed to coil during or after insertion to occupy a position closer to the modiolar wall of the cochlea where the spiral ganglion cells reside. These electrodes require a different insertion technique than the straight electrodes, and specialized insertion tools have been created to facilitate insertions. The potential advantages of perimodiolar electrodes include: (1) more selective stimulation of spiral ganglion cell subpopulations; (2) less current required for each stimulus thereby reducing the power consumption; and (3) less damage to the cochlear elements. These potential advantages may translate into better speech understanding using newer processing strategies, longer battery life, and preservation of residual hearing.

Cochlear Corporation Contour and Contour Advance Electrode

The receiver/stimulator should be seated in the well and secured prior to electrode insertion. The Contour Electrode is advanced into a 1.4-mm diameter cochleostomy until the middle hub is just inside the cochleostomy. At this point the electrode is gently held in place with a claw or forceps and the stylet is withdrawn entirely allowing the electrode to coil inside the cochlea. As the electrode contacts are only on the modiolar surface, correct orientation of the electrode in the scala tympani is important.

The Contour Advance electrode is inserted into the cochlea only to a marker on the antimodiolar side, ~11 mm. While holding the stylet firmly with a forceps in one hand, advance the electrode off the stylet into the cochlea using a forceps or claw. This maneuver allows the electrode to coil during insertion, thus reducing forces on the cochlear outer walls, obtaining a more consistent perimodiolar position. An insertion tool is under development but is currently not marketed. Reloading the stylet in both the Contour and Contour Advance electrode can be performed with an electrode-straightening tool. The maneuver requires delicate advancement of the stylet, taking care to not perforate the Silastic material.

Advanced Bionics Helix Electrode

The Helix electrode is packaged loaded onto a stylet and insertion tool tip. The receiver/stimulator should be secured first and then the electrode/tool tip combination is loaded onto a tool handle. The fins of the insertion tool are placed within a 1.6-mm diameter cochleostomy, and the footpad is engaged onto the cochleostomy inferior edge. The electrode is advanced off the stylet into the cochlea as the tool is pushed gently toward the cochleostomy. The electrode is then disengaged from the tool using a small claw or right-angle pick.

◆ The Obstructed or Malformed Cochlea

Making a cochleostomy in a patient with a malformed or obstructed cochlea requires modifications in the standard technique. Both CT scans and magnetic resonance imaging (MRI) studies are obtained in all of these patients. Thorough review of the imaging studies allows the surgeon to anticipate an abnormally positioned facial nerve, to evaluate the cochlear/vestibular malformations for intracavity septations, and to evaluate the fluid content and patency of the obstructed cochlea. Additionally, the nerve content of the internal auditory canal can be evaluated. This information may aid the implanting team in deciding which ear is best to implant.

The common cavity malformation is approached through the mastoid antrum in most cases. After delineating the cavity by removing air cells, the dome of the cavity is flattened and drilled until the endosteum is exposed for a 1-mm diameter. The endosteum is opened using a small right-angle pick. If a CSF gusher is encountered, the head of the bed is elevated and when the gusher stops the electrode is inserted. We utilize real time fluoroscopic guidance to avoid bending, kinking, intrameatal placement (in the internal auditory canal), and overinsertion of the electrode. Some surgeons prefer making a slot-like cochleostomy and introducing the electrode array as a slightly bent **U**-shape. In both techniques the cochleostomy must be packed tightly (like a champagne cork) to prevent postoperative CSF leak. The stimulable neural elements of the common cavity are most likely lying on the outer wall of the cochlea or attached to septations within the cochlea. Electrode insertion must be performed as delicately as possible so as to not disturb these elements.

Implanting the hypoplastic cochlea presents probably the most challenging cochlear implant electrode insertion. These cavities are usually only a few millimeters in diameter and are approached through a facial recess. Carefully analyzing the imaging studies facilitates determining the correct cochleostomy location. Cochleostomy size should be kept as small as possible. Removing the incus bar and the incus allows excellent visualization of the facial nerve and the middle ear. We also use intraoperative fluoroscopic guidance to locate and insert the hypoplastic cochlea. As in the common cavity malformation, the neural elements are undoubtedly on the outer cavity wall, and delicate insertion is paramount.

The obstructed cochlea presents an interesting challenge to the cochlear implant surgeon. We have adopted an algorithm for implanting the obstructed cochlea (**Fig. 9–21**). The basal turn of the cochlea is first explored via a normally placed cochleostomy. If fibrosis or new bone is encountered, attempts at removal are made. If a patent lumen of the scala tympani is found before or at the ascending turn of the cochlea, a scala tympani insertion is performed. Med-El provides a test electrode to probe the lumen prior to opening the actual device onto the sterile field. We have used a very small Boogie catheter for the same purposes. If the lumen remains obstructed, then the cochleostomy is extended superiorly to the scala vestibuli. This lumen is often patent in otosclerosis and postmeningitis cases, and a full scala vestibuli insertion

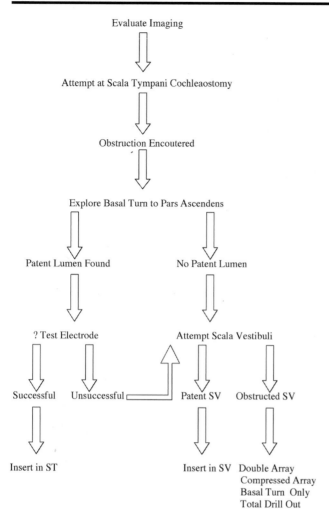

Evaluate Imaging

Attempt at Scala Tympani Cochleaostomy

Obstruction Encoutered

Explore Basal Turn to Pars Ascendens

Patent Lumen Found   No Patent Lumen

? Test Electrode   Attempt Scala Vestibuli

Successful   Unsuccessful   Patent SV   Obstructed SV

Insert in ST   Insert in SV   Double Array
Compressed Array
Basal Turn Only
Total Drill Out

Figure 9–21 Obstructed cochleae algorithm.

is desirable when the scala tympani is occluded. If the scala vestibuli is also obliterated, then a second cochleostomy is performed just anterior to the oval window. To facilitate access to this area the incus bar is taken down, the incus and stapes suprastructure is removed, and a cochleostomy is performed just anterior and lateral to the stapes footplate. Copious irrigation and caution is used to avoid heating or damaging the facial nerve in the postgeniculum region. The cochleariform process is used as a landmark for the superior limit of dissection. The cochleostomy opening is drilled until either a lumen is encountered or new bone is also encountered. If a lumen is found, a split or double array is used. One branch of the array is laid in the inferior basal turn

tunnel previously described, and the other branch is inserted in either an antegrade or retrograde manner in the superior cochleostomy. If new bone is obstructing the second turn, a careful superior tunnel is made with the 1- or 0.5-mm diamond burr or a rasp. This tunnel is directed slightly superiorly, toward the tensor tympani muscle, to avoid entering the modiolus and damaging the neural elements. The second branch of the array is then inserted in the superior tunnel. The electrodes should not be overinserted in either tunnel to avoid kinking or damaging the array. The cochleostomies are packed firmly with periosteum to secure the upper and lower array.

Electrodes for Malformed and Obstructed Cochleae

The straight Cochlear Corporation K electrode and the Med-El Combi 40+ electrode are best suited for the common cavity malformation and the hypoplastic cochlea. The electrode contacts are circumferential on the K electrode and on both sides of the electrode on the Combi 40+. Electrodes with modiolar facing contacts and coiling electrodes are not recommended in common cavity malformations. Med-El also manufactures a specific "common cavity" electrode, which has contacts only in the middle of the electrode and requires two cochleostomies for the recommended insertion technique. Med-El also manufactures a compressed electrode array where the contacts are compressed into a much shorter distance. This electrode may also be advantageous for the hypoplastic cochlea.

All available electrodes from all manufacturers can be potentially used for obstructed cochleae. The Med-El compressed or straight array, the Cochlear Corporation K electrode, or the Advanced Bionics J electrode can be used if a lumen is found in lower basal or ascending basal turns. The perimodiolar electrode arrays could also be used; however, the Helix electrode may not be desirable due to the larger diameter tip. Any of these electrodes might also be used in the scala vestibuli. The Med-El split electrode or the Cochlear Corporation double array is used with the dual cochleostomy technique. These devices have two separate electrode arrays with the number of contacts split between the arrays.

The cochleostomy and electrode insertion is probably the most important aspect of cochlear implant surgery. Optimal results with cochlear implantation depend on optimal electrode placement. Careful evaluation of the imaging studies and attention to device/electrode selection as well as a planned thoughtful operation should result in a favorable outcome.

References

1. Stevens SS. On hearing by electrical stimulation. J Acoust Soc Am 1937;8:191–195
2. Shah SB, Chung JH, Jackler RK. Lodestones, quackery, and science: electrical stimulation of the ear before cochlear implants. Am J Otol 1997;18:665–670
3. Jones RK, Stevens SS, Lurie MH. Three mechanisms of hearing by electrical stimulation. J Acoust Soc Am 1940;12:281–290
4. Graham JM. From frogs' legs to pieds-noirs and beyond: some aspects of cochlear implantation. J Laryngol Otol 2003;117:675–685
5. Spelman FA. The past, present, and future of cochlear prostheses. IEEE Eng Med Biol Mag 1999;18:27–33
6. Eisen MD. Djourno, Eyries, and the first implanted electrical neural stimulator to restore hearing. Otol Neurotol 2003;24:500–506
7. Michelson RP. Electrical stimulation of the human cochlea. Arch Otolaryngol 1971;93:317–323
8. Simmons FB. Electrical stimulation of the auditory nerve in cats: long term electrophysiological and histological results. Ann Otol Rhinol Laryngol 1979;88:533–539

9.   Simmons FB. Cochlear implants. Arch Otolaryngol 1969;89:61–69

10. Simmons FB, Mathews RB, Walker MG, White RL. A functioning multichannel auditory nerve stimulator. Acta Otolaryngol 1979;87:170–175

11. Michelson RP, Merzenich MM, Petit CR, Schindler RA. A cochlear prosthesis: further clinical observations; preliminary results of physiological studies. Laryngoscope 1973;83:1116–1122

12. House WF. Cochlear implants. Ann Otol Rhinol Laryngol 1976;85[suppl 27 (3Pt2)]:1–93

13. House WF, Urban J. Long term results of electrode implantation and electronic stimulation of the cochlea in man. Ann Otol Rhinol Laryngol 1973;82:504–517

14. Berliner KI, House WF. Cochlear implants: an overview and bibliography. Am J Otol 1981;2:277–282

15. Patrick JF, Clark GM. The Nucleus 22-channel cochlear implant system. Ear Hear 1991;12(4 suppl):3S–9S

16. Lai WK, Dillier N, Laszig R, Fisch U. Results from a pilot study using the Nucleus CI24M/SP5 cochlear implant system. Am J Otol 1997;18:S35–S36

17. Schindler RA, Kessler DK. Preliminary results with the Clarion cochlear implant. Laryngoscope 1992;102:1006–1013

18. Schindler RA, Kessler DK. Clarion cochlear implant: phase I investigational results. Am J Otol 1993;14:263–272

19. Kessler DK. The CLARION Multi-Strategy Cochlear Implant. Ann Otol Rhinol Laryngol Suppl 1999;177:8–16

20. Muller J, Schon F, Helms J. Fast-stimulator cochlear implant systems—the Wurzburg experience using the Med-El Combi 40: surgical considerations and preliminary results. Adv Otorhinolaryngol 1997;52:272–273

21. Helms J, Muller J, Schon F, et al. Evaluation of performance with the Combi 40 cochlear implant in adults: a multicentric clinical study. ORL J Otorhinolaryngol Relat Spec 1997;59:23–35

22. Zierhofer CM, Hochmair IJ, Hochmair ES. The advanced Combi 40+ cochlear implant. Am J Otol 1997;18:S37–S38

23. Fayad JN, Luxford W, Linthicum FH. The Clarion electrode positioner: temporal bone studies. Am J Otol 2000;21:226–229

24. Zwolan T, Kileny PR, Smith S, Mills D, Koch D, Osberger M. Adult cochlear implant patient performance with evolving electrode technology. Otol Neurotol 2001;22:844–849

25. Tykocinski M, Saunders E, Cohen LR, et al. The Contour electrode array: safety study and initial patient trials of a new perimodiolar design. Otol Neurotol 2001;22:33–41

26. Parkinson AJ, Arcaroli J, Staller SJ, Arndt PL, Cosgriff A, Ebinger K. The Nucleus 24 Contour cochlear implant system: adult clinical trial results. Ear Hear 2002;23:41S–48S

27. Leake-Jones PA, Walsh SM, Merzenich MM. Cochlear pathology following chronic intracochlear electrical stimulation. Ann Otol Rhinol Laryngol Suppl 1981;90(2 Pt 3):6–8

28. Leake-Jones PA, Rebscher SJ. Cochlear pathology with chronically implanted scala tympani electrodes. Ann N Y Acad Sci 1983;405:203–223

29. Miller JM, Sutton D, Webster DB. Brainstem histopathology following chronic scala tympani implantation in monkeys. Ann Otol Rhinol Laryngol Suppl 1980;89(2 Pt 2):15–17

30. Sutton D, Miller JM. Cochlear implant effects on the spiral ganglion. Ann Otol Rhinol Laryngol 1983;92:53–58

31. Linthicum FH Jr, Fayad J, Otto S, et al. Inner ear morphologic changes resulting from cochlear implantation. Am J Otol 1991;(suppl 12):8–10

32. O'Leary MJ, Fayad J, House WF, Linthicum FH. Electrode insertion trauma in cochlear implantation. Ann Otol Rhinol Laryngol 1991;100:695–699

33. Fayad J, Linthicum FH, Otto SR, Galey FR, House WF. Cochlear implants: histologic findings related to performance in 16 human temporal bones. Ann Otol Rhinol Laryngol 1991;100:807–811

34. Linthicum FH, Fayad J, Otto SR, Galey FR, House WF. Cochlear implant histopathology. Am J Otol 1991;12:245–311

35. Nadol JB Jr. Patterns of neural degeneration in the human cochlea and auditory nerve: implications for cochlear implantation. Otolaryngol Head Neck Surg 1997;117:220–228

36. Ketten D. Cochlear implant electrode position determined in vivo with computed tomography. Presentation at the Auditory Prosthesis Conference, Asilomar, CA, 1999

37. Tykocinski M, Cohen LT, Pyman BC, et al. Comparison of electrode position in the human cochlea using various perimodiolar electrode arrays. Am J Otol 2000;21:205–211

38. Gstoettner W, Franz P, Hamzavi J, et al. Intracochlear position of cochlear implant electrodes. Acta Otolaryngol 1999;119:229–233

39. Gstoettner W, Plenk H, Franz P, et al. Cochlear implant deep electrode insertion: extent of insertional trauma. Acta Otolaryngol 1997;117:274–277

40. Roland JT Jr. A model for cochlear implant electrode insertion and force evaluation: results with a new electrode design and insertion technique. Laryngoscope 2005;115:1325–1391

41. Roland JT Jr, Fishman AJ, Alexiades G, Cohen NL. Electrode to modiolus proximity: a fluoroscopic and histologic analysis. Am J Otol 2000;21:218–225

42. Kennedy DW. Multichannel cochlear implant electrodes: Mechanisms of insertion trauma. Laryngoscope 1987;97:42–49

43. Roland JT Jr, Magardino TM, Go JT, Hillman DE. Effects of glycerin, hyaluronic acid and hydroxypropyl methlycellulose on the spiral ganglion of the guinea pig cochlea. Ann Otol Rhinol Laryngol Suppl 1995;166:64–68

44. Cervera-Paz FJ, Linthicum FH Jr. Cochlear wall erosion after cochlear implantation. Ann Otol Rhinol Laryngol 2005;114:543–546

10

Complications of Cochlear Implant Surgery

Noel L. Cohen and

J. Thomas Roland Jr.

Surgical complications related to cochlear implants are classified as device related or medical-surgical. Device-related complications are mostly concerned with malfunctions and failures of the device or its various components, and may be due to faulty design, failure of electronic circuits or components, or external trauma. The trauma may have been caused by a blow to the head, a fall, or exposure to excessive current (as in a powerful electrostatic discharge or lightning strike). Although these complications are not caused by a medical or surgical condition, they require replacement of the device, and, therefore, additional surgery. Device failure, regardless of the underlying cause, is by far the most common reason for reimplantation.

Medical complications are not the result of conditions occurring due to the surgery or of the device itself. Otitis media may lead to infection under the flap, in the middle ear, or even the inner ear. Meningitis may also occur following cochlear implantation.

Surgical complications result directly from the operation itself, are largely avoidable, and may or may not compromise device function and the ability of the recipient to use or benefit from the implant. Surgical complications of multichannel cochlear implants are largely related to the incision and flap erosion and infection, electrode insertion, device migration, and facial nerve injury. These all have been steadily diminishing in frequency over time, in both adults and children.[1–6]

The avoidance of surgical complications begins with the thorough evaluation of the patient, continues through careful planning of the operation, and ends with meticulous surgery and postoperative observation.[7] A major goal of the evaluation process is to eliminate inappropriate candidates, such as those with useful hearing, active infection in the ear, or absence of a cochlea or eighth nerve. Anesthesia risk must also be considered. High-resolution computed tomography (CT) scanning and, when indicated, magnetic resonance imaging (MRI) are critical in the evaluation of the temporal bone anatomy and aid in both the evaluation of candidacy (e.g., aplasia of the cochlea) and surgical planning (e.g., cochlear dysplasia, aberrant facial nerve).

Whereas CT displays the anatomy of the mastoid, cochlea, vestibular apparatus, and associated structures such as the vestibular and cochlear aqueducts, the MRI shows soft tissue structures such as nerves and fluid such as cerebrospinal fluid (CSF) and perilymph/endolymph.[8,9] By thoroughly planning the surgery, especially in the potentially difficult case, many complications can be avoided. A special group within this category is the patient with a higher than average risk of meningitis following cochlear implant surgery.[10] The risk factors to be considered are children below the age of 24 months, adults above 65 years of age, those individuals with a prior history of meningitis or having a diminished immune capacity, and the presence of a dysplastic cochlea in the ear to be implanted.

These patients should be fully vaccinated against meningitis prior to surgery. In the case of children, the parents must be informed about the risk preoperatively. Meticulous surgical technique also is of major importance in this regard, in avoiding not only intraoperative problems but also postoperative events. Finally, careful follow-up is required to identify problems early and avoid true complications.

◆ Avoiding Complications During Surgery

Positioning and Anesthesia

The patient is placed on the operating table in the supine position, with the head turned away from the surgical site.[1,7] Facial nerve monitor electrodes are placed adjacent to the mouth and eye. Care should be taken that only short-acting paralytic agents are used for intubation to ensure that the monitor records any stimulation of the facial nerve. It is particularly important to use the monitor in operating on a dysplastic temporal bone, or in revising a case when the prior surgery was performed elsewhere.

Perioperative antibiotics are administered, in the form of a first-generation cephalosporin given just prior to incision. If the surgery should last more than 4 hours, a second dose is given. Perioperative antibiotics do not continue past this point unless a drain is placed or there is some reason to suspect an active infection. In this latter case, the implantation may need to be deferred.

Prep and Drape

A minimal amount of hair is shaved behind or above the ear to accommodate the incision. Often, in small children, no shave is needed. The area is then prepped and draped in routine fashion.

Incision

Planning the incision is critical for several reasons: it is imperative that the implants not abut the behind-the-ear speech processor commonly used (**Fig. 10–1**). The position of the device is chosen so that it lies on a relatively flat area of the skull with the takeoff of the electrode above the canthomeatal line. For adults, the long axis is at ± 45 degrees, but for small children it is more vertical. The incision must permit the safe insertion of the implant, and the flap outlined by the incision must have an adequate blood supply to prevent necrosis and breakdown. Because most surgeons have been using smaller incisions with excellent blood supply, flap-related complications have greatly diminished in frequency.[5,7] The use of infiltration with dilute (1:100,000 or 1:200,000) epinephrine and the monopolar cautery to make the incision limits blood loss during this phase of the surgery.

Raising the flap must also be done carefully, especially in the small child and the older (female) adult. The surgeon must dissect gently in the avascular plane deep to the scalp, avoiding drying of the flap and excessive retraction. When it is necessary to thin the flap of a heavy-set adult, care must be taken not to perforate the scalp or expose the roots of the hair follicles. Using the current short incision, starting at the mastoid tip, ascending behind the postauricular crease to the upper attachment of the auricle, then a short distance posterosuperior, we find that barbless fishhooks give sufficient retraction, and flap problems are routinely avoided. After retracting the flap posteriorly, we then raise a large anteriorly based Palva flap, exposing the areas for both the mastoidectomy and the well (**Fig. 10–2**). The flap will be closed over the proximal electrode at the end of the procedure.

We do not advocate the "minimally invasive" technique[11–13] since our standard incision for small children requires little or no shave, measures 4.0 to 4.5 cm in

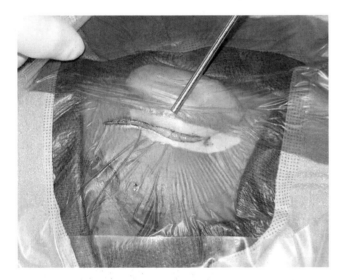

Figure 10–1 Placement of hardware and incision. The device is placed posterior to the behind-the-ear (BTE) speech processor and above the canthomeatal line. The incision is drawn and the center of the well is marked. The incision is usually made with the cutting current.

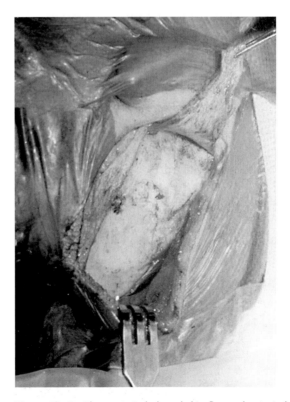

Figure 10–2 The posteriorly based skin flap and anteriorly based Palva flap are elevated and retracted with barbless fish hooks.

length, and permits both the drilling of a well and the tying down of the device. We do not think that any perceived cosmetic advantage should sacrifice safety.

The Well or Recess

The well may be created either prior to or following the mastoidectomy. We prefer the former because the location of the well or recess is very important as it determines the location of the device itself. Marking the center of the well with a single drop of methylene blue injected transcutaneously through the scalp prior to the incision simplifies this step. When creating the well, drilling down to dura is necessary in the case of a small child to lower the profile of the device as much as possible. The bone is thinned, and drilling to dura peripherally creates one or more bony islands. It is necessary to switch from cutting to diamond burrs to avoid trauma to the dura. If the dura is penetrated, it is closed by suturing a small piece of fascia or pericranium into the defect. The well for the Advanced Bionics (Valencia, CA) 90 K and the Nucleus 24 K and Contour devices (Cochlear

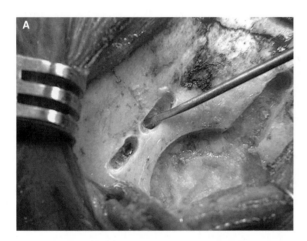

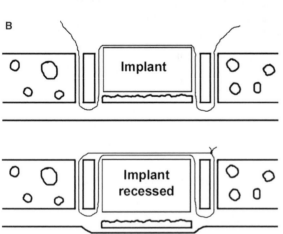

Figure 10–3 Well and tie-down holes. The well is drilled for the electronics of the Nucleus and Advanced Bionics devices and the entire body of the Med-El implants. **(A)** Tie-down holes for the Nucleus and ABC devices are drilled obliquely, whereas those for the Med-El devices are drilled vertically, and **(B)** a "sling" suture is placed.

Corporation, Sydney, Australia) is drilled to fit the protruding portion of the titanium case, including the electronics. Some surgeons drill the well sufficiently large for very small children so that the entire forward portion is recessed. The well for the Med-El Combi 40+ (Innsbruck, Austria) accommodates the entire ceramic case. After the well is created, tie-down holes are drilled in the adjacent bone to fix the device to the bone and to lower the profile as much as possible to diminish the chance of damage from external trauma (**Fig. 10–3**). This is particularly important in implanting a small child.

The Mastoidectomy

A simple mastoidectomy is performed in routine fashion, except that the superior and posterior cortex is not saucerized. Allowing some overhang creates an edge, under which the proximal electrode is placed. This keeps it below the level of the surface of the skull and eliminates tension, which might lead to electrode extrusion. For adults and older children with very well pneumatized mastoids, it is not necessary to drill out the periphery of the bone, such as a retrosigmoid, mastoid tip or zygomatic root cells. It is necessary to visualize the incus short process and the lateral canal as well as to thin the posterior external auditory canal wall, because these structures permit identification of the facial nerve and allow access to the facial recess. A channel is then drilled between the well and the mastoid cavity, sufficiently deep to allow the electrode or electrodes to lie deep to the surface of the bone, and in a gentle curve without angles or kinks.

The Facial Recess (Posterior Tympanotomy)

Opening the facial recess (performing the posterior tympanotomy) requires care since injury to the facial nerve, external auditory canal, and annulus of the tympanic membrane must be avoided. The facial nerve should routinely be identified but not exposed, whereas the chorda tympani may occasionally be sacrificed if the recess is very narrow. If the facial nerve has been exposed, every effort should be made not to cause either direct instrumental injury or thermal damage by the drill shaft while performing the cochleostomy. If the facial nerve has been exposed on its anterior surface, it should be protected at the end of the surgery by placing a piece of Silastic sheeting between the electrode and the nerve. If the anatomy is difficult or the surgeon unsure or inexperienced, the facial recess may be opened from above by sacrificing the incus bar and removing the incus. If the external auditory canal wall is perforated, it should be reconstructed with bone and fascia prior to the end of surgery. This will help to prevent a retraction pocket in the future. The annulus and drum should also be grafted with fascia and, if they have been injured, supported from within by Gelfoam pledgets.

The facial recess should be wide enough so that the round window niche, stapedius tendon, and posterior promontory are visualized. Some surgeons remove the bone forming the roof of the round window niche to visualize the round window membrane itself.

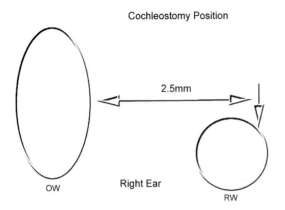

Cochleostomy Position

2.5mm

OW

Right Ear

RW

Figure 10–4 The cochleostomy position is anterior and inferior to the midpoint of the round window membrane.

The Cochleostomy

Prior to opening the scala tympani, all bone dust should be thoroughly irrigated out of the wound, and the surgeon should check that all preliminary steps have been completed. The cochleostomy technique is preferred over taking down the round window membrane. It is easier to access, enters the cochlea past the "hook" area, and is easier to pack to prevent a perilymph fistula. A point on the promontory immediately anterior to the middle and inferior third of the round window niche is taken as the center of the cochleostomy (**Fig. 10–4**). This allows placement of the electrode into the scala tympani, and avoids damage to the basilar membrane. It is safer to begin the cochleostomy too low than too high. It is excavated with a 1.5-mm diamond burr down to a depth of ~1.5 mm or until the white endosteum is seen. Care is taken to use sufficient irrigation to avoid heating the cochlea. Contact with the bone over the facial nerve by the revolving drill shaft must be avoided, since this will heat the bone and may result in a thermal injury to the facial nerve itself. The 1.0-mm diamond burr is then used to complete the cochleostomy down to endosteum. A sharp needle is used to open the latter, and stapes footplate instruments (such as the McGee rasps) are used to smooth the bony edges to allow easy insertion of the electrode. The diameter of the cochleostomy varies from 1.0 to 1.5 mm depending on the electrode used and the need for an insertion tool. The endosteum is opened, taking care not to suction on the endolymph. If desired, a lubricant such as Healon (Advanced Medical Optics, Santa Ana, CA) or 50% glycerin is deposited at the cochleostomy, but not injected into the scala tympani.

Device Placement

The body of the device is now placed in the well. For the Nucleus and Advanced Bionics devices, the posterior portion is placed in a pericranial pocket and the anterior portion is placed in the well. The Med-El device is placed entirely in the well, and covered by the Palva flap. We believe that suturing the device to bone prevents later migration and possible extrusion. Nonabsorbable soft material such as Tevdek (Teleflex Medical, Mansfield, MA) or Ticron (Tyco Healthcare, Mansfield, MA) is excellent for this purpose. Some surgeons may prefer to insert the electrode prior to placing the body of the implant.

Electrode Insertion

Regardless of the type of electrode, it is important to aim the tip toward the middle of the scala tympani in order to avoid the basilar membrane, osseous spiral lamina, or stria vascularis. The Med-El electrode is placed free-hand and generally can be deeply inserted without problems. The Clarion Hi Focus I and Helix electrode are placed with the use of an insertion tool. The Nucleus Contour electrode with its stylet is placed manually. It seems likely that occasionally electrodes may penetrate the basilar membrane,[8,9] and all manufacturers are devising techniques intended to minimize this potential damage. This is particularly important since patients with an appreciable amount of residual hearing are being implanted.

Electrophysiologic Testing

Electrode impedances should be checked at this point. One or two electrodes with high impedances are usually caused by air or N_2O bubbles, are transient, and require no action. However, multiple electrodes with high impedances or any short circuits are of concern, and the manufacturer should be contacted. This may indicate significant damage to the electrode and require use of the backup device. We also check the electrical acoustic reflex (EAR) and neural response telemetry (NRT; for Nucleus devices) or neural response imaging (NRI; for Clarion devices) to be sure of device integrity.

Packing the Cochleostomy

It is very important that the cochleostomy be packed with soft tissue such as pericranium or fascia strips placed around the electrode within the bony cochleostomy. This serves to prevent perilymph leakage and may help to avoid postimplant meningitis. Bone pate, bone wax, and cement are not appropriate substitutes.[14,15] A blunt or ball-tip probe is useful for inserting the packing atraumatically between the electrode array and the bony edge of the cochleostomy, and avoids damage to the electrode.

Closure

The Palva flap is closed over the proximal electrode lead as close as possible to its exit from the body of the device (**Fig. 10–5**). It may also cover the body of the device, especially the Combi 40+. This technique contains the electrode in the bony channel, protects it from external trauma, and interposes a second layer of tissue between the device and the skin closure. We typically use 3–0 chromic catgut or Vicryl for tacking the Palva flap down. Hemostasis is

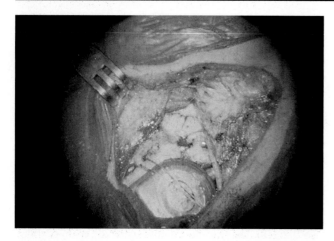

Figure 10–5 The proximal electrode is protected by the sutured Palva flap.

achieved with the use of the bipolar cautery, because the monopolar cautery must be turned off and disconnected once the implant is in contact with the patient.

The skin is closed in layers using chromic or Vicryl followed by staples for older children and adults or a subcuticular suture and Steri-Strips for small children. A drain is rarely ever needed, but, if placed, a closed system drain such as an Axiom (Axion Medical Inc., Rancho Dominguez, Torrence, CA) for children or Jackson-Pratt (Zimmar Inc., Warsaw, IH) drain for adults is used. It should be removed the following morning.

X-Ray

At some point between electrode insertion and applying the dressing, it is advised that a single portable transorbital or Stenvers x-ray be taken in the operating room (**Fig. 10–6**). This documents the location of the electrode, depth of insertion, and absence of kinking.[16,17] If the electrode is

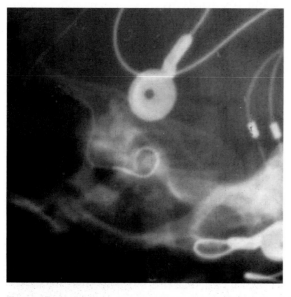

Figure 10–6 An intraoperative anteroposterior (AP) transorbital or modified Stenvers x-ray demonstrates the electrode in good position.

seen to be extracochlear (the hypotympanum is the most common location) or badly kinked, it should be removed and correctly reinserted or the backup device should be used.

Dressing

A mastoid dressing is applied and the patient is sent to the recovery room. The dressing should not be excessively tight since this might lead to flap necrosis.

◆ Special Cases

Dysplastic Cochlea

Congenital dysplasias require thorough evaluation, careful operative planning, and a candid discussion with the parents[10] due to the increased risk of perilymph fistula, facial nerve injury, partial electrode insertion, and less than optimum benefit from the implant. Patients with classical Mondini dysplasia may have a perilymph "gusher" on opening the scala tympani, and packing the cochlea firmly can control it. The hearing results are generally very satisfactory in these cases. The more severe the anomaly, the greater the likelihood of intraoperative problems and the less optimum the benefit. The common cavity often is accompanied by an incomplete lateral end of the internal auditory canal (IAC), and a major CSF gusher. This is dealt with by raising the head of the table, patiently suctioning the fluid from the middle ear, inserting of the electrode, and firmly packing circumferentially around the electrode, using the technique of a champagne cork, with pericranium or fascia packed well within the scala tympani. A spinal drain is seldom needed for dealing with the gusher. Even in the worst cases, such as the common cavity or hypoplastic cochlea, at least partial electrode insertion can be achieved, and the child is likely to derive significant benefit from the device.

Obliterated Cochlea

The obliterated cochlea, usually the result of meningitis and labyrinthitis ossificans, also represents a challenge.[18,19] Patients with a diagnosis of deafness following meningitis should be evaluated as expeditiously as possible. Imaging should consist of both CT and MRI, and surgery should be performed, if possible, promptly to avoid (further) ossification. Granulation tissue, noncalcified osteoid, and proximal new bone can usually be removed or drilled through to achieve full insertion. These patients generally do well if full intraluminal insertion has been accomplished. Complete ossification requires a special technique and leads to less satisfactory results. This may include partial insertion, the use of a split or double array, or a basal turn or perimodiolar circumferential drill-out.

Revision Surgery

Revision surgery, most often required due to device failure, but occasionally resulting from complications of prior surgery, may also be challenging. Typically in younger children there is bone growth around the body of the device and the proximal lead, all of which must be drilled out. The cochleostomy site is usually scarred and may require enlargement to accommodate the new electrode. The facial nerve may be exposed. All of these problems can be anticipated and successfully dealt with at the time of revision. Fortunately, the functional results tend usually to be as good as those originally obtained.[20]

"Soft" Versus "Hard" Failure

Most cochlear implant failures are exactly that: the device ceases to function and the recipient derives no benefit. These "hard" failures are dramatic, clear-cut, easy to diagnose, and usually result in an abnormal integrity test. They may be caused by external trauma or by failure of internal components such as the integrated circuit, seepage of fluid into the case, short-circuits, or a variety of other modes. They clearly require reimplantation, and the patient typically does well with the replacement device. On the other hand, an occasional recipient experiences adverse events, such as excessive loudness of sound, harsh noises, or intermittent signals, while on trouble-shooting the device seems to be functioning properly. In these cases, the integrity test often is normal. This situation has come to be considered a "soft" failure.[21] Another still more difficult scenario is one in which the patient does not experience any adverse effect, but the performance on speech testing decreases from a previous higher level. Again, the integrity test in these cases is usually normal. These also are considered by many to be "soft" failures, and are appropriately treated by replacement of the device. Note that this diagnosis requires a demonstrable decrease in patient performance, not merely dissatisfaction with test result. In all cases of suspected device failure, a thorough medical and radiographic workup must be performed before the device is presumed to have failed. All explanted devices are returned to the manufacturer for analysis of the failure mode. Unfortunately, just as the integrity test is often unremarkable, the final failure analysis may also be unrevealing. This points out the potential difficulty in making this diagnosis, and the importance of further developing both the integrity tests and the failure analyses by the cochlear implant manufacturers. The surgery for all categories of failed devices tends to be quite straightforward, but replacing a thinner electrode with a thicker one (e.g., Nucleus 22 with the Contour) requires enlargement of the cochleostomy.

The Very Young Child

Cochlear implant surgery in the child below the age of 12 months creates several theoretical and practical problems.[12,13,22,23] Labyrinthitis ossificans is the best medical indication for implantation at this age, and may in fact be a reason to consider bilateral simultaneous implantation. However, most implants at this early age are performed because of the firm diagnosis of a profound bilateral loss, lack of benefit from amplification, and parental desire to proceed with implantation as soon as possible. A frank discussion with the parents must include the risks of

potential airway problems, blood loss, immature thermal regulation, lack of mastoid development, and facial nerve injury. These concerns are balanced by the parent's desire to help their deaf child and the fact that the child will presumably start to hear and develop speech at an earlier age.

◆ Meningitis

A word about meningitis is in order.[14,15,24] This postoperative complication of cochlear implantation was thought to be very uncommon, but events in the spring of 2002 revealed what appeared to be a rather sudden increase in such cases in both North America and Europe. Governmental agencies in many countries worked with cochlear implant manufacturers and clinicians to understand and deal with this serious problem. In the United States, this led to a survey of all implant centers in North America[15] and a searching inquiry by the Food and Drug Administration (FDA) and the Centers for Disease Control and Prevention (CDC).[24] As a result of these inquiries, several risk factors for meningitis were recognized. These include the very young child, the dysplastic cochlea, a past history of meningitis, and diminished immune status. Due to concerns about the role that they might have played in the etiology of meningitis, cochlear implants with two-part electrodes (positioners) were voluntarily withdrawn from the market by the manufacturer. Furthermore, a vaccination protocol against *Streptococcus pneumoniae* was promulgated by the FDA and CDC, and surgical technique has emphasized packing of the cochlea to prevent perilymph leakage. The sum of these efforts is expected to be a return in the frequency of meningitis to its previously low level, but there is evidence that there have still been cases of meningitis and fatalities reported in both 2003 and 2004. Cochlear implant surgeons have been cautioned to ensure appropriate vaccination of all implant candidates at risk, to be aware of factors that increase the risk, to pack the cochleostomy circumferentially with soft tissue, and to report all complications to the manufacturer and/or the FDA.

◆ Fluoroscopy

We advocate the use of intraoperative fluoroscopy in implanting the obstructed cochlea, major dysplasias, such as common cavity, and cochlear hypoplasia, and in complex revision surgery. Positioning and using the fluoroscopy unit takes time, and care must be taken to minimize radiation exposure of the patient as well as the surgical team, but these inconveniences are justified by the results.[8,16,17]

◆ Conclusion

Cochlear implant technology continues to improve, surgical techniques continue to evolve, candidacy becomes less restrictive, and the results of implantation have become much more gratifying for both adults and children. As part of the evolutionary series of changes, the incidence and nature of surgical complications have improved and will continue to improve if we understand that the principle must be not merely to be able to treat complications but even more importantly, to prevent them. Most complications can be avoided by the combination of thorough evaluation, careful surgical planning, meticulous operative technique, and conscientious follow-up. If complications arise, they should be recognized promptly and treated actively and without delay.

References

1. Cohen NL, Roland JT, Alexiades G. Cochlear implants. In: Bluestone CD, ed. Surgical Atlas of Pediatric Otolaryngology. New York: BC Decker: 2002:222–249

2. Cohen NL, Hoffman RA. Complications of cochlear implant surgery. In: Eisele DW, ed. Complications in Head and Neck Surgery. St Louis: Mosby-Year Book, 1993:722–729

3. Hoffman RA, Cohen NL. Complications of cochlear implant surgery. Ann Otol Rhinol Laryngol Suppl 1995;166:420–422

4. Roland JT. Complications of Cochlear Implant Surgery. In: Waltzman SB, Cohen NL, eds. Cochlear Implants. New York: Thieme, 2000:171–175

5. Wang RC, Parisier SC, Weiss MH, et al. Cochlear implant flap complications. Ann Otol Rhinol Laryngol 1990;99(10 pt 1):791–795

6. Webb RL, Lehnhardt E, Clark GM, et al. Surgical complications with the cochlear multiple-channel intracochlear implant: experience at Hannover and Melbourne. Ann Otol Rhinol Laryngol 1991;100:131–136

7. Cohen NL. Surgical techniques to avoid complications of cochlear implants in children. Adv Otorhinolaryngol 1997;52:161–163

8. Roland JT Jr, Fishman AJ, Alexiades G, Cohen NL. Electrode to modiolus proximity: a fluoroscopic and histological analysis. Am J Otol 2000;21:218–225

9. Kennedy DW. Multichannel intracochlear electrodes: mechanism of insertion trauma. Laryngoscope 1987;97:42–49

10. Hoffman RA, Downey LL, Waltzman SB, Cohen NL. Cochlear implantation in children with cochlear malformations. Am J Otol 1997;18:184–187

11. O'Donoghue GM, Nikolopoulos TP. Minimal access surgery for pediatric cochlear implantation. Otol Neurotol 2002;23:891–894

12. James AL, Papsin BC. Cochlear implant surgery at 12 months of age or younger. Laryngoscope 2004;114:2191–2195

13. Gibson WP. A surgical technique for cochlear implantation in very young children. Adv Otorhinolaryngol 2000;57:78–81

14. Cohen NL, Roland JT Jr, Marrinan M. Meningitis in Cochlear Implant Recipients: the North American Experience. Otol Neurotol 2004;25:275–281

15. O'Donoghue G, Balkany T, Cohen N, Lenarz T, Lustig L, Niparko J. Meningitis and cochlear implantation. Otol Neurotol 2002;23:823–824

16. Fishman AJ, Roland JT Jr, Alexiades G, Mierzwinski J, Cohen NL. Fluoroscopically assisted cochlear implantation. Otol Neurotol 2003;24:882–886

17. Fishman AJ, Holliday RH. Principles of cochlear implant imaging. In: Waltzman SB, Cohen NL, eds. Cochlear Implants. New York: Thieme, 2000:79–107

18. Balkany T, Gantz BJ, Stevenson RL, et al. A systematic approach to electrode insertion in the ossified cochlea. Otolaryngol Head Neck Surg 1996;114:4–11

19. Balkany T, Gantz B, Nadol JB Jr. Multichannel cochlear implants in partially ossified cochleas. Ann Otol Rhinol Laryngol Suppl 1988;135:3–7

20. Alexiades G, Roland JT Jr, Fishman AJ, Shapiro W, Waltzman SB, Cohen NL. Cochlear reimplantation: surgical techniques and functional results. Laryngoscope 2001;111:1608–1613

21. Waltzman SB, Roland JT, Waltzman M, Shapiro W, Lalwani AK, Cohen NL. Cochlear reimplantation in children: soft signs, symptoms, and results. Cochlear Implants Int 2004;5:138–145

22. Young NM. Infant cochlear implantation and anesthesia risk. Ann Otol Rhinol Laryngol Suppl 2002;189:49–51

23. Kempf HG, Johann K, Lenarz T, Complications of pediatric cochlear implant surgery. Eur Arch Otorhinolaryngol 1999;256:128–132

24. Reefhuis J, Honein MA, Whitney CG, et al. Risk of bacterial meningitis in children with cochlear implants. N Engl J Med 2003;349:435–445

11

Device Programming

William H. Shapiro

The ultimate goal of device programming is to adjust a device so that it can effectively convert acoustic input into a usable electrical signal for each electrode stimulated. The more accurate this conversion process, the greater the potential for the patient to achieve the ultimate goal of open-set speech perception. There are basic psychophysical measures that the programming audiologist must obtain independent of the device used to achieve this goal. The method used and the degree of difficulty in obtaining these psychophysical measures can vary considerably depending on several factors (e.g., patient chronological age, mental status, length of deafness, other handicapping conditions, etc.). This chapter focuses on device programming in general, programming techniques specific to children, a brief overview of the programming parameters of the three most widely used, commercially available multichannel cochlear implant systems—Clarion device (Advanced Bionics Corporation, Valencia, CA), Med-El Combi 40+ (Innsbruck, Austria), and Nucleus C124RCS (Cochlear Corporation, Sydney, Australia)—and how these various parameter manipulations can affect perception and, finally, objective programming techniques.

◆ Programming

Device programming typically begins approximately 2 to 4 weeks following cochlear implantation. Prior to the initial stimulation, it can be quite helpful for the audiologist to obtain a copy of the operative or intraoperative monitoring report (discussed later in the chapter). This can provide useful information regarding the number and the integrity of electrodes inserted intracochlearly. Avoidance of the stimulation of extracochlear electrodes during the initial stages of programming can prevent nonauditory side effects, which can delay the smooth transition to the use of the device, especially in children.

Traditionally, regardless of the device, two measures need to be obtained to create a program: electrical thresholds (T levels) and most comfortable levels (C/M levels). More recently, programming for the Advanced Bionics and Med-El devices have not necessitated acquiring of T levels, as these levels have been obtained through automatic software manipulation (discussed later in the chapter). Electrical threshold (minimal stimulation level), although defined differently by different cochlear implant manufacturers, is typically the softest sound that can be reliably identified by the patient 100% of the time. Electrical comfort level (maximum stimulation level) is defined as the loudest sound that can be listened to comfortably for a sustained period of time. These two measures must be obtained in order for a channel to be activated. The ease with which the programming audiologist can obtain these values and the type of conditioned response observed vary with the patient's age, among other variables. For children, many of the techniques used to obtain these responses are similar to those used by pediatric audiologists.

Because threshold and comfort levels can be affected by the speech-encoding strategy used, it is important to set the speech encoding strategy prior to collecting T- and C-level data. Encoding strategies can be defined as the method by which a given implant translates the incoming acoustic signal into patterns of electrical pulses, which in turn, stimulate the existing auditory nerve fibers. Strategies, in general, provide the listener with either salient cues regarding spectral or envelope information (SPEAK) or temporal information [continuous interleaved sampling (CIS)/high resolution (HiResolution)]. Even though the number of encoding strategies has increased over the years, as have their methods of implementation, the clinician is still required to obtain the same basic measures (thresholds and comfort levels) on each electrode that will eventually be activated.

Historically, another important parameter that needed to be determined prior to obtaining T and C levels was the selection of stimulation mode. Stimulation mode refers to the electrical current flow; that is, the location of the indifferent (reference) electrode, relative to the active (stimulated) electrode. In monopolar refers to a remote ground located outside of the cochlea, whereas bipolar refers to all stimulation occurring within the cochlea. The Advanced Bionics and Nucleus devices can be programmed in a monopolar or bipolar mode, and the Med-El can be programmed in a monopolar mode only. Typically, a wider stimulation mode (monopolar) results in lower threshold values due to a larger physical separation of active and ground electrode, which may, in turn, extend the battery life for behind-the-ear (BTE) speech processor users. Additionally, the use of monopolar stimulation allows for a more consistent threshold value for adjacent electrodes due to the wider spread of current. This consistency throughout the array can allow for interpolation of threshold and comfort level values of adjacent electrodes not obtained through actual behavioral testing. This can be especially beneficial where time is critical, as in programming children. Initial concerns that monopolar stimulation would not be place specific proved unfounded. Research suggests that patients in monopolar stimulation can pitch rank and perceive a monotonic decrease in pitch as the stimulating electrode is moved from the base to the apex of the cochlea (American Speech-Language Hearing Association, 2004). For these reasons, over the past few years, monopolar stimulation has been the desired stimulation mode.

Once the (T and C/M levels) measures have been obtained, loudness balancing of the adjacent electrodes at 100% and 50% of the dynamic range is often performed. Equal loudness across the electrode array has been suggested to be important for optimal speech perception and production. Loudness balancing in an adult or patient with an auditory memory is not a difficult task; however, obtaining loudness information in a congenially hearing impaired 2-year-old can be a truly challenging task. Studies have demonstrated that despite their inability to loudness balance, young children can obtain open-set discrimination; therefore, loudness balancing, at least in the very young, should not be considered a mandatory step in the programming process.

After the T and C/M levels have been obtained and loudness balancing achieved, a program is created. The program provides patients with their first exposure to live speech stimuli. Based on the individual's initial reaction to the stimuli, various parameter manipulations (specific device programming procedure section) can be instituted to achieve a comfortable and effective signal.

◆ Device Programming in Children

Preprogramming

The goal of preprogramming is to prepare the child for the initial stimulation. This can be accomplished by training auditory concepts in a child who may have had limited exposure to sound. Responsibility for training these concepts usually lies within the domain of the speech therapist working with the child, the audiologist evaluating the child, and, most importantly, the parent. The fitting of an appropriate sensory aid is integral to the preprogramming process. The type of sensory aid can range from a high-powered postauricular aid to an frequency modulated (FM) system. Many large cochlear implant centers have instituted loaner hearing aid/FM programs both to assist in determining candidacy and to fill the gap between the time of diagnosis and surgery. Cross-modality training, including vibrotactile stimulation, to assist in the conditioning of a child to respond to auditory stimulation is sometimes used. This method can be helpful when a child has either a total hearing loss or limited exposure to auditory stimuli. The amount of preprogramming varies depending on the auditory needs of the specific child.

Intraoperative Monitoring

Intraoperative monitoring consists of a battery tests typically performed by an audiologist in the operating room. These tests include, but are not limited to, impedance telemetry, electrical stapedial reflex thresholds, and neural response telemetry/imaging. Although monitoring can be time-consuming and costly, it provides the implant team with important information regarding the implanted device. Specifically, intraoperative monitoring provides information about the electrical output of the device and the patient's auditory system response to stimulation. Additionally, monitoring can provide the clinician with preliminary psychophysical measures as an adjunct to programming at initial stimulation. Finally, providing the family member with information regarding device function immediately postsurgery can be a powerful tool in cultivating the relationship between the professional and the patient.

Through Intranet connections, it is now possible for an audiologist to monitor implant surgery from remote locations. An individual such as a resident, nurse, or fellow is identified in the operating room as responsible for setting up the laptop and all connections to the Intranet. When the surgeon is ready for device monitoring the audiologist is contacted over a "landline" and "takes over" the computer in the operating room via the Intranet and commences with the monitoring. The use of a speakerphone can facilitate communication between the operating room and the audiologist at the remote location.

Initial Stimulation

Establishing a comfortable programming environment is critical to the success of programming during the initial stages, especially with children (Shapiro and Waltzman, 1998).

The room should be equipped with appropriately sized chairs and tables. For children, the presence of two audiologists is optimal: one to condition the child and the other to operate the computer. It is important to have a variety of toys on hand to help condition the children. Toys should be changed often because measurements can become unreliable as a child adapts to a particular toy. Parents should be encouraged to bring the child's favorite toy to the programming session.

The initial stimulation can be a time of anticipation and apprehension for both the young child and the accompanying parents. It is of utmost importance that the programming audiologist conveys a sense of calm to the parents and the child. Whenever possible, it is recommended that the child separate from the parents during the programming sessions so that a rapport develops between the child and the audiologist.

The videotaping of program sessions can provide additional information regarding the child's response style, which can then be used to modify the conditioning methods and the responses obtained and to document progress. Basic as well as advanced programming techniques are essential to the implementation of a viable children's cochlear implant program. Although experience in programming adults should be a prerequisite, there is no substitute for the experience gained by programming large numbers of children.

The initial stimulation is typically scheduled over a 2- to 3-day period, consisting of approximately 2 or 3 hours each day. It is important to note that the length of the initial stimulation phase can vary depending on the child. The time spent during these visits can be divided into two main categories: (1) psychophysics—obtaining T and C levels (i.e., device tuning) with subsequent modifications; and (2) device orientation for child and parents. Historically, with a young child, half the electrode array of the Nucleus 24-channel device was programmed on the first day with the remaining electrodes on the second day. The third day, if required, may be used for programming modifications (Cochlear Corporation, 1996). The Clarion and Med-El devices, which have fewer electrodes, required a little less time. With the greater use of objective testing techniques and streamlined fitting procedures (explained later in this chapter), however, device programming time has been reduced significantly without a compromise in performance for all devices. As a result of these procedures, the full array can typically be programmed at the initial visit. Modifications can consist of creating additional programs for the speech processor. These programs, at least during the initial period of stimulation, might be devoted to increases in C levels (i.e., each successive program having increased power). When it is believed that true C levels have been approximated during the initial stimulation phase, other modifications, which will be discussed later in this chapter, are attempted. The use of multiple programs can be implemented with the Nucleus 24RCS, Med-El Combi-40+, and Clarion device.

Obtaining T and C levels on young children can be both challenging and difficult. One cannot assume that the T and C levels obtained during the initial stages of programming are ideal. During the first few months, as the child adjusts to this novel acoustic signal, the comfort levels typically increase (Henkin et al, 2003). Alternatively, it is important to note that overly ambitious maximum levels may introduce distortion to an otherwise clear signal. Second, physiologic changes occur that are reflected in changes in the T during the initial few months of stimulation. Typically, the more accurate the T and C levels, the better the performance with the program.

The initial response of the pediatric patient to electrical stimuli can differ greatly from the response to acoustic stimuli. Reactions can range from no response to crying. Although the older child can be conditioned to raise his or her hand or use play audiometry, conditioned orientation reflex audiometry, behavioral observation audiometry, or visual reinforcement audiometry needs to be used to obtain T on the younger child. Obtaining C levels in a young child is more subjective and can require greater clinical acumen on the part of the audiologist. Commonly the child will not respond until the electrical current is too high, at which point he or she will react adversely. During the initial phases of stimulation, setting conservative/dynamic range (i.e., reduced spread between T and C levels) is the preferred approach so as not to frighten the child with a loud sound.

During the initial stages of programming, it is important that parents understand what should and should not be expected of the child. It is not uncommon for a child who previously had some auditory detection and discrimination to have difficulty maintaining the same level of performance during the early poststimulation phase. Parents need to be prepared for this scenario and to be reassured that over time the child's performance will improve.

Although the initial pediatric programming techniques vary among audiologists, generally accepted procedures are followed. A gross estimate of the child's behavioral response is obtained via standardized procedures at an apical electrode, quickly skipping three or four electrodes toward a more basal area electrode, and continuing this process until the whole electrode array has been stimulated. Once the gross estimates of thresholds have been determined, more definitive measures should be obtained. While the young child is engaged in some activity, comfort levels are set, either psychophysically (tones or bursts) or through live voice stimulation for each of the electrodes. During the setting of C levels, the audiologists are responsible for closely monitoring the child for any adverse reactions. Underestimating C levels initially can allow for a smooth transition to the implant by reducing loud auditory sensations.

Daily Care, Maintenance, and Troubleshooting

A portion of time during the initial stimulation is devoted to the daily care and maintenance of the device and understanding how to troubleshoot the external equipment. Parents and patients should be encouraged to ask questions and read the user manual supplied by the manufacturer. Of particular importance during the initial phases of programming is a daily check of the skin under the headset magnet to assess the skin integrity. It is common for parents in particular to tighten the magnet sufficiently to ensure that the coil never falls off. In the most extreme of circumstances, this can lead to skin necrosis under the magnet. Parents and adult patients should be advised that during the first few weeks it is not uncommon for the headset to fall off and should be reassured that over time the expectation is that the child (adult) during the "bonding" process with the device, will learn to put the headset back on by him/herself and that the constant magnetic attraction will eventually lead to a more secure coupling.

Although the speech processor, headset and cables are robust, breakdowns can occur. For adult cochlear implant users having spare parts such as batteries, cables, and possibly a headset, should be adequate to solve most of the hardware problems. Parents should maintain an even greater supply of parts for their child and provide the school with some as well. Numerous counseling sessions regarding device troubleshooting offered by the cochlear implant center in conjunction with comprehensive troubleshooting guidelines provided by the manufacturers is usually sufficient for problem solving; however, if all attempts to resolve the problem fail, the implant center should be contacted immediately. Regularly scheduled in-servicing of the school personnel by the child's cochlear implant center is crucial to maintain a high functional level. The failure rate of the internal portion of the cochlear implant is low; however, should a failure occur, reimplantation should be performed as quickly as possible.

Electrostatic discharge (ESD) can pose a problem for cochlear implant users. The transfer of static electricity to the implant system can corrupt or eliminate a stored program in the speech processor and, on rare occasions, be responsible for the breakdown of the internal electronics package. Device manufacturers suggest removal of the externally worn parts prior to exposure to high levels of static electricity, such as plastic slides. It should be noted, however, that with the advent of more robust electronics, ESD has become a less significant problem.

◆ Device-Specific Programming

One of the more powerful tools in current devices is the ability to provide the user with multiple-program, multiple-strategy options. Although the multiple-program option should not serve to lengthen the time between programming visits, it can provide a more flexible, efficient transition during the initial stimulation period. More importantly, the multistrategy option allows clinicians and researchers to determine which particular speech-coding strategy may be optimal for an individual patient by allowing the patient access to these different strategies in different programs. Because time is necessary to determine the best strategy for a particular individual, it is advisable to allow a significant and equal amount of time with each strategy.

From an historical perspective, the Clarion multistrategy cochlear implant with the CI ICS and the body-worn processor was able to provide the patient with two speech-coding strategies: continuous interleaved sampling (CIS) or simultaneous analog stimulation. These two strategies represented significantly different approaches to decoding and encoding the incoming electrical signal. This original device (versions 1.0 and 1.2) consisted of 16 intracochlear electrodes arranged in eight closely spaced, independent parallel output circuits, oriented radially. Over time, further changes included the enhanced bipolar stimulation pattern, which stimulated the medial electrode in one pair relative to the lateral electrode in the next most apical electrical pair. The wider electrode spacing resulted in lower T and maximum C levels with a maximum of seven independent stimulation sites within the cochlea. In an attempt to further reduce current requirements, a Silastic positioner was used to "push" the electrode contacts closer to the modiolus. In October 2002, the Clarion device was voluntarily removed from the market due to concerns regarding an increased rate of bacterial meningitis in this population. The CII ICS was then introduced and referred to as the Bionic Ear. This version had 16 independent output circuits that could stimulate each of the 16 electrode contacts simultaneously, nonsimultaneously, or in various combinations. The newest internal device to be introduced, the 90K, is the first Advanced Bionics device that does not use a ceramic case to house the electronic components; instead a Silastic type material allows for the surgical removal of the internal magnet without disturbing the electrode array in the cochlea. This device, as well as the CII, is used in conjunction with the SoundWave software platform (discussed later in the chapter).

The Advanced Bionics device, featuring continuous bidirectional telemetry, allows electrode impedances to be measured during each fitting, thus enabling the clinician to determine the integrity of each electrode. Electrodes with impedances outside of the normal range (5 to 150 K ohm) are automatically disabled at initiation of programming. This continuous two-way telemetry also allows for an audible alarm to sound when the headset is not linked to the internal receiver-stimulator. The T and most C levels prior to Soundwave software were determined channel-by-channel using pulsatile (CIS) or sinusoidal compressed analog (CA) stimulation. Upper-limit comfort levels (ULCLs) are measured using live speech only. Following the loudness balancing procedure, the clinician adjusts the most comfortable level (M) using live voice in real time. Because the M levels are subjective and can vary depending on a variety of factors, they can be adjusted with the volume dial on *speech processor*. The volume dial shifts the patient's dynamic electrical range by increasing or decreasing the M level. The upper limit of comfort levels is set by the upper volume range. Volume range is the percentage of the electrical dynamic range above Ms, and the lower volume range is defined as the percentage below Ms. The clinician can set both of these ranges with the volume dial during live-voice speech or manually without stimulation (Advanced Bionics Corporation, 1995). This is especially important in programming children because the audiologist can limit the range in which the volume dial can be manipulated. The sensitivity dial interacts with the volume dial by increasing and decreasing the audio gain. Raising the sensitivity dial will allow an increased perception of loudness because the incoming signal is mapped higher in the patient's electrical dynamic range.

Various general programming parameters are available to the audiologist, including a gain adjustment palette and input dynamic range (IDR). The gain adjustment consists of an emphasis/de-emphasis tool palette. The emphasis/de-emphasis tool allows for the adjustment of the sound level of the individual frequency band associated with each channel. This parameter can be helpful in troubleshooting (e.g., if a patient complains of a boomy quality, the lower frequencies can be attenuated). IDR specifies the electrical range of sounds that is transmitted to the patient from the M levels down to T levels. The default IDR is set to capture the full intensity range of speech sounds. Decreasing the IDR will exclude low-level sounds and noise along with the possibility of losing certain speech information (e.g., quiet fricatives). Increasing the IDR can increase the perception of noise. The specific parameters available in a CIS encoding strategy are envelope detection and cutoff frequency, repetitive rate, pulse width, and firing order. Additional suggested parameter manipulations can be used depending on the specific complaints of the patient.

As the complexity of speech coding strategies have evolved from a diffuse broad-band signal found in single channel devices to transmission of significantly more detailed information as found in multichannel devices, so has the device programming time. Clinicians are faced with more programming decisions due to increased number of channels, use of bilateral implants and parametric options. The greater amount of time spent on device programming has reduced the amount of time the clinician has to focus on other tasks, such as counseling and rehabilitation (Garber et al, 2002). In 2003, the Food and Drug Administration (FDA) approved a new speech processing strategy referred to as "Hi-Resolution Sound." This strategy, along with a new software platform called SoundWave Professional Suite, introduced a new fitting methodology geared toward reducing fitting time while maintaining optimal patient performance. This fitting strategy can be used with the CII or 90K device. The basis of HiResolution programming is the use of "speech bursts" during psychophysical testing. This new feature more accurately represents dynamic real-time input. "Speech bursts" (white noise) are created when complex stimuli are delivered to the processing system, and transmitted through the same filter's amplitude detections, averaging a logarithm utilized for incoming acoustic sound. This allows for more representative real-time stimulation. With speech bursts, three to four channels are programmed simultaneously. Preliminary studies have demonstrated equivalent performance between single-channel programming and HiResolution programming (Advanced Bionics Corporation, 2003). This reduces the number of loudness adjustments during programming sessions, reduces programming time, and may serve to reduce patient fatigue.

The SoundWave platform employs a different approach for setting threshold levels (minimal audible levels), called "Auto T." Historically, the obtaining of T levels was not a requirement in all processing strategies, such as the simultaneous analog strategy (SAS) (Kessler, 1999). Testing of HiResolution programs, with T levels and without T [T = 1 cu (clinical units) for all channels, showed equivalent performance. SoundWave auto sets T levels at M/10 based on the average dynamic range (20 dB) of CII Bionic Ear users programmed with HiResolution Sound. This automatic setting can be adjusted as needed globally or for individual channels in real-time stimulation. Loizou et al (2000) demonstrated that a clinician could optimize performance by jointly varying pulse rate and pulse width. Automatic pulse width (APW) and rate adjustment is a parameter in SoundWave that optimizes each patient program to maintain the narrowest pulse width and fastest stimulation rate based on the patient's own stimulation levels required to achieve adequate loudness growth. With SoundWave, the APW algorithm is able to monitor voltage compliance to limit distortion. The SoundWave software uses two strategies for delivering HiResolution technology: HiResolution-P (two channels simultaneously paired) and HiResolution-S (two channels stimulated sequentially). The APW will continue to maintain the narrowest pulse width and fastest rate possible within each strategy option. The Power Estimator (PoEM) is responsible for managing the radiofrequency (RF) power, obviating the need for the clinician to optimize RF at the end of the session. This allows a program created on the body device platinum speech processor (PSP) to be downloaded directly to the BTE speech processor with automatic RF adjustment.

Med-El

The Med-El Combi 40+ hardware system consists of an implanted stimulator driving a 12-electrode-pair, intracochlear scala tympani array. It can provide the patient with two separate and distinct speech coding strategies: CIS and number of maxima (n of m) spectral peak speech extractor. As is the case with the Advanced Bionics device, one can obtain voltage differences between an active or nonactive electrode and the remote ground (electrode impedance) via telemetry modes. The coupling mode of the Med-El implant is monopolar, which avoids the high current densities that would be necessary for the fast pulsatile stimulation in bipolar mode. The CIS-PRO processor (body device) features a four-position switch of off and programs 1 through 3, which allows for multiple programs. An LED indicator system (one red, one green) allows five speech processor conditions to be programmed and a volume dial is used for controlling the amplitude of the stimulation signal. An external input connection is used for interfacing approved accessory equipment, such as FM systems. The more widely used Tempo+ BTE employs a three-program switch along with a three-program volume control that allows the user to have as many as nine separate programs. Additionally, a sensitivity control allows for greater flexibility. This device, which is presently the standard device, offers a wide array of wearing configurations that make it ergonomically appropriate for young children. The speech processing strategy continues to be either a sequential or simultaneous processing strategy, that is, a new version of the CIS strategy, called CIS+, in addition to n-of-m.

The typical psychophysical measures that need to be obtained are T and M levels, with C levels loudness balanced. Recently, however, research has focused on the automatic setting of T levels at 10% of the maximum comfort level (MCL) for several reasons, including reduced programming time, reduced audibility of low-level noise, and enhanced peak to valley ratio for formant perception. In 2005, Spahr and Dorman studied 15 subjects implanted with the Combi 40+. The purpose of the study was to determine whether any difference in performance occurred between assigning a threshold of M/10 as compared with the actual setting of minimum stimulation levels to behavioral thresholds. The results showed equivalent scores between both procedures, in quiet, and in noise at low input levels. Parameters other than T and M levels that can be manipulated to achieve a desired auditory effect include the map-law, channel order, volume mode, and bandpass filters. Map-law controls the shape of the amplitude growth function and its compression characteristics and can change in real time. The growth function can be logarithmic or linear. The four log functions provide signal expansion at the lower part of the dynamic range and signal compression at the upper part. The default Combi 40 mapping law coefficient is 500. Channel order specifies the sequence of interleaved stimulation for the CIS processor strategy. The default for an eight-channel CIS strategy is $1-5-2-6-3-7-4-8$. This is referred to as staggered sequence. An apex-to-base or base-to-apex sequence is the default for the *n*-of-*m* peak extraction strategy. Staggering is not the preferred sequence due to the continuously changing channel selection. The range of the volume control can be adjusted through software manipulation. In addition, two different volume modes can be selected in software for the manual control knob on the speech processor: the IBK (Innsbruck) mode and the RTI (Research Triangle Institute, Research Triangle Park, NC) mode. The RTI mode allows the patient to control stimulation amplitude at threshold, whereas the IBK mode does not (Med-El Corporation, 1997).

Med-El's present version of software, CI Studio, a Windows-based system, can be used to program all previous generation Med-El devices and differs from the older DOS version in certain aspects. In terms of dynamic range, this software allows for interpolation between channels, and features "drag and drop" functions. The pulse duration can vary per channel and the pulse rate can be changed in steps of 1.7 μs. The maplaw controls the shape of the amplitude growth function and its compression characteristics. As for maplaw, the **S**-slope can reduce unpleasant background noise, although the **S**-slope maplaws cannot be exported. It is now possible to create nonstandard maplaw with text files. The bandpass filter now has an extended frequency band (200–8500 Hz).

Med-El's newest device, the Pulsar[100] contains electronics and an application-specific integrated circuit (ASIC) that provides the user with up to 5 days of battery life, with a flexible platform design for future cochlear implant technology. Currently, the Pulsar CI[100] cochlear implant is programmed via CI Studio+ 2.01. It continues to use a CIS speech-coding strategy with Hilbert transformation, and has the potential for simultaneous stimulation to enhance acoustic detail and clarity without the disadvantages of channel interaction using intelligent parallel stimulation (IPS). It is hoped that parallel stimulation without channel interaction may be able to provide the user with more detailed information and signal replication leading to improved performance in difficult listening situations. The new software also offers simultaneous fitting, that is, a split screen and dual interfaces for use with bilateral implants, QuickFit programming, a interactive task that can provide a quick and accurate estimation of MCLs based on data derived from electrical stapedial reflex threshold (ESRT) measures, and a test button within the interface configuration function to be used to confirm communication between the programming interface and the computer.

Nucleus

The Nucleus 22-channel cochlear implant, the antecedent to the Nucleus 24, like the two previously described multichannel implants, can be programmed to fit the requirements of the individual implant recipient. Although not currently used in the United States, it merits some discussion because of its similarities to the Nucleus 24 and the large number of recipients still using the device. Dedicated software is used to deliver electrical stimulation and to measure T and C levels for each of the 22 implanted electrodes. The parameters are then combined with a predetermined speech-processing strategy to create a program or "MAP". T and C level values can be affected by several important parameters, one of which, stimulation mode, determines the current flow within the cochlea. The wider the current spread, the more reduced the electrical T and C levels and, therefore, the fewer the electrode pairs available for stimulation. It is preferable to provide stimulation at as low an electrical level as possible because elevated stimulation levels reduce the overall efficiency of the system by slowing down the stimulation rate and reducing usable auditory information (Cochlear Corporation, 1996). Although monopolar stimulation is not available in the Nucleus 22 system, common ground stimulation is available. This mode allows any of the 22 electrodes to be used as active. When an active electrode is designated, all of the other electrodes are connected to form a single indifferent electrode, which will result in a more diffuse current flow. The common ground mode is useful as a diagnostic mode when checking the integrity of individual electrodes independently because it allows the clinician to select and stimulate individual electrodes to determine if an electrode can generate a response or if the response generated results in loudness growth. Common ground is often used during the initial stimulation of a young child with limited exposure to auditory input because it provides a more conservative approach to programming, as all electrodes are linked together in "common ground." This increases the likelihood of aberrant electrodes being detected and therefore decreasing the possibility of unpleasant sound sensations. Common ground is not recommended for partial insertions because current will flow outside the cochlea and possibly cause a nonauditory stimulation.

The frequency-to-electrode allocation parameter allows the audiologist to assign a particular bandwidth to a given electrode. The allocation will depend on the speech-processing strategy used and the number of electrodes available for stimulation. For the spectral peak (SPEAK) strategy, the frequency bands are linearly distributed in the low frequencies to ~1850 Hz and logarithmically distributed thereafter. The default frequency allocation table (electrode-to-bandwidth allocation) for 20 active electrodes as determined by the software is 9. Skinner et al (1994, 1997) suggested that a default frequency allocation table of 7 results in improved phoneme, word, and sentence perception possibly due to an increased number of electrodes assigned to frequencies below 1000 Hz, which allows for the more accurate perception of the change in formant frequencies for diphthongs and the recognition of the phoneme / m / as different from / l /.

In the SPEAK strategy each of the 20 programmable filters in the speech processor has a default gain of 8. Because the gain is applied to each filter prior to maximum selection, the gain settings affect which maximum is determined. Reducing the gain on a particular filter will de-emphasize that filter output.

The amplitude mapping algorithm is a nonlinear function determined by the interaction of the base level and the Q value. The base level controls the minimum input level that will produce electrical stimulation. The default value of the base level is 4 and is rarely changed. Increasing the base level increases the level of sound required to initiate electrical stimulation. The base level may be changed if a patient complains of unwanted environmental noise or perceives an internal electrical noise generated by the speech processor. In the past few years, improved speech processor design, with its reduced internal noise, has obviated the need to manipulate this parameter. When the function knob in the speech processor is set to the S position, the base level is automatically raised to 10. This serves to reduce the acoustic dynamic range of the processor from 29.5 dB (base level = 4) to 22.7 dB. Therefore, the patient should be advised to use caution when manipulating this parameter because speech perception can be adversely affected.

The Q value controls the steepness of the amplitude growth and determines the percentage of the patient's electrical range devoted to the top 10 dB at the speech processor's input range. As the clinician reduces the Q value, the amplitude growth function at the lower end of the speech processor's input range becomes steeper. Reducing the Q value can serve to make soft sounds seem louder, including background noise. Increasing the Q value reduces the background noise but may result in the patient not hearing soft voices or speakers at a distance. Additionally, global modifications in the T or C levels can also result in louder or softer sound sensations. Increasing T levels globally results in louder sound sensations for the low-level acoustic signals, and may serve to reduce tinnitus. Conversely, decreasing T levels globally results in softer sound sensations for low-level input. Certainly increasing or decreasing C levels by a fixed percentage of the dynamic range results in louder or softer sound sensations. Research recently has focused on the effect of increased T levels on speech perception. Skinner et al (1998) compared methods for obtaining minimum stimulation levels (T levels) used in programming the Nucleus 22 cochlear implant with subjects using the SPEAK strategy. The study looked at the differences in speech perception, at different input levels, as a function of

the method of setting minimum stimulation levels. Two programs were created; one at raised thresholds ($m = +2.04$ dB) and one at threshold (clinical default value) to determine if raised levels would improve recipients understanding of soft speech sounds with the SPEAK speech coding strategy. Results obtained suggested that use of a raised level program for the Nucleus 22 device users has the potential of improving speech perception at lower intensity levels.

The Nucleus C124M device has 22 active electrodes implanted within the cochlea and two remote grounds: a ball electrode implanted under the temporalis fascia muscle and a plate (ground) near the receiver-stimulator, which permits programming in a common ground, bipolar, or monopolar stimulation mode. Shortly after the Nucleus CI24M was introduced, a modification of this system called the Nucleus 24 Contour (CI24RCS) was introduced that had a precoiled electrode array. Using an array that "hugged" the modiolus allows for the possibility of closer proximity to the auditory nerve fibers. The goal was the reduction of current requirements and current spread, while increasing battery life and enhancing place specificity.

The SPRint (body) speech processor (Cochlear Corporation, Englewood, CA) holds four separate and distinct programs, allowing for flexibility in programming and has a personal or public audible alarm to alert others to device manipulations, especially important in the pediatric population because of the tendency for children to play with equipment.

The SPRint supports three different encoding strategies: advanced combination encoder (ACE), a hybrid strategy designed to combine SPEAK (large number of stimulation sites, dynamic channel selection, moderate rate, and improved frequency representation) with CIS (high stimulation rate, fixed channel selection, and improved resolution) (Cochlear Corporation, 1998a–d). The C124RCS offers a choice of a 4-, 6-, 8-, or 12-channel CIS coding strategy from over 22 sites of stimulation. The Esprit (BTE) speech processor, which implements the SPEAK strategy, is capable of storing two separate programs, but cannot support the more advanced encoding strategies (CIS and ACE). The newer two-program ESPrit 3G now allows for the use of the CIS and ACE strategies, which make this device a more attractive choice for older children and adults than the body device.

Prior to initial stimulation, telemetry can be used to ensure the integrity of the electrodes. The C124RCS is capable of various types of telemetry to assess the internal functioning of electrodes as well as to measure the response of the whole nerve action potential (neutral response telemetry, discussed later in this chapter). Electrode impedance is used to detect short- and high-impedance electrodes that should not be used in MAP. If an electrode has high impedance, a voltage compliance problem may occur, which in turn will affect loudness growth. Under these circumstances reducing T and C levels by increasing the pulse width or using another stimulation mode (monopolar) can resolve the problems. If this fails, the electrode should be deactivated because the MAP will not convey appropriate loudness information.

After assessing electrode integrity, the speech-encoding strategy is chosen and a stimulation rate is selected. Generally, a decrease in T levels will occur with increasing rate. Patients should be encouraged to remain in a specific strategy for several weeks to allow for an adjustment period prior to fine-tuning secondary parameters. These secondary parameters for CIS and ACE include channel/electrode allocation (i.e., electrode set), gain/frequency response shaping, frequency table, order of stimulation, jitter, and Q value. Manipulating the electrode set may provide the most efficient means of affecting changes in sound quality. Sound quality complaints of uncomfortably high pitch can be improved by lowering the stimulation rate, incorporating a more apical electrode in the electrode set, and adjusting the low/high-frequency gain settings (Cochlear Corporation, 1997). Taking advantage of the multiprogramming strategy, especially in ACE, can be useful by fitting the patient with multiple programs of varying stimulation rates and maximums.

Managing the deleterious effects of background noise is a dilemma. The 3G (BTE) features the "whisper" setting, which is a fast-acting compression circuit that increases the range of input signal intensities coded by the speech processor. Clinical trials have shown a 15% improvement in scores for words presented at a reduced level in quiet, without a decrement in performance in noise. The Sprint (body) processor also employs adaptive dynamic range optimization (ADRO), which is a preprocessing scheme that continuously adjusts the gain in each frequency band to optimize the signal in the output dynamic range. This often results in improved overall sound clarity through better detection of soft speech, while maintaining comfort level for loud sounds.

Managing nonauditory side effects such as facial nerve stimulation, pain, and dizziness, irrespective of device, can be a challenging task and is the subject of ongoing research. For the Advanced Bionics device, lowering clipping levels or deactivating the channel can accomplish the desired effects. For the Nucleus device, these side effects can usually be programmed out by reducing current levels on a given electrode (reducing maximum stimulation level), bypassing that electrode, or using a variable-mode programming strategy to widen the stimulation mode. Variable mode allows the clinician to specify both the active and the indifferent electrode (i.e., channel of stimulation). This flexibility of combining different bipolar modes in the same MAP can result in a greater number of active channels than actual electrodes available for stimulation. Pseudo-monopolar mode, a form of variable mode, can be useful in partial insertions because it uses an extracochlear electrode as the indifferent electrode for all other intracochlear electrodes. Unlike typical stimulus flow configuration, this mode couples an indifferent electrode that is located basally, usually outside of the cochlea, to the active electrode.

Double-electrode MAPping also can be clinically useful with patients who have a partial insertion of the electrode array or a limited number of usable channels available for stimulation because it increases the overall frequency range that the speech processor analyzes. For example, if a patient has 12 stimulable channels, the overall bandwidth would be 240 to 4926 Hz using the default frequency allocation. Double electrode MAPping of the eight most basal channels increases the upper bandwidth limit by more than twofold, which can serve to improve the sound quality of high-frequency phonemes. The clinician, of course, may choose to double-electrode MAP the apical electrodes instead. All programming manipulation, however, should ultimately be based on the patient's sound quality judgments.

Much has been discussed in the cochlear implant (CI) community "creative programming," that is, the ability of clinicians to work "out of the box" in attempting to improve patient outcomes through innovative tweaking. For instance, Skinner et al (1998) demonstrated that using counted Ts during psychophysical testing can improve a patient's perception of soft speech. The technique of requiring the patient to actually count the number of stimulations will typically raise the threshold level. Furthermore, a recent article by Fourakis et al (2004) showed that manipulation of the frequency allocation table (FAT) by shifting more electrodes toward the lower frequency range could improve vowel perception without compromising consonant recognition in adult Nucleus 24 users. Manipulation of T levels or gains at a formant frequency level have been employed by a handful of CI audiologists to reduce substitution errors. This technique requires that F0F1F2 of both misinterpreted sounds be identified in order to determine where the frequency differs. The audiologist would then increase the T levels of the electrodes responsible for these differences in an attempt to make the differences more apparent. This technique, on occasion, may have the desired effect possibly due to the correction of "T tails" (nonlinear growth of loudness on a particular electrode), a common phenomenon in psychophysical testing. This tweaking of different parameters can occur independently of or in combination with other parametric changes. This author would urge caution with this technique because overmanipulation might increase errors for other phonemes. Furthermore, there have been with no publications in the scientific literature that demonstrate efficacy with use of this procedure.

Because the Nucleus 24 uses monopolar stimulation there is less variability in T and C levels between adjacent electrodes. Plant and Psarros (2000) investigated the feasibility of measuring every second and fifth electrode while interpolating intermediate electrodes. The study was done at three different stimulation rates, and the results were compared with those obtained using a standard behavioral device programming technique. They found no significant T and C level differences for all stimulation rates as compared with behaviorally obtained (T/C) levels at every electrode. Minor adjustments of T and C levels were suggested, however, when increasing the distance between measured channels. Based on this work, a study was designed by Cochlear Americas (Denver, CO) to systematically evaluate some of the newer "streamlined" programming techniques and compare them to the traditional behavioral technique whereby every electrode was measured. The objectives of the study were threefold: to demonstrate equivalent speech perception outcomes between three streamlined programming techniques and traditional behavioral programming, to evaluate the clinician's time during the objective versus the behavioral technique, and to provide the clinician with a more standardized programming approach for both adults and children.

Three techniques were used: first fit behavioral, first fit integrated OR, and first fit integrated initial activation (IA). The first technique involved interpolation of five behaviorally measured T levels with C levels set in live voice; the second technique involved using 5 NRT values obtained intraoperatively to set an overall profile with absolute T and C levels determined in live voice mode; and the third technique was identical to the second except that NRT was obtained at initial activation, not intraoperatively. Preliminary data suggest that it takes less time to create a first fit integrated OR or behavioral streamlined MAP as compared with a traditional behavioral programming MAP in adults (Chute and Popp, 2004). For the majority of subjects, however, there were few performance differences between the traditional behavioral and streamlined programming technique.

◆ Managing Programming (MAPping) Complaints

Most patient complaints can be effectively managed simply by manipulation of the T and C levels, as these measures are the "building blocks" by which all additional manipulation is accomplished. One cannot, however, underestimate the effectiveness of counseling in the remediation of various complaints or misperceptions. At present, many cochlear implant centers maintain a large caseload and the counseling portion of their program may suffer from a lack of time. Counseling should be integrated into the entire CI process, by the entire implant team, during all time periods. This is especially important during presurgical counseling and the early stages of stimulation, as the clinician attempts to juxtapose a patient's expectations with performance. It is not uncommon for a patient to feel that progress has been too slow during the initial stages of programming, and it is incumbent upon the team to help the patient through this time. Auditory training (critical for children, recommended for adults) can be a powerful tool in this process. Over the last few years, aural rehabilitation for adults has become more commonplace, either in the form of one-to-one therapy or through the use of computer technology.

Another issue that often arises during the course of programming is that a patient who has been making progress reaches a performance plateau. This may in some patients signal the need for a more aggressive parameter change, for example, speech coding strategy, repetition rate, etc. The programming audiologist should not be reluctant to institute such changes while closely monitoring the patient for any performance degradation. This process needs to be incorporated with the close collaboration of the patient's therapist. There are occasions where a patient might best be served by seeing another audiologist at the center to offer a different perspective; taking a fresh approach to a patient's programming issues often can be helpful.

One of the most common issues arising in the early stages of programming is the patient's inability to effectively manipulate and understand the different functions of the volume and the sensitivity controls. The audiologist must explain, often repeatedly, that the comfort level (C/M level) is directly related to the volume control and that any manipulation by the volume control will influence loudness and that the sensitivity control can influence distance hearing and perception in noise. Additionally, as the process matures, parents, patients, and therapists must understand the appropriate use of the multiple program approach; that is, evaluating the performance of an individual with multiple programs should be done in a structured listening environment and is often performed by the child's speech therapist. Each of the programs, usually differing by a single parameter (gain, maxima, input dynamic range, etc.), is assessed during a therapy session to determine the program that provides maximum speech understanding. Failure to do so can result in the use of a "stale" MAP, that is, with inappropriate T and C/M levels at the time a particular MAP is used.

There are auditory (MAPping) complaints that are universal, including, but not limited to, speech or environmental sounds being too loud/soft, other voices or the patient's own voice having increased echo, background noises being inappropriately loud in relation to the speech signal, and voices being too high/low pitched. Actions for each of these scenarios are clearly outlined in the manufacturers' technical service manuals, in addition to an extensive manufacturer support system for the programming audiologist.

◆ Device Failures (Hard/Soft)

As the number of cochlear implant recipients has increased over the past 25 years, so has the number of device failures. Although failures still represent a very small percentage of the user population, the absolute numbers are large enough to require mention in this chapter. The speed at which a device failure is accurately diagnosed and corrected is critical to the process. Device failures can be divided into two categories: hard failures, where the internal device ceases to function entirely, and soft failures, where a device functions suboptimally, but a suspected mechanical or electronic malfunction exists that cannot be determined with current clinical diagnostic tools. Prior to suspecting a device failure, the clinician should check and replace the external hardware, and the device should be reprogrammed. With the advent of bidirectional telemetry, hard device failures have become relatively easy to diagnose. Following the initial diagnosis of a hard failure a device integrity test is typically performed, either by the CI audiologist or manufacturer representative. An integrity test measures the voltages generated by the biphasic current pulses at the electrode array, which can be accomplished by the use of surface electrodes. Concurrently, a plain film is obtained to assess electrode position and to compare this to the film taken intraoperatively.

Soft failures can be subdivided into long-term progressive or short-term progressive failures, which may be more elusive to diagnose. It is quite possible that an integrity test may *not* diagnose a soft failure and the implant team may need to consider explantation in the absence of electrophysiologic data to support device failure. Progressive failures may include electrode migration, intermittent electrode shorting, or open circuits, which may manifest in progressively poorer speech perception for the patient. This underscores the need for periodic speech perception evaluations to objectively compare pre- and postevent performance. This often expedites insurance approval for reimplantation. From an auditory standpoint, patients may complain of atypical tinnitus, buzzing, loud intermittent noises, clicking, roaring, etc. This may be manifested from a MAPping perspective by facial nerve stimulation, fluctuant T and C levels, reduction in usable channels, frequent manipulation of pulse width, narrow dynamic ranges, wide variation in impedance or compliance measures, and the need for frequent MAPping. For patients unable to provide valuable feedback, such as children, behavioral issues may be evidenced, such as pulling the device off, aggressive behavior, inexplicable crying, etc. More sophisticated diagnostic tools are required to more effectively diagnose device failures (hard and soft), so that appropriate measures may be taken in a more timely fashion. Reimplantation should occur as quickly as possible following the failure determination so performance is not compromised (Waltzman et al, 2004).

Objective Programming Techniques

As the criteria for selection for cochlear implant candidates broaden over time to include lowering of the age of implantation and the implantation of the developmentally delayed or disabled, the use of objective electrophysiologic measures to assist in device programming has taken on an increasingly important role. Historically, electrophysiologic measures have been used throughout the cochlear implant process: preoperatively, intraoperatively, and/or postoperatively (Shallop, 1993). They have been used preoperatively as a possible predictor of postoperative performance (Waltzman et al, 1991) or ear selection (Kileny et al, 1992) (promontory stimulation); intraoperatively, to assess device integrity and neural stimulation [electrically evoked auditory brainstem response (EABR), averaged evoked voltages (AEV), electrical stapedial reflexes (elicited acoustic reflex threshold, EART), neural response telemetry/imaging (NRT, NRI), and electrical impedances)]; and postoperatively, to assess device integrity (AEV and EABR) and to program the device (EABR, EART, and NRT/NRI). The following subsections focus on electrophysiologic measures as they related to postoperative device programming.

Evoked Auditory Brainstem Response

Several researchers have investigated the relationship between EABR thresholds and behavioral measures of T and C levels in Nucleus 22 channel cochlear implant users (Kileny, 1991; Mason et al, 1993; Shallop et al, 1990, 1991) and have found varying degrees of correlation between these measures. Shallop et al (1991) studied the relationship between intraoperative EABR thresholds and behavioral measures of thresholds and maximum comfort levels for 11 patients implanted with the Nucleus 22 device. They found EABR to more closely approximate the maximum C levels rather than the behavioral T levels, and on occasion to exceed behavioral C levels by more than 20 programming

units. They suggested that differences between EABR thresholds and behavioral T levels might be partially due to differences in the rate of stimulation used for the two procedures. Mason et al (1993) studied the relationship between intraoperative EABR thresholds and the behavioral T levels for 24 children. They reported that EABR thresholds consistently overestimated T levels by an average of 35 programming units. The use of correction factors to improve this predicative model was moderately successful. Factors that confound these correlations include postoperative changes in the EABR growth function over time and reduction in impedance during the first few months of electrical stimulation.

In 1994, Brown et al studied the relationship between EABR thresholds obtained both intraoperatively and post-stimulation and behavioral T and C levels in 26 subjects—12 postlingually deafened adults and 14 perilingually deafened children. These results suggest a strong correlation between EABR thresholds and behavioral T and C levels in those EABR thresholds that consistently fell within the behavioral dynamic range. Additionally, there was a correspondence between the configuration of the EABR thresholds and the configuration of the MAP, although there was no correspondence between EABR thresholds and the T or C levels. They concluded that, although EABR thresholds cannot be used as a predictor of behavioral T or C levels, they can be used as a conditioning tool in the difficult-to-program child. Because the configuration of the EABR thresholds versus electrode curve is a good indication of the configuration of the MAP, the programming audiologist can interpolate T and C levels on electrodes not obtained through behavioral methods. Gordon et al (2004b) confirmed that EABR could be reliably measured in children using the Nucleus 24 device and did not note any significant change in levels in the first 6 to 12 months of implant use. In summary, EABR if interpreted cautiously may provide a valuable starting point in the difficult to test population.

Elicited Acoustic Reflex Threshold

The feasibility of using electrically elicited acoustic reflex threshold (EART) as a tool in programming the difficult-to-test population has also been explored. Jerger et al (1986) determined that it was indeed possible to elicit a stapedial reflex by electrical stimulation in a patient who received the Nucleus multichannel cochlear implant. In a follow-up study involving seven adult subjects (Jerger et al, 1988), behavioral C levels were close to the electrical reflex threshold and below reflex saturation in all subjects. These results have been echoed by others who have found good agreement between EART and behavioral C levels in adult cochlear implant users. In 1990, Hodges studied six patients in an attempt to correlate EART thresholds with C levels in Nucleus patients. She demonstrated a strong correlation between the measured EART and C levels. At the same time, Battmer et al (1990) studied the amplitude growth function of the EART in 25 subjects with the Nucleus 22. They reportedly were able to elicit an EART in 76% of patient studied. Amplitude growth was in agreement with the Jerger findings in that saturation was near the C level.

In 1994, Spivak and Chute studied the relationship between behavioral C levels and EART in 35 Nucleus cochlear implant patients. The results suggested that the relationship between EART and C levels could vary considerably among subjects. First, EART were obtained for 69% of subjects (12 adults and 12 children); these results were similar to those of Battmer. Second, for the 31% of subjects for whom no EART was seen, no middle ear pathology was seen, which would suggest another mechanism might be responsible for the lack of response. Third and most importantly, close agreement between EARTs and C levels were seen in only 50% of subjects with an EART, while significantly overestimating or underestimating C levels for the other 50%. They postulated that the EART might prove to be a long-term predictor of the stable C levels that are reached within the first 6 to 9 months poststimulation; however, no data exist to support this hypothesis.

Gordon et al (2004a) proposed a method of obtaining comfortable stimulation through the use of EART, in Nucleus 24 users that who could not provide behavioral responses. Buckler and Overstreet (2003) demonstrated a systematic relationship between speech burst EARTs and HiResolution programming units. They found that speech burst EARTs are "highly correlated" with speech burst M levels in patients using HiResolution sound processing. This information, they further conclude, can be useful in setting M levels in populations where behavioral information is difficult to obtain (younger, long-term deafness, cognitively impaired, etc.). Several limitations of using EART as a tool for programming include, but are not limited to, the prevalence of middle ear disease, which can obliterate a response, and the need for the child to remain motionless during the 15 minutes it takes to obtain the EART for 20 electrodes. Despite some drawbacks, however, the use of an EART can provide the clinician with a starting point for psychophysical testing and provide information regarding maximum stimulation level.

Evoked Compound Action Potential

In 1990, Brown and Abbas demonstrated the ability to directly measure the electrically evoked compound action potential (ECAP) in Ineraid cochlear implant users. Until recently, the primary method of directly recording this potential was either through an Ineraid percutaneous plug or a temporary electrode in the cochlear (Brown and Abbas, 1990, 1996), and therefore did not find widespread application. The Nucleus C124M cochlear implant features an NRT system that allows for the measurement of whole-nerve action potentials. The system as described by Brown and Abbas (1990) "allows the voltage in a specific electrode pair to be recorded by a neighboring electrode after a stimulation pulse is presented." This voltage is amplified and digitized and transmitted back to the stimulating computer, where it is averaged and the response waveform displayed. The NRT response is characterized by a single negative peak (N1) that occurs with a latency of about 0.2 to 0.4 ms following the stimulation set and a positive peak (P2). As the stimulus level is increased, the EAP amplitude increases. Growth and recovery of response can them be systematically evaluated. The ECAP has several advantages over the EABR assessing

the response of the auditory system. First, the response is much larger than the EABR. Second, the intracochlear location of the recording electrode results in less contamination from muscle artifact (obviates the need for sedation). The lack of contamination by muscle artifact allows for incorporation of these tools into routine postoperative evaluation of an implanted child (American Speech-Language Hearing Association, 2004).

Brown et al (1994) studied the relationship between ECAP thresholds and MAP T and C levels in 22 postlingually deafened adults. They found that 36% (eight of 22) of the subjects had evoked action potential (EAP) thresholds that fell within ~5 programming units of C levels; 50% (11 of 22) of the subjects had EAP thresholds that typically fell in the top half of the dynamic range; and 14% (three of 22) of the subjects had EAP thresholds that were 10 or more programming units higher than their C levels for the majority of electrodes tested. Brown et al (1997) demonstrated the ability to reliably record EAP responses for 17 of 19 adults and five of six children tested. No responses were obtained for one child who required a surgical drill-out and did not perceive any auditory stimulation with the device. They also found a strong correlation between EAP threshold and behavioral thresholds. Hughes et al (1998) suggest that, with the exception of initial stimulation, EAP thresholds in children using the C124M consistently fall within the MAP dynamic range, that is, between the T and C levels. Several other investigators have demonstrated that the ECAP is typically recorded at levels where the programming stimulus is audible to the child (DiNardo et al, 2003; Franck et al, 2001; Gordon et al, 2004a). Researchers have demonstrated that the contour of the ECAP thresholds across electrodes often follows the contour of the behavioral measures of M levels (Brown et al, 2000). Gordon et al (2002) assessed the ECAPs of 37 children who underwent implantation of the Nucleus 24 device between the ages of 12 and 24 months. They found the ECAPs to be of large amplitude, with tNRIs. If one draws a line through the input–output function and extrapolates down to the stimulus level that would elicit a threshold ECAP response, that level is the tNRI (Koch and Overstreet 2003) between behavioral T and C levels. A correction factor applied to the ECAP thresholds provided a useful prediction of T levels. They concluded that NRT could be used to ensure adequate auditory stimulation at initial stimulation even in this age group. Gordon et al (2004b) demonstrated that EABR and ECAP thresholds did not significantly change over the first 6 and 12 months of implant use, respectively, whereas ESRT thresholds increased. Hughes et al (2001) performed a longitudinal study to investigate the relationship among electrode impedance, ECAP, and behavioral measures in Nucleus 24 cochlear implant users and concluded that beyond the 1- to 2-month visit, children exhibited significant increases in electrode impedance, ECAP thresholds, slope, and MAP T levels, whereas these same measures in adults, remained stable.

Kaplan-Neeman (2004) evaluated the efficacy of NRT-based cochlear implant programming versus behaviorally based programming on MAP T and C levels and speech perception abilities in 10 congenitally deafened children between the ages of 12 and 39 months. The results suggest no significant differences between NRT-based versus behaviorally based MAPs. In fact, all studies suggest that if ECAP thresholds are to be used to assist in device programming, it is prudent to obtain those measures at the same visit as device programming rather than use measures previously obtained. Objective programming is currently so widespread that NRT data can be imported directly from a linked software application and used to generate objective MAPs. Three different techniques for using NRT data to generate MAP are built into the Nucleus software: progressive preset MAP, set T and C profile, and determine T/C offset. Advanced Bionics Corporation has recently developed a technique to measure the ECAP, referred to as neural response imaging (NRI). In contrast to the NRT in the Nucleus device, which uses a masker probe technique to cancel the stimulus artifact, NRI uses an alternating polarity approach to cancel out the rather large stimulus artifact. Investigations of 19 subjects who participated in the HiResolution clinical trial suggest that the average first NRI was at 85% of the M level, whereas tNRI was at 65% of the M level (Koch and Overstreet, 2003). Koch and Overstreet (2003) showed that the average levels required to elicit an ECAP, after appropriate conversion factors are applied, are similar across devices.

In summary, NRT and NRI are noninvasive, can be acquired in awake patients, and do not require commercial evoked potential averaging equipment, making them valuable tools in programming a variety of patients including children and the difficult-to-test. Further investigations are underway involving NRT/NRI to assess channel interactions and neural growth functions. Additionally, comparing NRI responses to evoked potentials from higher auditory centers may shed light on the entire auditory pathway in cochlear implant users (Koch and Overstreet, 2003).

◆ Follow-Up Programming

Regardless of age, accurate electrical thresholds and comfort levels continue to be a main contributor to postoperative performance. Research has demonstrated that electrical thresholds can fluctuate during the first year following initial stimulation, emphasizing the need to set up a comprehensive programming schedule to ensure maximum benefit from the device. The following first year schedule has been suggested for children after initial stimulation: at 1 to 2 weeks, 4 to 5 weeks, 3 months, 4 to 5 months, 6 months, twice between 6 months and 12 months, and at 12 months. Subsequent visits usually occur at 3-month intervals (Shapiro and Waltzman, 1995). Additional programming sessions should be scheduled if certain changes in the child's auditory responsiveness or speech production occur. These changes include, but are not limited to, changes in auditory discrimination, increased request for repetition, addition and/or omission of syllables, prolongation of vowels, and change in vocal quality. The actual length of time it requires for a child to adjust to a new program can vary greatly. It is therefore important that his or her therapist, teachers, and parents monitor the child's speech perception/production to provide input to the programming audiologist, and the programming audiologist should provide the therapist with a copy of the changes made to the program so that they can work together to maximize performance. Although an important relationship exists between speech perception and speech production, a change in a child's speech production may actually have little correlation with the need for a program adjustment. Additionally, all professionals involved with the child need to appreciate the limits of a cochlear implant; that is, not everybody will be an excellent performer. Typically, however, the most effective program is the one that requires minimal manipulation; obtaining accurate psychophysical measures will usually lead to optimal performance.

The programming timetable for adults is often not as strict and comprehensive as for children and should allow for greater autonomy on the part of the patient. The typical first year follow-up schedule for adults, after the initial stimulation is 10 days, 6 weeks, 3 months, 6 months, and 12 months, with visits once to twice per year thereafter, depending on the patient.

Device program changes are not the only determinants that contribute to postoperative performance. Age at implantation, family support, duration of deafness, communicative approach, cognitive ability, and length of device usage are but a few of the other variables that can affect performance, and ongoing counseling of patients/parents regarding all issues can lead to a more satisfied and optimal user.

References

Advanced Bionics Corporation. (1995). Clarion Device Fitting Manual. Sylmar, CA: Advanced Bionics

Advanced Bionics Corporation. (2003). New methodology for fitting cochlear implants. Valencia, CA: Advanced Bionics

American Speech-Language Hearing Association. (2004). Technical report: cochlear implants. ASHA Suppl 24:1–35

Battmer RD, Laszig R, Lehnhardt E. (1990). Electrically elicited stapedius reflex in cochlear implant patients. Ear Hear 11:370–374

Brown CJ, Abbas PJ. (1990). Electrically evoked whole-nerve action potentials: Data from human cochlear implant users. J Acoust Soc Am 88:1385–1391

Brown CJ, Abbas PJ. (1996). Electrically evoked whole-nerve action potentials in Ineraid Cochlear implant users: Responses to the different stimulating electrode configurations and comparison to psychophysical responses. J Speech Hear Res 39:453–467

Brown CJ, Abbas PJ, Fryauf-Bertschy H, Kelsay D, Gantz B. (1994). Intraoperative and postoperative electrically evoked auditory brainstem responses in Nucleus cochlear implant users: Implications for the fitting process. Ear Hear 15:168–176

Brown CJ, Hong SH, Hughes M, Lowder M, Parkinson W, Abbas PJ. (1997). Comparisons between electrically evoked whole nerve action potential (EAP) thresholds and the behavioral levels used to program the speech processor of the Nucleus C124M cochlear implant. Presented at the 7th symposium on cochlear implants in children, Iowa City, IA

Brown CJ, Hughes M, Luk B, Abbas P, Wolaver A, Gervais J. (2000). The relationship between EAP and EABR thresholds and levels used to program the Nucleus 24 speech processor: data from adults. Ear Hear 21:151–163

Buckler L, Overstreet E. (2003). Relationship Between Electrical Stapedial Reflex Thresholds and Hi-Res Program Settings: Potential Tool for Pediatric Cochlear-Implant Fitting. Valencia, CA: Advanced Bionics

Chute PM, Popp A. (2004). Preliminary results of mapping procedures in cochlear implant centers in North America. Streamlined Programming News. Denver, CO: Cochlear Americas

Cochlear Corporation. (1996). Technical Reference Manual. Englewood, CO: Cochlear Corporation

Cochlear Corporation. (1997). Clinical Bulletin. Englewood, CO: Cochlear Corporation

Cochlear Corporation. (1998a). Encoder Optimization Study. Englewood, CO: Cochlear Corporation

Cochlear Corporation. (1998b). Recommended ACE Fitting Strategy for SPEAK Conversion Patients. Englewood, CO: Cochlear Corporation

Cochlear Corporation. (1998c). Recommended CIS Fitting Strategy for SPEAK Conversion Patients. Englewood, CO: Cochlear Corporation

Cochlear Corporation. (1998d). Win DPS Programming Summary. Englewood, CO: Cochlear Corporation

Di Nardo W, Ippolito S, Quaranta N, Cadoni G, Galli J. (2003). Correlation between NRT measurement and behavioral levels in patients with the Nucleus 24 cochlear implant. Acta Otorhinolaryngol Ital 23: 352–355

Fourakis MS, Hawks JW, Holden LK, Skinner MW, Holden TA. (2004). Effect of frequency boundary assignment on vowel recognition with Nucleus 24 ACE speech coding strategy. J Am Acad Audiol 15:281–299

Franck KH, Norton SJ. (2001). Estimation of psychophysical levels using the electrically evoked compound action potential measured with the neural response telemetry capabilities of Cochlear Corporation's CI24M device. Ear Hear 22:289–299

Garber S, Ridgely MS, Bradley M, Chin KW. (2002). Payment under public and private insurance and access to cochlear implants. Arch Otolaryngol Head Neck Surg 128:1145–1152

Gordon KA, Ebinger KA, Gilden JE, Shapiro WH. (2002). Neural response telemetry in 12- to 24-month old children. Ann Otol Rhinol Laryngol Suppl 189:42–48

Gordon K, Papsin BC, Harrison RV. (2004a). Programming cochlear implant stimulation levels in infants and children with a combination of objective measures. Int J Audiol 43(suppl 1):S28–S32

Gordon K, Papsin BC, Harrison RV. (2004b). Toward a battery of behavioral and objective measures to achieve optimal cochlear implant stimulation levels in children. Ear Hear 25:447–463

Henkin Y, Kaplan-Neeman R, Muchnik C, Kronenberg J, Hildesheimer M. (2003). Changes over time in electrical stimulation levels and electrode impedance values in children using the Nucleus 24M cochlear implant. Int J Pediatr Otorhinolaryngol 67:873–880

Hodges AV. (1990). The relationship between electric auditory evoked responses and psychophysical percepts obtained through a Nucleus 22 channel cochlear implant. Ph.D. Dissertation, University of Virginia, Charlottesville, VA

Hughes ML, Abbas PJ, Brown CJ, et al. (1998). Using neural response telemetry to measure electrically evoked compound action potentials in children with the Nucleus C124M cochlear implant. Presented at the 7th symposium on cochlear implants in children. Iowa City, IA

Hughes ML, Vander Werff KR, Brown CJ, Abbas PJ, Kelsay DMR, Teagle HFB, Lowder MW. (2001). A longitudinal study of electrode impedance, EAP, and behavioral measures in Nucleus 24 cochlear implant users. Ear and Hearing 22:471–486.

Jerger J, Jenkins H, Fifer R, Mecklenburg D. (1986). Stapedius reflex to electrical stimulation in a patient with a cochlear implant. Ann Otol Rhinol Laryngol 95:151–157

Jerger J, Oliver TA, Chimel RA. (1988). Prediction of dynamic range from stapedius reflex in cochlear implant patients. Ear Hear 9:4–8

Kessler DK. (1999). The CLARION Multi-Strategy Cochlear Implant. Ann Otol Rhinol Laryngol Suppl 1999;177:8–16

Kileny PR. (1991). Use of electrophysiologic measures in the management of children with cochlear implants: brainstem, middle latency, and cognitive (P300) responses. Am J Otol 12(suppl):37–42

Kileny PR, Zwolan TA, Zimmerman-Phillips S, Kemink JL. (1992). A comparison of round-window and transtympanic electric stimulation in cochlear implant candidates. Ear Hear 13:294–299

Koch D, Overstreet E. (2003). Neural response imaging; measuring auditory-nerve responses from the cochlea with the Hi-resolution bionic ear system. Advanced Bionics Technical paper, pp. 1–5

Loizou PC, Poroy O, Dorman M. (2000). The effect of parametric variations of cochlear implant processors on speech understanding. J Accoust Soc Am 108(2):790–802

Mason SM, Shepparp DS, Garnham CW, Lutman ME, O'Donoghue GM, Gibbin KP. (1993). Improving the relationship of intraoperative EABR thresholds to T-level in young children receiving the Nucleus cochlear implant. Paper presented at the 3rd International Cochlear Implant Conference, Innsbruck, Austria

Med-El Corporation. (1997). CIS PRO + Audiologist Manual. Vienna, Austria: Med-El

Plant K, Psarros C. (2000). Comparison of a standard and interpolation method of T- and C-level measurement, using both narrowly-spaced and widely spaced electrodes. Nucleus Technical Paper. Englewood, CO: Cochlear Corporation

Shallop JK. (1993). Objective electrophysiological measures from cochlear implant patients. Ear Hear 14:58–63

Shallop JK, Beiter AL, Goin DW, Mischke RE. (1990). Electrically evoked auditory brain-stem response (EABR) and middle latency response (EMLR) obtained from patients with the Nucleus multichannel implant. Ear Hear 11:5–15

Shallop JK, Van Dyke L, Goin D, Mischke R. (1991). Prediction of behavioral thresholds and comfort values for the Nucleus 22 channel implant patients from electrical auditory brainstem response test results. Ann Otol Rhinol Laryngol 100:896–898

Shapiro WH, Waltzman SB. (1995). Changes in electrical thresholds over time in young children implanted with the Nucleus cochlear implant prosthesis. Otol Rhinol Laryngol Suppl 104:177–178

Shapiro WH, Waltzman SB. (1998). Cochlear implant programming for children: the basics. In: Estabrooks W, ed. Cochlear Implants for Kids, pp. 58–68. Washington, DC: AG Bell

Skinner MW, Holden LK, Holden TA. (1999). Comparison of two methods for selecting minimum stimulation levels used in programming the Nucleus 22 cochlear implant. J Speech Lang Hear Res 42:814–828

Skinner MW, Holden LK, Holden TA. (1994). Effect of frequency boundary assignment on speech recognition with the Speak speech-coding strategy. Ann Otol Rhinol Laryngol Suppl 104(suppl 166):307–311

Skinner, MW, Holden, LK, Holden, TA. (1997). Parameter selection to optimize speech recognition with the Nuclear implant. Otolaryngol Head Neck Surg 117:188–195

Skinner, MW, Holden, LK, Holden, TA. (1998). Comparison of two methods for selecting minimum stimulation levels used in programming of the Nucleus 22 cochlear implant. Presented at the American Academy of Auditory Implants

Spahr AJ, Dorman MF. (2005). The effects of minimum stimulation settings for the Mel EL Tempo+ speech processor on speech understanding. Ear Hear 26(4 suppl):2S–6S

Spivak LG, Chute PM. (1994). The relationship between electrical acoustic reflex thresholds and behavioral comfort levels in children and adult cochlear implant patients. Ear Hear 15:184–192

Waltzman SB, Cohen NL, Shapiro WH, Hoffman RA. (1991). The prognostic value of round window electrical stimulation in cochlear implant patients. Otolaryngol Head Neck Surg 103:102–106

Waltzman SB, Roland JT, Waltzman MN, et al. (2004). Cochlear reimplantation in children: sot signs, symptoms and results. Cochlear Implants International 5:138–145

12

Speech Perception in Children with Cochlear Implants

Susan B. Waltzman

Multichannel cochlear implants were first used in children in the United States in 1987. Early results mainly focused on the ability of children with implants to obtain benefit when the prosthesis was used as an adjunct to speech reading or in situations where a finite number of alternatives were available as response choices (closed set). Postimplantation improvement was observed for suprasegmental features, consonant and vowel recognition, and word and sentence perception on closed-set tests (Osberger et al, 1991; Staller et al, 1991). Subsequently, numerous investigators examined the results over time in children who were both younger at time of implantation and congenitally/prelingually hearing impaired. Concurrently, the focus shifted from postoperative performance on closed-set tests to the ability to perform on open-set measures where no alternative choices are provided and the results, therefore, are more closely aligned to unrestricted environmental listening conditions. Over the last several years, however, improvements in diagnosis of hearing loss, implant technology, processing strategies, surgical technique, programming options, and intervention approaches have proven that cochlear implants are a safe and effective treatment for children with sensorineural hearing loss leading to expanded criteria for implantation.

Children 2 years of age and older have been receiving implants since the late 1980s. The outcome of numerous investigations documented that pre- and postlinguistically deaf children of all ages could achieve significant open-set phoneme, word, and sentence recognition following cochlear implantation with a multichannel cochlear prosthesis beyond what could be achieved with conventional amplification. These results, coupled with advancements in cochlear implant technology and postoperative care, led to the implantation of children below 2 years of age. Again, performance in this age group revealed an increase in access to auditory stimuli leading to enhanced speech perception and oral language development. Despite the positive outcomes reported, the studies also revealed a wide range of performance. Postoperative auditory comprehension extended from the capability of using audition as the sole means of receptive communication to an ability to understand speech under restricted conditions to the need to augment auditory cues with sign language (Gantz et al, 1994; Waltzman et al, 1997). Indeed, monosyllabic word scores on tests designed for the pediatric population showed scores ranging from 0% to 100% at 1 year postimplantation, with pediatric cochlear implant recipients continuing to outperform children without implants using hearing aids on measures of speech perception (Meyer et al, 1998). Nevertheless, despite the use of less sophisticated speech processing schemes as compared with the current strategies, recent studies on long-term outcomes in the pediatric population have been surprisingly good. Waltzman et al (2002a) and Haensel et al (2005) reported continued improvement in speech perception over time with no deleterious effects in children implanted for 5 to 13 years.

◆ Factors Affecting Speech Perception in Children with Cochlear Implants

Despite the numerous positive results in pediatric cochlear implantation, published data still indicated a wide range of performance among implant recipients. Because the first

Table 12–1   Factors that Can Influence Speech Recognition by Children with Cochlear Implants

1. Implant technology
2. Surviving neural population
3. Auditory (sensory) deprivation
4. Auditory pathway development
5. Plasticity of the auditory system
6. Length of deafness
7. Age at time of implantation
8. Etiology of deafness
9. Preoperative selection criteria
10. Preoperative hearing level
11. Preoperative auditory speech perception
12. Measures of speech perception (preoperative and postoperative)
13. Preoperative linguistic level: spoken language/manual language
14. Other handicaps
15. Surgical issues
16. Device programming
17. Device/equipment malfunctions
18. Mode of communication
19. Auditory input
20. Frequency/type of training
21. (Pre) school environment/education setting
22. Parental/family motivation, social issues

question of parents of pediatric implant candidates often is "Which device is best for my child?," there remains a need to study the possible variables that could account for the diversity of performance and affect ultimate outcome. An appreciation of the possible factors that influence results is critical to both the professionals dealing with the parents and to the parents/guardians themselves. It is not the purpose of this chapter to extensively review previously published results but rather to present for consideration a variety of factors, some of which have already been shown to influence outcome and others that warrant attention. Categorizing these determinants increases the ability of clinicians to offer educated preoperative prognoses to the families and might potentially allow for manipulation of variables in an attempt to achieve the best possible outcome. **Table 12–1** is a list of possibilities. The task of considering 22 potential intertwining variables becomes less daunting when one realizes that many of them are closely aligned and can be grouped together as units. The first variable, however, stands alone as to significance and influence.

Implant Technology

Since initial research began on the development of cochlear implants, numerous designs and strategies have emerged. In the past, the prostheses had either single or multiple electrodes and channels. The electrode array was either long or short (6–30 mm) and could be positioned either in or out of the cochlea. Although there are design differences among devices, the basic implant system consists of an implanted electrode array and receiver-stimulator, and an externally worn microphone, transmitter, and processor. Currently, the most widely used devices are multielectrode/multichannel and use a straight or precoiled electrode array and transcutaneous transmission. The single most affecting difference, however, is the processing strategy,

which ultimately determines the nature of the stimulation of the electrodes. The variable factors include rate of stimulation, simultaneous or sequential stimulation, analog or pulsatile stimulation, fewer or more channels, and variations of waveform or speech feature extraction of the incoming signal.

A review of coding strategies and resultant performance used in early versions of cochlear implants can be found in a variety of publications. The most obvious result of advances in coding methodology can be found in the studies that have compared postoperative performance following speech processor upgrades using updated approaches to signal processing. The investigations showed markedly improved adult subject performance on open-set stimuli when continuous interleaved sampling (CIS) replaced simultaneous analog, when Spectral Peak (SPEAK) supplanted its predecessor MPEAK, when Multi Peak (MPEAK) succeeded its antecedent, and so forth. Those improvements in children that can be attributed to technology are somewhat more difficult to determine. The assessment of speech perception in very young children is particularly difficult because the measures are language based and therefore not appropriate for young congenitally/prelinguistically deaf children. The same group of children who are 4 to 5 years old may still not be linguistically competent to perform a perception task where the language has been standardized on hearing children. Despite the obvious evaluation dilemmas, children of all ages with implants have shown increased speech recognition skills with each successive technological evolution. It is not, then, unreasonable to assume that future alterations in processing regimens would further enhance subject outcome in both adult and child implantees.

Concurrently, research related to electrode design and its ultimate impact on performance is being conducted. The goal of electrode research is to design an array that (1) is the least traumatic to the region; (2) may be sufficiently atraumatic as to preserve residual hearing; (3) can get close to the neural elements to reduce the power needed for stimulation; (4) can stimulate a more selective cell subpopulation; and (5) can deliver lubricants, antiinflammatory agents, and neurotrophic growth factors should they be proven beneficial. Manufacturers have also provided various types of arrays so that patients with a Mondini deformity common cavity and other anatomic deformities can be successfully implanted.

In summary, dynamic technological advancements in implant design and processing not only alter absolute postoperative scores but also influence the interactions and correlations among all of the variables that affect outcome with a cochlear implant.

Surviving Neural Population, Auditory Deprivation, Auditory Pathway Development, Plasticity of the Auditory System, Length of Deafness, and Age at Time of Implantation

The second variable subset involves the physiologic manifestation of ganglion cell survival and the effects of the lack of auditory input to the system over a period of time. Investigators have demonstrated that chronic electrical stimulation in neonatally deafened kittens resulted in the preservation of spiral ganglion cells that, without stimulation, would follow a pattern of continuous neuronal degeneration (see Chapter 3). Although numerous studies have shown that early sound deprivation does result in negative effects on the central auditory system, a finite critical period has not yet been defined; however, deprivation at later times during development does not have the same severe consequences as early deprivation, confirming the existence of an as yet unspecified critical period. Similar neutralizing effects of electrical stimulation have been found on neurons in kittens that were deafened as adults.

Ponton et al (1996) and Sharma et al (2002) provided further support for the detrimental effects of deprivation with concomitant positive effects of the introduction of stimulation, although the effects may be limited (Ponton et al, 1999, 2001). In the Ponton study, evoked cortical responses were obtained from groups of normal hearing and deaf children. Although the rate of development of P1 was similar in the deaf and normal-hearing groups, the development of P1 was delayed by the length of deafness prior to implantation of the deaf children. Latencies of the P2 component reached adult levels at a very young age in the normal-hearing group, but the P2 component did not appear to develop at all in the deaf group despite implantation. On the basis of these results, it is possible to postulate that the auditory pathways do not evolve without stimulation. Nevertheless, maturation of P1 does occur following the introduction of sound. The lack of development of P2, however, might indicate some selective plasticity, confined to certain portions of the pathways. The data from the Sharma et al study, which examined P1 latencies in congenitally deaf children implanted at ages ranging from 1 to 17 years, suggested that there is a period of ∼7 years in which the human auditory system is plastic to different degrees. Beyond age 7, the plasticity of the system is reportedly greatly reduced.

We can hypothesize that the clinical correlates of deprivation and plasticity and their consequences are related to length of deafness and age at implantation and their effects on performance with a cochlear implant. Fryauf-Bertschy et al (1997) showed that children who received implants before age 5 performed better on open-set recognition tasks than did those who received implants after 5 years of age. Additionally, the above age 5 group had a greater number of inconsistent implant users than the younger group, presumably due, at least in part, to their reduced benefit. More compelling was the fact that of five children whose length of deafness was at least 10 years, only one child uses the device consistently.

In several studies, Waltzman and colleagues examined the effects of age and length of deafness on implant performance. In the initial study in 1994, results on open-set tests on children who received implants before the age of 3 were found to be better than for results reported by Miyamoto et al (1993) on children whose mean age at implantation was 6.1 years. Although the majority of children in both studies were congenitally deaf, the mean length of deafness for those with acquired prelingual hearing loss was 4.8 years in the Miyamoto study and 1.5 years in Waltzman's New York University (NYU) study. Another NYU study by Waltzman and Cohen (1998) compared the development of auditory

skills in children who received implants before the age of 2 to those who received implants between 3 and 5 years of age. The results suggested that the younger children achieved levels of auditory performance equal to or greater than the older group with comparable duration of usage. In fact, recently it has been shown that children implanted at a young age achieve auditory skills that can allow them to develop oral fluency in several languages (McConkey Robbins et al, 2004b; Waltzman et al, 2003).

Universal newborn hearing screening, however, has enabled the early detection of significant hearing loss worldwide and consequently an interest in implanting children below the age of 2 and most recently below 12 months of age. The rationale for earlier implantation is rooted in the fact that these children have significant delays in oral language skills relative to their normal-hearing peers despite the use of hearing aids and appropriate intervention. Results in these children have been very encouraging. Waltzman and Cohen (1998), Govaerts et al (2002), Kirk et al (2002), Geers et al (2003a,b), McConkey Robbins et al (2004a), Svirsky et al (2004), and Zwolan et al (2004) found that children implanted between the ages of 12 and 24 months attained better speech perception scores and oral language capability than those who received implants above the age of 2. (This chapter is focused on speech perception; for a more in-depth discussion of language development, see Chapter 13.) Although these and other studies too numerous to mention have discussed the relative benefits of implantation below the age of 2, data regarding the safety and efficacy of implantation in children below the age of 12 months are just beginning to emerge. Although James and Papsin (2004) and Waltzman and Roland (2005) reported that implant surgery was shown to be safe in children under 12 months, the authors caution that special attention needs to be paid to issues related to anesthesia, blood loss, flap breakdown, etc. The potential speech perception and linguistic advantages of implantation below 12 months of age versus implantation between 12 and 24 months, however, are still in the early stages of exploration. Lesinski-Schiedat et al (2004) reported on a small number of children implanted under 12 months of age and followed for 2 years and found better performance on the Infant Toddler Meaningful Auditory Integration Scale (IT-MAIS) in this group than for children implanted between 12 and 24 months. Similar results on a slightly larger group of children were described by Waltzman and Roland in the 2005 study. In that report, results on the IT-MAIS for young implanted children followed for 1 year were found to be in the same range as for normal-hearing children. Svirsky (2005), however, in a presentation at the CI2005 pediatric meeting in Dallas, found no difference in language development for the short term in a small number of subjects implanted below 12 months of age versus implantation in the 12- to 24-month age group, although both groups performed better than those implanted above the age of 2. These data are surely preliminary and it remains to be seen whether implantation below 12 months of age is truly more beneficial for oral language development in the long term compared with implantation at 12 to 24 months of age.

With so much focus on younger children, the inference should not be made that later-implanted children do not derive considerable benefit from devices. As technology evolves, outcomes for the congenitally deaf later-implanted group have shown substantial improvement. Dowell et al (2002a,b), Schramm et al (2002), and Waltzman et al (2002b) found significant improvement in open-set speech understanding in congenitally deaf children implanted between the ages of 8 and 18, and similar results have been shown with long-term deafened adults. Because research in the early 1990s did not reveal improvement in auditory performance following implantation in the long-term deafened population, it is not unreasonable to assume a connection between newer processing strategies and improved functioning, nor is it unreasonable to assume that future coding strategies might allow for greater achievements.

The effects of these results on our understanding of the plasticity of the auditory system are as yet unclear but would indicate a more complex interaction between physiologic plasticity and electrical stimulation.

Preoperative Hearing Level and Preoperative Auditory Speech Perception

As Chapter 6 indicated, criteria for implantation have expanded to include those with greater amounts of residual hearing. Several investigators have noted that children with higher (better) hearing levels preoperatively obtain better results postimplantation when compared with children with greater amounts of preoperative hearing loss (Dowell et al, 2004; Gantz et al, 2000; Mondain et al, 2002). Although preoperative hearing levels and speech perception skills appear to contribute to postoperative performance, the effects of technology upgrades and length of usage, which permit a global improvement in scores, may reduce the influence of preoperative open-set speech recognition. More in-depth studies over a protracted period of time are needed to define the contribution of baseline hearing.

Additional Handicaps

Hearing impairment in a child is sometimes one of several sequelae associated with a particular syndrome or etiology, the presence of which can affect the outcome with a cochlear implant. Moreover, a child with no other apparent physical or cognitive issues can have other soft sign disabilities manifest themselves after they start school similar to their normal-hearing peers. For instance, children without hearing loss are often diagnosed with a variety of conditions including learning disabilities or attention deficit disorders only after they have entered elementary school. The same is certainly true of hearing-impaired children. The preoperative implant counseling sessions should alert the family to this possibility and to the adverse effects these and other issues, related to the hearing loss or not, can have on the ability of a child to make use of the signal provided by the implant. Reports on handicapped children using cochlear implants have confirmed that many show substantial improvement in auditory, linguistic, and communication skills following

implantation, although the degree of gain is largely based on the extent of the disability not related to the hearing loss (Donaldson et al, 2004; Fukuda et al, 2003; Hamzavi et al, 2000; Knutson et al, 2000; Waltzman et al, 2000). Disabilities include blindness, CHARGE syndrome (coloboma of the eye, heart anomaly, atresia choanae, retardation, and genital and ear anomalies), attention deficit/hyperactivity disorder (ADHD), cerebral palsy, pervasive developmental disorder (PDD), autism, and many others. The parents of children with other issues often want to believe that the presence of the implant will "cure" the child. It is important to gently reduce their expectations without completely discouraging them.

There are two conditions that warrant special comments: deafness from meningitis and auditory neuropathy. The results associated with postmeningitic hearing loss are often dependent on the amount of ossification in the cochlea and the additional sequelae associated with meningitis. If bony growth is in place in the cochlea, a partial insertion of the electrode array or drill-out procedure (see Chapter 10) is not unusual. In these cases, prognosis should be guarded. Moreover, if the child had additional problems resulting from the meningitis, the outcomes can also be compromised (Francis et al, 2004).

Auditory neuropathy/dyssynchrony is a type of hearing impairment in which the outer hair cells are functional but neural transmission is impaired and the hearing loss can vary from near normal to severe. A few of the defining characteristics are the presence/absence of a significant hearing deficit, presence of otoacoustic emissions, but abnormal auditory brainstem response (ABR) recordings. The speech perception ability of these children varies from expected performance levels commensurate with the level of sensorineural hearing loss to little or no speech understanding despite good auditory thresholds. Results with cochlear implants, however, have been promising. Shallop et al (2001) matched a group of children diagnosed with auditory neuropathy to an implanted group with other etiologies and found no difference in benefit between the two groups; similar results are being reported by other clinicians (Peterson et al, 2003; Rance et al, 2002, 2004). Although preliminary, these data suggest that cochlear implantation is a viable treatment option for children diagnosed with auditory neuropathy.

Surgical Issues

The goal of cochlear implant surgery is to insert the entire electrode array into the scala tympani with as little damage as possible to the structure of the inner ear. Various factors can affect the ability of the surgeon to fully insert the electrode array: severe Mondini dysplasia or common cavity bone growth (labyrinthitis ossificans) leading to obstruction within the cochlea, properties of the electrode array itself, and surgical experience. Additional surgical issues include kinking or other surgical trauma to the electrode, facial nerve injury, and postoperative flap problems, including breakdown or infection that might lead to extrusion. For a complete review of surgical issues and complications, see Chapter 9.

The importance and seriousness of the surgical procedure and potential complications should not be minimized. Experienced otologic and implant surgeons are far less likely to encounter surgical complications, particularly in anatomically compromised cochleae. The accuracy of electrode and device placement is crucial to the process and dependent on the surgeon's ability to accurately position the internal portions without damage or kinking. Although general surgical procedures are the same for all implants, differences between electrode arrays and insertion tools require that surgeons familiarize themselves with the techniques associated with the individual devices.

Device Programming

A very important influence on performance is the manner in which the speech processor is programmed. Behavioral responses in adult implant recipients were sufficient to obtain accurate electrical threshold and comfort levels for the majority of patients. Although presumed reasonably accurate at the time of programming, thresholds and comfortable loudness levels have been shown to vary over time both in adults and children (Henkin et al, 2003; Lee et al, 2000; Shapiro & Waltzman, 1995; Skinner et al, 1995; Waltzman et al, 1986). These shifts can be indicative of measurement technique, physiologic changes brought about by electrical stimulation, or greater familiarity with the stimulus on the part of the patient. The need for accurate psychophysical measures is simple: If electrical thresholds and comfort levels are incorrect, the access to sound is flawed, leading to both poorer postoperative performance and possible nonuse by the patient. Skinner et al (1997) advocated specific subjective procedures and periodic programming sessions in an attempt to decrease the effects of programming issues on outcome, while over the years numerous investigators have advocated objective techniques including evoked stapedius reflex (ESR) to establish device thresholds. Although this and other objective methods did not supersede behavioral approaches for the adult population, implanting devices in very young children provided a more pressing need to examine the applicability of objective measures in implant programming. Loudness scaling techniques and averaged electrical voltages, in addition to ESR, have been used in an attempt to obtain valid and reliable electrical threshold and comfort levels suitable for use in a processor program. Most recently, neural response telemetry (NRT) in the Nucleus device (Cochlear Corporation, Sydney, Australia) and neural response imaging (NRI) in the Clarion device (Advanced Bionics, Valencia, CA) have been implemented to assist with device programming. These bidirectional systems enable the measurement of electrical action potentials from within the cochlea. Information is gathered about the response of the auditory nerve to both electrical stimulation and the functioning of the prosthesis (see Chapter 8). These techniques are becoming increasingly more popular as the age of implantation of children decreases and as the capabilities of the systems within each device increase in both reliability and efficiency and are being advocated by numerous clinicians. Nevertheless, behavioral programming techniques are still commonly and successfully used to program children of all ages. When used appropriately, both methods employed in tandem can be useful and time saving, especially with multiply-handicapped or difficult-to-test children.

Programming, however, is not simply the determination of thresholds and comfort levels; programming dilemmas often arise. Labyrinthitis ossificans, Mondini deformities, and other inner ear abnormalities often result in a partial insertion of the electrode array, thereby limiting the number of electrodes available for programming. Pseudomonopolar, variable-mode, and double-electrode mappings are some of the special condition strategies used in challenging programming situations. For a complete discussion of behavioral and objective programming techniques, see Chapters 8 and 11.

To a much smaller extent, device reliability plays a role in outcome. Although current implants are reliable and device failures infrequent, there are cases of internal receiver/stimulator or external equipment failure that remain undetected due to either intermittence or an inability to diagnose the defect. These problems, while discomfiting and distressing, do not usually have a long-term effect on performance. Temporary decreases in speech perception and production may be observed until the equipment is replaced, and recent studies have shown that reimplantation of an electrode array does not have an adverse affect on performance; the same or better results can be achieved following reimplantation (Alexiades et al, 2001; Ray et al, 2004; Waltzman et al, 2004).

Mode of Communication, Auditory Input, Frequency/Type of Training, Educational Setting, and Goals and Expectations

The trend is clear: implanted children obtain speech perception benefit no matter what type of communication mode is used; however, the ability to understand open-set speech stimuli and develop competence in oral language is far greater when oral communication (OC) is the primary mode of communication. Several studies have shown that when oral-only intervention and oral education were employed, children achieved higher levels of speech perception and oral language skills (Geers et al, 2002, 2003a,b; Hodges et al, 1999). It is, however, important to remember that children who use total communication (TC) do benefit from implants and, in fact, many have become oral communicators following implantation. For in-depth information on the effects of mode of communication, see Chapters 15 and 16.

It is unquestionably challenging to assimilate all of these confounding factors and their impact on outcome. However, any prognosis related to postoperative speech perception should include a discussion of the possible effects of all of the variables, including age at implantation, length of deafness, communication mode, and so forth. Although the interactions are not fully known, the preliminary evidence is clear: the wide range of performance reported among implanted children is associated in part with components external to the implant and not solely the implant as an independent entity. This fact becomes crucial during the preoperative counseling of parents regarding expectations. Parents, siblings, and extended family members are central to the process. Much depends on the knowledge they have accumulated prior to surgery and their ability to be flexible as the child's auditory and linguistic skills begin to emerge. A key factor in this process is the availability of the information necessary for them to make educated decisions. Preoperatively, they need information regarding the available devices so that a choice can be made based on fact rather than hearsay. They need to be apprised of all aspects of implantation, not just device choice, and its ramifications so that they can be certain about the decision to implant. Concurrently, choices need to be made regarding training and educational placement. Flexibility is key: the preoperative auditory and linguistic levels usually dictate the initial communication and school settings, but the course of emerging skills postoperatively often requires a change in the type of training the child is receiving. Depending on the progress, a child who began in a total communication setting may switch to an oral/aural setting or vice versa. It is important that the family not expect immediate or rapid changes in the communication skills of the children. They need to be patient and consistent about follow-up regarding programming and training to maximize the potential for long-term success.

It is hoped that this chapter has inspired contemplation about the complicated ongoing process of pediatric cochlear implantation. The intermeshing of all the variables that might affect outcome is complex, symbiotic, and, to some degree, obscure. But as clinicians and investigators, we would be remiss if we did not attempt to study and clarify the nature of these interactions: undoubtedly, they are dynamic and will change based on technological advancements and expanding criteria.

References

Alexiades G, Roland JT, Fishman AJ, et al. (2001). Cochlear reimplantation: surgical techniques, and functional results. Laryngoscope 111:1608–1613

Donaldson A, Heavner K, Zwolan T. (2004). Measuring progress in children with autism spectrum disorder who have cochlear implants. Arch Otolaryngol Head Neck Surg 130:666–675

Dowell R, Dettman S, Blamey P, Barker E, Clark G. (2002a). Speech perception in children using implants: prediction of long-term outcomes. Cochlear Implants International 3:1–18

Dowell R, Dettman S, Hill K, Winton E, Barker E, Clark G. (2002b). Speech perception outcomes in older children who use multichannel cochlear implants: older is not always poorer. Ann Otol Rhinol Laryngol Suppl 189:97–101

Dowell R, Hollow R, Winton E. (2004). Outcomes for cochlear implant users with significant residual hearing. Arch Otolaryngol Head Neck Surg 130:575–586

Francis H, Pulsifer M, Chinnici J, et al. (2004). Effects of central nervous system residua on cochlear implant results in children deafened by meningitis. Arch Otolaryngol Head Neck Surg 130:604–611

Fryauf-Bertschy H, Tyler RS, Kelsay DM, Gantz BJ, Woodworth GG. (1997). Cochlear implant use by prelingually deafened children: the influences of age at implant and length of device use. J Speech Hear Res 40:183–199

Fukuda S, Fukushima K, Maeda Y, et al. (2003). Language development of a multiply handicapped child after cochlear implantation. Int J Pediatr Otorhinolaryngol 67:627–633

Gantz BJ, Rubinstein JT, Tyler RS, et al. (2000). Long-term results of cochlear implants in children with residual hearing. Ann Otol Laryngol Suppl 2000;185:33–36

Gantz B, Tyler R, Woodworth G. (1994). Results of multichannel cochlear implants in congenital and acquired prelingual deafness in children: five year follow-up. Am J Otol 15:1–7

Geers A, Brenner C, Davidson L. (2003a). Factors associated with development of speech perception skills in children implanted by age 5. Ear Hear 24:24S–35S

Geers A, Brenner C, Nicholas J, Uchanski R, Tye-Murray N, Tobey E. (2002). Rehabilitation factors contributing to implant benefit in children. Ann Otol Rhinol Laryngol Suppl 189:127–130

Geers A, Nicholas J, Sedey A. (2003b). Language skills of children with early cochlear implantation. Ear Hear 24:46S–58S

Govaerts P, De Beukelaer C, Daemers K, et al. (2002). Outcome of cochlear implantation at different ages from 0 to 6 years. Otol Neurotol 23:885–890

Haensel J, Engelke J, Ottenjann W, Westhofen M. (2005). Long-term results of cochlear implantation in children. Otolaryngol Head Neck Surg 132:456–458

Hamzavi J, Baumgartner WD, Egelierier B, Franz P, Schenk B, Gstoettner W. (2000). Follow-up of cochlear implanted handicapped children. Int J Pediatr Otorhinolaryngol 56:169–174

Henkin Y, Kaplan-Neeman R, Muchnik C, Kronenberg J, Hildesheimer M. (2003). Changes over time in electrical stimulation levels and electrode impedance values in children using the Nucleus 24M cochlear implant. Int J Pediatr Otorhinolaryngol 67:873–880

Hodges AV, Dolan Ash M, Balkany TJ, Schloffman JJ, Butts SL. (1999). Speech perception results in children with cochlear implants: contributing factors. Otolaryngol Head Neck Surg 12:31–34

James A, Papsin B. (2004). Cochlear implant surgery at 12 months of age or younger. Laryngoscope 114:2191–2195

Kirk KL, Miyamoto RT, Lento CL, Ying EE, O'Neill T, Fears B. (2002). Effects of age at implantation in young children. Ann Otol Rhinol Laryngol Suppl 189:69–73

Knutson JF, Ehlers SL, Wald RL, Tyler RS. (2000). Psychological predictors of pediatric cochlear implant use and benefit. Ann Otol Rhinol Laryngol Suppl 185:100–103

Lee M, Kim S, Huh M, Kim L. (2000). Changes in electrical thresholds and dynamic range over time in children with cochlear implants. Adv Otorhinolaryngol 57:339–342

Lesinski-Schiedat A, Illg A, Heermann R, Bertram B, Lenarz T. (2004). Paediatric cochlear implantation in the first and second year of life: a comparative study. Cochlear Implants Int 5:146–159

McConkey Robbins A, Green JE, Waltzman SB. (2004a). Bilingual oral language proficiency in children with cochlear implants. Arch Otolaryngol Head Neck Surg 130:644–647

McConkey Robbins A, Koch D, Osberger M, Zimmerman-Phillips S, Kishon-Rabin L. (2004b). Effect of age at implantation on auditory skill development in infants and toddlers. Arch Otolaryngol Head Neck Surg 130:570–574

Meyer TA, Svirsky MA, Kirk KI, Miyamoto RT. (1998). Improvements in speech perception by children with profound prelingual hearing loss: effects of device, communication mode and chronological age. J Speech Lang Hear Res 41:846–858

Miyamoto R, Osberger M, Robbins A, Myres W, Kessler K. (1993). Prelingually deafened children's performance with the Nucleus multichannel cochlear implant. Am J Otol 14:437–445

Mondain M, Sillon M, Vieu A, et al. (2002). Cochlear implantation in prelingually deafened children with residual hearing. Int J Pediatr Otorhinolaryngol 63:91–97

Osberger M, Miyamoto R, Zimmerman-Phillips S, et al. (1991). Independent evaluation of the speech perception abilities of children with the Nucleus 22 channel cochlear implant system. Ear Hear 12:66S–80S

Peterson A, Shallop J, Driscoll C, et al. (2003). Outcomes of cochlear implantation in children with auditory neuropathy. J Am Acad Audiol 14:188–201

Ponton CW, Eggermont JJ. (2001). Of kittens and kids: altered cortical maturation following profound deafness and cochlear implant use. Audiol Neurootol 6:363–380

Ponton C, Eggermont J, Waring M, Kwong B, Masuda A. (1996). Auditory system plasticity in children after long periods of complete deafness. Neuroreport 8:61–65

Ponton CW, Moore JK, Eggermont JJ. (1999). Prolonged deafness limits auditory system developmental plasticity: evidence from an evoked potentials study in children with cochlear implants. Scand Audiol Suppl 51:13–22

Rance G, Cone-Wesson B, Wunderlich J, Dowell R. (2002). Speech perception and cortical event related potentials in children with auditory neuropathy. Ear Hear 23:239–253

Rance G, McCay C, Grayden D. (2004). Perceptual characterization of children with auditory neuropathy. Ear Hear 25:34–46

Ray J, Proops D, Donaldson I, Fielden C, Cooper H. (2004). Explantation and reimplantation of cochlear implants. Cochlear Implants Int 5:160–167

Schramm D, Fitzpatrick E, Seguin C. (2002). Cochlear implantation for adolescents and adults with prelinguistic deafness. Otol Neurotol 23:698–703

Shallop JK, Peterson A, Facer GW, Fabry LB, Driscoll CL. (2001). Cochlear implants in five cases of auditory neuropathy: postoperative findings and progress. Laryngoscope 111:555–562

Shapiro W, Waltzman S. (1995). Changes in electrical thresholds over time in young children implanted with the Nucleus cochlear prosthesis. Ann Otol Rhinol Laryngol Suppl 166:177–178

Sharma A, Dorman M, Spahr A. (2002). A sensitive period for the development of the central auditory system in children with cochlear implants: implications for age of implantation. Ear Hear 23:532–539

Skinner M, Holden L, Demorest M, Holden T. (1995). Use of test-retest measures to evaluate performance stability in adult cochlear implant users. Ear Hear 16:187–197

Skinner M, Holden L, Holden T. (1997). Parameter selection to optimize speech recognition with the Nucleus implant. Otolaryngol Head Neck Surg 117:188–195

Staller S, Dowell R, Beiter A, Brimacombe J. (1991). Perceptual abilities with the Nucleus 22 channel cochlear implant system. Ear Hear 12:34S–47S

Svirsky M, Holt R. (2005). Speech perception and language in congenitally deaf children implanted in the first year of life. Paper presented at the Tenth Symposium on Cochlear Implants in Children, March 2005, Dallas, Tx

Svirsky M, Teoh S, Neuberger H. (2004). Development of language and speech perception in congenitally, profoundly deaf children as a function of age at implantation. Audiol Neurootol 9:224–233

Waltzman S, Cohen N. (1998). Cochlear implantation in children younger than 2 years of age. Am J Otol 19:158–162

Waltzman S, Cohen N, Gomolin R, et al. (1997). Open-set speech perception in congenitally deaf children using cochlear implants. Am J Otol 18:342–349

Waltzman S, Cohen N, Green J, Roland JT. (2002a). Long-term effects of cochlear implants in children. Otolaryngol Head Neck Surg 126:505–511

Waltzman S, Cohen N, Shapiro W. (1986). Long-term effects of multichannel cochlear implant usage. Laryngoscope 96:1083–1087

Waltzman SB, Cohen NL, Shapiro WS. (2004). Use of a multichannel cochlear implant in the congenitally and prelingually deaf population. Laryngoscope 102:395–399

Waltzman S, Robbins AM, Green J, Cohen N. (2003). Second oral language capabilities in children with cochlear implants. Otol Neurotol 24:757–763

Waltzman S, Roland JT, Cohen N. (2002b). Delayed implantation in congenitally deaf children and adults. Otol Neurotol 2002;23:333–340

Waltzman SB, Roland JT. (2005). Cochlear implantation in children younger than 12 months. Pediatrics 116:e487–e493

Waltzman S, Roland JT, Waltzman M, Shapiro W, Lalwani A, Cohen N. (2004). Cochlear implantation in children: soft sign, symptoms and results. Cochlear Implants International 5:138–145

Waltzman S, Scalchunes V, Cohen N. (2000). Performance of multiply handicapped children using cochlear implants. Am J Otol 21:329–335

Zwolan T, Ashbaugh C, Alarfaj A, et al. (2004). Pediatric cochlear implant patient performance as a function of age at implantation. Otol Neurotol 25:112–120

13

Language Development in Children with Cochlear Implants

Amy McConkey Robbins

"Language is the light of the mind." John Stuart Mill

This chapter addresses issues related to language development in children with cochlear implants. Language is more than the words we speak. It is a complex enabler. It allows us to participate, to understand, and to interact with the world around us. In short, it enables us to communicate (Froehlinger, 1981). Because language skills are essential for learning almost anything, those who are deficient in such skills face difficult challenges in many other aspects of achievement. Conversely, a well-developed language foundation provides the potential for success in other achievement areas. It is this potential for enhanced life achievement that cochlear implants offer to children with profound deafness.

A cochlear implant (CI) is not a cure for deafness, but it is a powerful technology that allows many profoundly deaf children to function as well as hard-of-hearing children (Blamey et al, 2001; Boothroyd and Eran, 1994; Boothroyd-Turner and Boothroyd, 1998; Eisenberg et al, 2004). Such a transformation greatly improves the chances of achieving high levels of speech perception, good language competence, intelligible speech, and the ability to succeed in a mainstream educational setting, to name a few. This transformation also allows a deaf child the possibility of developmental equivalences with hearing individuals, the outcome measure that health agencies seek as evidence for effectiveness of an intervention (Yoshinaga-Itano et al, 2004).

◆ Effects of Profound Deafness on Language Development

Early-onset profound hearing loss has been shown to have devastating consequences for the development of language. [For the purposes of this chapter, we confine our discussion to the development of English-language skills in spoken and signed forms. Although the issues regarding development of American Sign Language within a deaf culture context are important ones, they are beyond the scope of this chapter. The reader is referred to Curtiss (1989) for a review of this topic.] During the critical period for language learning, falling between birth and about 7 years of age, children with normal hearing master almost all of the essential elements required for being a competent communicator in their language. The presence of profound hearing loss dramatically alters children's ability to extract linguistic cues from the auditory language models around them (Carney and Moeller, 1998). These children are also deprived of one of the primary sources of language information; that is, the linguistic models that are available during "overhearing" language via various sources in the environment are drastically reduced.

English-Language Achievement of Profoundly Deaf Children

Children with prelingual onset of profound deafness have been shown to experience substantial delays and deviances in their mastery of all aspects of communication including vocabulary (Boothroyd et al, 1991; Osberger et al, 1986) grammar (Geers and Moog, 1994; Power and Quigley, 1973), concepts (Davis, 1974), and pragmatics (Kretschmer and Kretschmer, 1994), in both the receptive and expressive domains. Over the past several decades, substantial advances in traditional hearing aid technology, tactile aid development, and teaching methodologies for children with profound hearing loss have taken place. Unfortunately, these advances have not translated into dramatic improvements in the overall language or academic attainment levels of deaf children. Remarkably similar language achievement levels have been documented by researchers studying children from a variety of educational settings and using different communication methodologies (Levitt et al, 1987; Moog and Geers, 1985; Osberger, 1986). Although much variability is seen across students, the average profoundly deaf child without a CI has been shown to acquire language at a rate that is approximately half of that expected from normal hearing children (Carney and Moeller, 1998; Osberger, 1986; Robbins et al, 1997).

The ability to read and write is based strongly on the foundation of language. Thus, delays in language resulting from hearing loss typically interfere with the child's development of literacy skills. Many profoundly deaf children reach the end of high school having attained only third-grade reading levels (Holt et al, 1997), a factor that severely limits their options for postsecondary education and job placement. An economic analysis (Mohr et al, 2000) estimated that the average cost to society of an individual with prelingual severe to profound hearing loss exceeded $1 million over the lifetime of that individual. The authors concluded that "interventions aimed at children, such as early identification and/or aggressive medical intervention may have a substantial payback."

The Cognitive-Linguistic Gap

Normally developing children acquire cognitive and linguistic skills concurrently wherein language milestones are intimately tied to cognitive ones. Deaf children typically acquire cognitive skills at a normal rate but are delayed in their acquisition of language, a phenomenon known as the cognitive-linguistic gap. This gap reflects the developmental asynchrony between nonverbal cognitive skills and linguistic skills in deaf children (Boothroyd, 1982). When a significant hearing loss exists, nonverbal cognitive skills emerge normally but linguistic development lags behind because of the sensory impairment. In other words, deaf children (excluding those with intellectual impairment) have the cognitive readiness to understand and use linguistic constructs, but the sensory deficit interferes with access to these constructs. This gap may actually work to the deaf child's benefit in the following way. These children, although delayed in language, have more sophisticated nonverbal comprehension strategies and means of organizing their experiences than their language level indicates (Moeller and McConkey, 1984) (i.e., their language skills are more like those of younger children with normal hearing, whereas their

cognitive skills are age-appropriate). This means that the deaf child can capitalize upon underlying knowledge of the world to accelerate language learning, *provided the child gains access to the linguistic code.* It is this linguistic access, and the best way to provide it, that is at the heart of the controversy surrounding communication methodologies for deaf children. Cochlear implants are allowing such linguistic access to many prelingually deaf children, providing a growing body of compelling evidence regarding the usefulness of these devices in the pediatric population.

◆ Benefits of Cochlear Implants for Language Development

Measuring Language Benefit in Children with Cochlear Implants

Aspects of Language Assessed

Language is a complex entity made up of two domains, comprehension and production; and many components, such as vocabulary, syntax, morphology, and pragmatics. Most research studies have investigated only one component at a time. Depending on the component(s) assessed, children with CIs may compare more or less favorably to their age peers with normal hearing. The component that has been studied most often in children with cochlear implants is single-word vocabulary comprehension. In normal-hearing children, vocabulary comprehension correlates strongly with verbal IQ. However, it is well documented that in children with hearing loss, an imperfect relationship exists between single-word vocabulary and overall language competence and that receptive vocabulary scores may over- or underestimate overall language skills in this population (Moeller et al, 1983). Moreover, single-word identification tasks give no insights into the child's lexical organization or knowledge in context, both of which are skills essential to reading comprehension (Johnson et al, 1982). Assessments should include tests that more closely resemble real-world communication, most notably tests of connected language, not only single words.

In addition, some aspects of language, such as everyday use of grammatical elements, can only be judged adequately using a spontaneous language sample. Grammatical elements, such as finite morphemes (e.g., third person singular, –s; past tense, –ed,) are highly vulnerable in hearing children and persist longer than deficits in other language areas in children with specific language impairment (Goffman and Leonard, 2000; Rice et al, 1998). The same appears to be true for children with cochlear implants. Assessment of language competence can be best accomplished using a battery of language tests that sample many aspects of communication. If a single component of language has been tested, statements pertaining to performance should be limited to the skill actually assessed (i.e., vocabulary comprehension) and not extended to overall language competence.

Methods of Analysis

One of three measurements is generally employed in studies of language development. First, performance may be expressed as an age-equivalent score (or language age) if a test standardized on children with normal hearing is used to assess language skills. Second, language quotients are often utilized as the measurement technique. Age-equivalent scores are used to obtain this measurement. A language quotient is determined by dividing a child's language age by his or her chronological age and multiplying by 100. A "normal" language quotient of 100 is obtained if language age is equivalent to chronological age. An advantage of using language quotients with implanted children is that one may observe the size of the gap between language and chronological age. Studies of implanted children utilizing language quotients measure this gap and assess if it is stable or closes over time.

A third approach to quantifying language development involves measurement of the rate of language change that occurs over a specified period of time following implantation. This approach provides information about the change measured in language skills relative to the period of time during which the change occurred. The absolute language levels of the children are not considered in this type of analysis. Rather, the goal is to observe the rate of language learning over time (**Fig. 13–1**). Some studies have utilized a combination of these analysis methods as a way of viewing the data from several perspectives.

Evidence from the Literature

In the last 5 years, there has been a dramatic increase in published investigations regarding the language of children using a CI. Variables often studied include effect of age at implantation, effect of communication mode, and comparison of the language of children with CIs to that of children with either normal hearing (NH) or hearing loss. A representative sample of studies is reviewed below.

In the most comprehensive study to date, the performance of 181 prelingually deaf 8- and 9-year-olds who received a CI by age 5 was evaluated (Geers et al, 2003); 157 of the children had performance IQs within the average range and therefore were administered a battery of language measures. On several measures including those of verbal reasoning and narratives, more than half of the children exhibited language skills that were similar to age-matched peers with normal hearing. This proportion of profoundly deaf children scoring within the average range is a landmark finding and far exceeds those reported in previous studies of similar children using hearing aids. When language measures were examined separately for expressive and receptive tasks, there was no difference between students using oral communication (OC) and those using total communication (TC) on the receptive syntax measure, but a significant expressive language advantage for children from OC settings. A similar finding was reported by Kirk et al (2002), who evaluated language skills in 73 implanted children and compared results in: (1) children implanted before 3 years of age to those implanted at 3 years or older, and (2) children using OC to those using TC. The children who received implants before 3 years of age had significantly faster rates of language development than did the children with later implantation. In addition, among the early-implanted children, OC children were acquiring age-appropriate expressive language skills whereas TC children were not. Even after 4 years of CI use, the early-implanted TC children's expressive language lagged behind their chronological age.

Hammes et al (2002) compared language development in 47 children implanted by 48 months of age. They found that children implanted under 18 months of age had substantially better language outcomes than those implanted after 18 months of age. The majority of the subjects used TC prior to implantation, yet a strong shift to spoken language was observed after implantation, depending on age at CI. All of the children implanted under 18 months of age made successful transitions to spoken language. As age at implantation increased, fewer and fewer children became competent users of spoken language. In fact, of 22 children who received their CI between 31 and 48 months, more than half remained dependent on sign language, even after 9 years of implant use. This study also looked at the differential effects of early identification/intervention and early implantation. Even among children identified, aided, and enrolled in intervention prior to 6 months of age, those who received implants earlier out-performed the early-identified, later-implanted children. This important finding suggests that although early identification and intervention are necessary, they are probably insufficient alone in producing children with age-appropriate, intelligible spoken language.

Blamey et al (2001) studied a group of 87 children with hearing loss, including 47 with cochlear implants, using single-word vocabulary Peabody Picture Vocabulary Test (PPVT) and Clinical Evaluation of Language Fundamentals (CELF) tests. The average rate of language improvement (0.56 to 0.63) was considerably less than the rate reported by several other investigators (Bollard et al, 1999; Dawson

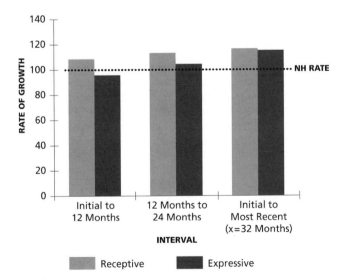

Figure 13–1 Average language learning rates on the Reynell Developmental Language Scales for 18 prelingually deafened children with Clarion (Advanced Bionics, Sylmar, CA) implants at three time intervals. Learning rate was calculated by dividing the change in language age equivalent scores at two intervals by the time between intervals and multiplying by 100. Calculations from the initial period were made from the time of initial stimulation. A normal-hearing child would make 12 months of progress in 12 months' time, yielding a learning rate of 100, as noted by the horizontal line.

et al, 1995; Miyamoto et al, 1997; Robbins et al, 1997). Some children in the Blamey et al (2001) study had received their CI at ages as late as 8 years, a factor that likely accounts for the slower rate of language growth.

Connor and Zwolan (2004) found that in 91 children who had received cochlear implants, earlier age at implantation was positively correlated with higher reading scores when the children were school-aged. Preimplant mode of communication (OC or TC) was not correlated with reading outcomes in this study.

Superior grammatical skill development was documented in children implanted by age 3 versus at age 4 years or older by Nikolopoulos et al (2004). Svirsky et al (2004) found that implantation before the age of 2 resulted in higher speech perception and language scores. Using a single-subject design, Miyamoto et al (2003) obtained language scores from a subject implanted at 6 months of age. The child's language scores at 2 years of age were nearly equivalent to those achieved at the age of 5.5 years by children implanted at later ages.

Studies have found a positive effect of early implantation even on prelinguistic communication behaviors. Houston et al (2003) used the Preferential Looking Paradigm (PLP) to assess the pre–word-learning skills of infants and toddlers who either had normal hearing or a cochlear implant. Children implanted between 7 and 15 months of age performed similarly to the children with normal hearing after 2 to 6 months of CI experience. In contrast, children who received their implants at later ages (16 to 25 months of age) did not demonstrate learning of the associations within the context of the study. The authors emphasize the possible role of intersensory redundancy, that is, that babies with normal hearing are exposed to language from birth, receiving combined auditory and visual input. Evidence suggests that early auditory deprivation impairs the development of neural pathways connecting the auditory cortex to other cortices (Kral et al, 2000; Ponton & Eggermont, 2001). Later age at implantation delays the onset of auditory input and, therefore, of neural pathway development.

Another study of early communication behaviors compared infants and toddlers who received a CI at the age of 12 to 18 months, 19 to 23 months, or 24 to 36 months (Robbins et al, 2004c). The children also were divided into three groups based on age at CI: 12 to 18 months ($n = 45$), 19 to 23 months ($n = 23$), and 24 to 36 months ($n = 30$). Scores from the Infant-Toddler Meaningful Auditory Integration Scale (IT-MAIS), a parent interview schedule (Zimmerman-Phillips et al, 2001), were compared with the normative IT-MAIS scores reported by Kishon-Rabin et al (2001). The most impressive gains were demonstrated by the children implanted between 12 and 18 months of age. Over half of the children in the youngest age group achieved auditory milestones approximating those of hearing peers after only 6 months of device use. For the children implanted between 19 and 23 months, only about one fourth attained scores within the broad normal range after 6 months of device use. Although they showed impressive progress with their CI, only a handful of children implanted between 24 and 36 months achieved scores comparable to their peers with normal hearing at the 6-month follow-up visit. Based on these data, a child's IT-MAIS score may be assigned a NH age equivalent score (**Table 13–1**).

Table 13–1   Conversion of IT-MAIS Scores to Normal-Hearing (NH) Age Equipments

IT-MAIS Score (% correct)	NH Age Equivalent
10%	1 month
20%	2 months
30%	3 months
40%	4.5 months
50%	6 months
60%	7.5 months
70%	10 months
80%	13 months
90%	17 months
100%	26 months

The studies cited above provide research evidence regarding the effects of cochlear implants on communication development in children. Several findings characterize the results of these studies.

Earlier Age at Implantation Results in Superior Language Benefit

The trend for better performance in children implanted younger also has been documented in speech perception and speech production studies (see Chapters 12 and 14). Many factors favor early age at implantation, including neural plasticity and the notion of critical periods. Researchers have used the latency of the P1 cortical auditory evoked potential as a measure of the maturity and function of central auditory pathways (Sharma et al, 2002) and found that children implanted at 3.5 years or younger show age-appropriate latency responses within 6 months of implantation. The authors concluded, "In the absence of normal stimulation there is a sensitive period of about 3.5 years during which the human central auditory system remains maximally plastic."

There is also an additive effect of early implantation and superior speech processing strategies. In one study that failed to find a significant advantage for children implanted at age 3 or younger (Geers, 2004), the author acknowledged the possibility that less sophisticated speech processing schemes used by the earliest implanted children may have provided insufficient auditory input during the early period of device use. When two powerful influences come together, that is, state-of-the-art technology and early age at implantation, the language benefit derived by deaf children is unparalleled. Another potent force that must be factored in is the ability of younger children to learn language incidentally, a topic addressed later in this chapter.

Children with Cochlear Implants Outperform Their Profoundly Deaf Peers Who Use Hearing Aids

In studies comparing the language performance of implanted children to that of their nonimplanted peers with profound hearing loss, faster rates of language learning and higher overall language achievement levels have been seen in the implant subjects (Geers and Moog, 1994; Robbins et al, 1997; Tomblin et al, 1999). The average profoundly deaf child learns language at about half the rate of normal-hearing children (i.e., 6 months of language in 1 year's time) (Svirsky et al, 2000).

Cochlear Implants Allow Many Deaf Children to Begin to Learn Language at a Rate Equivalent to that of Normal-Hearing Children

Several studies, including Robbins (2003b), have demonstrated that the average child who receives a CI learns approximately 1 year of language in 1 year's time (**Fig. 13–1**). This effect seems to be particularly true for those implanted in the first 2 years of life. Recall that, while the *average* child with CI demonstrates a normal learning rate, some children with CI demonstrate more than 1 year of growth in a year's time, whereas others demonstrate a considerably slower rate of language growth.

Many Children Remain Delayed in Their Language Skills Even After Implantation

This finding appears to be the case largely because of the significant delays that already exist in children's language at the time they receive their implants, as shown in **Fig. 13–2** (Robbins, 2003b). To avoid this continued delay, children must either learn language at a faster-than-normal rate after implantation to "catch up" to their hearing peers (Bollard et al, 1999), as some appear to be doing (see **Fig. 13–3** for one subject's data from Robbins, 2003b), or must receive their implants early enough to prevent a unclosable gap from forming between language age and chronological age. In addition, up to 40% of deaf children have additional developmental or learning disabilities (Parrish & Roush, 2004; Yoshinaga-Itano et al, 1998). Among that group, a rate of language development equivalent to that of NH children would be the exception, rather than the rule.

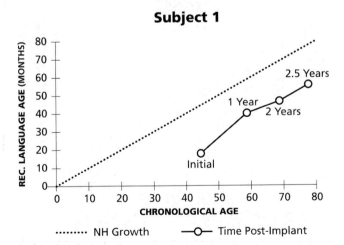

Figure 13–2 Individual Reynell data for one subject wearing the Clarion implant. Chronological age is plotted against receptive (Rec.) language age at each test interval. The dotted diagonal line represents language growth expected from a normal-hearing (NH) child; that is, the change in chronological age equals the change in language age. The gap between this child's language and that of normal-hearing peers has not closed over time.

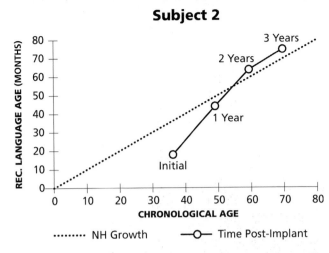

Figure 13–3 Individual Reynell data for one subject wearing the Clarion implant. Chronological age is plotted against receptive (Rec.) language age at each test interval. The dotted diagonal line represents language growth expected from a normal-hearing child; that is, the change in chronological age equals the change in language age. This child has learned language at a faster-than-normal rate since implantation, allowing the gap between his language and that of normal-hearing peers to close.

A Wide Range of Language Benefit Is Observed Across Children

Virtually every study of the performance of implanted patients, whether adults or children, has yielded a wide range of performance outcomes. The studies of language enhancement in this population are no exception (Spencer et al, 2003). The attempt to tease out what factors might account for this variability is ongoing. It is important to keep this large performance variance in mind, especially when reviewing data that have been averaged across subjects.

Morphosyntactic Development, Particularly in Expressive Language, Lags Behind Other Language Skills in Children with Cochlear Implants

Even in children with CIs whose comprehension of language is age-appropriate, expressive use of morphological markers is often delayed (Geers et al, 2003; Kirk et al, 2002; Nikolopoulos et al, 2004; Tomblin et al, 1999). Difficulties with these markers also persist longer than deficits in other language areas in NH children with specific language impairment (Goffman and Leonard, 2000; Rice et al, 1998).

Both Oral- and Total-Communication Children Improve in Their Language Skills After Implantation, but Oral-Communication Children Outperform Total-Communication Children on Most Expressive Language Skills

When some aspects of language are assessed, OC and TC children have demonstrated equivalent language benefit from the CI (Connor et al, 2000; Robbins et al, 2000). However, enhanced benefit to OC children becomes apparent when certain aspects of language are assessed. Many implanted children who use OC separate from their TC counterparts when morphosyntactic aspects of language are assessed, including use of bound morphemes, utterance length, and narrative form. Geers et al (2003) found no significant differences in language comprehension or verbal reasoning between the scores of children who were in OC educational programs and those in TC programs. Implanted children in OC programs outperformed their TC counterparts when spontaneous language samples were analyzed for lexical diversity, use of bound morphemes, utterance length, syntactic complexity, and use of the narrative form. *These advantages were apparent whether or not the children were credited with signed productions in addition to spoken language.*

◆ Mechanisms by Which Cochlear Implants Improve Language in Prelingually Deaf Children

The investigations cited before confirm that cochlear implants provide measurable language enhancement to children, particularly young children, who receive them. What is less certain is the mechanism by which this enhancement takes place. At the present time, one can only hypothesize about the nature of these mechanisms.

Access to the Spoken Language Code

For a profoundly deaf child with limited hearing aid (HA) benefit, more of the cues necessary to interpret the spoken language code are available via a CI than via HAs. Even the best CI users, however, do not hear normally; the signal they receive is degraded. Still, state-of-the-art CIs provide a rich enough signal to give "linguistic access" in many of the children who receive them. Data from studies cited earlier confirm that congenitally deaf children are able to learn spoken language via information from their CI.

Use of Audition to Monitor One's Environment

Most profoundly deaf children without a CI do not have adequate residual hearing to use audition as a way of monitoring their environment. This means they must periodically look up from the task at hand to monitor their surroundings. For a student in a classroom, this means that his attention to the book in front of him or the arithmetic problem on the board is interrupted as the child looks around, then returns to the task at hand. If the CI allowed the child to develop a listening mechanism for monitoring his environment, the child could concentrate on his work while processing auditory signals around him (i.e., "That is the sound of the water fountain at the back of the room; that is the sound of someone throwing paper in the wastebasket. I can ignore those sounds").

Ability to Cue into a Speaker

Children with hearing loss who use speech reading often miss the first parts of sentences spoken by others in conversation. This occurs because they are not visually cued into the speaker as he or she begins to talk. Anecdotal reports suggest that the CI ameliorates this problem because listeners are immediately aware when someone is speaking and can direct visual attention to that speaker. This means that, rather than processing only the second half of a message, the CI user has full access to the whole conversation, even if the user relies heavily on speech reading for language comprehension.

Potential for Incidental Language Learning

Incidental language learning is the avenue by which a child with normal hearing learns language. It occurs when (1) the child has adequate (not necessarily perfect) access to the speech code of the language and (2) what is heard takes on meaning. Traditionally, auditory language learning in deaf children was viewed as a process of *auditory training*. The approach mandated that the child be didactically *trained* to achieve each of the listening skills along the hierarchy of auditory development. This approach was based on the assumption that whatever the child needed to learn would have to be directly taught. This was not an unreasonable assumption prior to the advent of CIs, because many profoundly deaf children received only minimal auditory cues or patterns through their hearing aids. These pattern perceivers did not hear enough of the auditory code to use listening as their primary source of linguistic input. In order for these children to learn spoken language a direct, systematic approach to training was required. As one textbook advised, "It is important to remember as we work with hearing-impaired children that language skills need to be overtly learned" (Froehlinger, 1981). Deaf children were, in large part, unable to make use of incidental learning, such as through the overhearing of conversation, as a means of acquiring language. Incidental learning is the most efficient and perhaps the only way to truly master a spoken language code.

Even with the improved signal provided by the CI, children require intervention to develop age-appropriate language skills, but the focus of that intervention must take into account the child's enormous potential for learning language incidentally. If teachers assume that a CI child's learning is completely dependent on didactic instruction, many opportunities for incidental learning will be lost. In addition, failure to adopt an emphasis on incidental learning lessens the effectiveness of parents to utilize "teachable moments" at home to foster their child's communication development.

A child's potential for incidental learning and generalization is greatest in the early years and slowly decreases with age. All things being equal, the younger the child at the time of implantation, the greater the influence of incidental language learning. Conversely, the older the child at the time of implantation, the greater the need for didactic instruction to foster language development. Although children who are older at the time of implantation may still benefit from incidental learning, it is likely that their curriculum will need to be heavily weighted with didactic instruction if they are to learn new skills at an adequate rate.

◆ Clinical Management of Language Skills in Children with Cochlear Implants

Four issues regarding the clinical management of language skills in children with CIs are presented in this section. These are the selection of assessment tools, principles for developing language, birth-to-age-3 interventions in natural environments, and special populations of implanted children.

Selecting Tools for Measuring Language Skills

Establishing a baseline of English-language skills preoperatively and monitoring ongoing development after implantation are vital to assessing implant benefit and making appropriate educational recommendations for implanted children. The purpose of assessing language is to reveal the child's underlying competence in abstract linguistic knowledge (in our case, English). For this reason, it is typical to assess a child's language in his or her preferred communication mode, which may include spoken English alone, simultaneous spoken and signed English, or spoken English and cued speech. For a child using total communication, such an assessment yields information about underlying language abilities, not necessarily *spoken* language. It is also important to assess spoken language in every child with a CI, even those who typically communicate with signs, because spoken language skills are predictors of device benefit and impact decisions such as educational inclusion. Both formal and informal assessment procedures are useful when evaluating the language skills of implanted children. Recommended procedures and rationales for their use are found in the following subsection. Clinicians may also use the criterion-referenced red flag procedure to identify children who are making slower-than-average progress after implantation (**Table 13–2**). These red flags are based on data from published studies and reflect average performance for three different groups of children based on preimplant characteristics (Robbins, 2005).

Formal Assessment Procedures

A battery of language tests is recommended that sample communication behaviors across several subskills in the most time-efficient way. Receptive and expressive language skills should be evaluated independently, rather than inferred from one another. Tests should sample the broad areas of vocabulary, connected language, grammar, concepts, and pragmatics. The tests listed in **Table 13–3** meet several important assessment criteria: (1) they provide normative data for comparison to hearing peers; (2) they are relatively brief to administer; (3) they can be used with a broad age

Table 13–2   Red Flags that May Indicate Inadequate Progress in Children Implanted by 36 Months of Age

Full-time implant use not accomplished 1 month after initial activation

No change in quality or quantity of vocalizations after 3 months of device use

Child not spontaneously alerting to own name 25% of time after 3 months of device use

Child not spontaneously alerting to own name 50% of time after 6 months of device use

Lack of spontaneous alerting to some environmental sounds 6 months postactivation

Skills from audiological testing not observed in everyday settings after 9 months of use

No evidence of meaning being derived from sound after 12 months of device use

Major improvement in language not observed after 12 months of device use

range of children, an important factor when performing longitudinal assessments; and (4) they have all been used with deaf children and found to be appropriate for this population (Moeller et al, 1983; Osberger, 1986; Waltzman et al, 2003). A spontaneous language sample has always been an important part of a test battery and recent studies of children with CIs (Geers et al, 2003), which suggests that spontaneous samples identify morpho-syntactic weaknesses that are not revealed by other tests.

As infants and toddlers receive CIs with greater frequency, communication assessment remains vital for children at the prelinguistic stage, as revealed in findings by Kane et al (2004). These investigators correlated preimplant Communication and Symbolic Behavior Scales (CSBS) scores with postimplant Reynell scores in a group of early-implanted children. Results suggested that very low performance on the CSBS preimplant was a red flag for low Reynell scores after 2 years of device use. Preliminary results suggest that if children lack appropriate prelinguistic behaviors, the development of age-appropriate formal language is at risk.

If time permits, an assessment of pragmatics and verbal problem solving reveals how the child uses language to "put it all together." Suggestions include the Test of Problem Solving and the Preschool Language Assessment Instrument, both for problem solving and conversational pragmatics.

Informal Assessment Procedures

Informal testing allows the clinician to vary the difficulty, length, and complexity of language input to assess the child's ability to handle linguistic information. In this regard, informal procedures are akin to diagnostic teaching, which allows the clinician not just to assign a "pass" or "fail" to a test item, but to determine what methods work best with a child. Some formal tests identify primarily what the child *cannot* do, whereas informal procedures permit the flexibility to explore what the child *can* do, and under what conditions. Both are needed to paint a complete picture of the child's communicative competence. Robbins (2000) provides suggestions for informal procedures with children wearing a CI.

Table 13–3 Test Battery for Assessing Children with Cochlear Implants

Test Instrument	Skill Assessed
Receptive Language	
CSBS	Pre- and early-communication behaviors
MacArthur Communicative Inventories	Single-word vocabulary and word combinations
Peabody Picture Vocabulary Test (PPVT)	Single-word vocabulary
Reynell Developmental Language Scales (RDLS)	Connected language
Test of Language Development (TOLD-P)	
Grammatic Understanding subtest	Syntax and morphology
Oral and Written Language Scales (OWLS)	Concepts and grammar; connected language
Expressive Language	
CSBS	Pre- and early-communication behaviors
MacArthur Communicative Inventories	Expressive vocabulary and word combinations
Woodcock-Johnson Psychoeducational Battery	
Picture Vocabulary subtest	Single-word vocabulary
Antonyms-Synonyms subtest	Concepts; "thinking with language"
Analogies subtest	
Reynell Developmental Language Scales	Connected language
Spontaneous Language Sample*	Syntax and morphology
Oral and Written Language Scales (OWLS)	Grammar, vocabulary, idioms, pragmatics

*Analyzed formally using D.S.S., LARSP, IPSyn, etc., to evaluate structural complexity.

Principles for Developing Language in Children with Cochlear Implants

This section contains suggestions for the design of language learning programs for implanted children. Rather than being a prescribed curriculum, the following principles may be incorporated into an existing language program.

Establish a Foundation for Generalization Learning in the Early Stages of Implant Use

The foundation for establishing generalization and utilizing incidental learning should be built from the earliest days of cochlear implant use and embedded in the therapy program. The first weeks and months of device use are critical in establishing either a pattern that encourages generalization or one that emphasizes isolated training that may lead to "greenhoused" communication skills (Robbins, 2000). A model for building such a foundation is found in Robbins and Kirk (1996). The model includes using communication sabotage, teaching the child to recognize and label the absence of sound, and emphasizing name recognition. Even at the earliest stages of implant use, the emphasis is placed on behaviors that have relevance to real-world communication.

Emphasize the Suprasegmental Patterns of Spoken Language

Most children are delayed in language at the time they receive their CI, creating a sense of urgency to make up for lost time and close the language gap. Some parents and clinicians concentrate too heavily on single-word productions to close the gap, ignoring the vital role that suprasegmentals play in language development. "But affect is information and prosody conveys" (Locke, 1993). During the first year of life, an NH infant latches onto suprasegmental features in the parents' speech: the prosody and intonation that communicate feelings and intentions. Via cues from a human voice, the listener knows the speaker's identity (we are revealed through our voiceprint), his emotional state (is the speaker happy, worried, angry?), and the speaker's intent (is he telling me something, asking me something, commanding that I do something?) all before factoring in the linguistic content of the words and grammar. Cues about speaker identity, emotional state, and speaker intent are well transmitted by the CI, meaning that the early-implanted child can learn communication intent and linguistic correctness as a gestalt, just as NH babies do (Robbins, 2003a).

Help All Implanted Children, Whether Oral- or Total-Communication, Move as Far Along the Auditory Continuum as Possible

The way language is organized and processed by deaf children falls along a continuum from fully visual to fully auditory. Most CI children are somewhere in between these two, relying both on auditory and visual cues during communication interaction. Our goal in language instruction with CI children is to move each child as far down the auditory continuum as possible for that child. How far down the continuum a given child moves is dependent on many factors, including age at implantation; etiology of deafness; presence of additional handicaps; parental support; educational environment; and x-factors (Head, 1983), which are the characteristics unique to each child, including temperament, tolerance for frustration, personality traits, and internal motivation to master tasks. Many of these factors, perhaps most of them, might be internally operating and not amenable to change. After implantation, some children may become almost completely auditory, relying on visual cues only in extremely noisy situations, whereas others remain highly dependent on vision to augment what they hear.

It should not be assumed that every child who uses TC prior to implantation will remain a visual learner after implantation. TC children can move far down the auditory continuum, but generally require radical changes in their educational programs and in parent expectations for listening and speaking skills to do so (Robbins, 1998a). Even if a TC child remains primarily a visual learner following implantation, the contributions that auditory input can make to his language development are profoundly important, provided the child learns to derive meaning from this input. There is ample clinical evidence to suggest that a child who is given an implant and then placed in a home or school environment where audition and speech are not valued, worked on, or naturally reinforced will demonstrate very little benefit from his implant in real-world communication situations. Successful children with implants may be found in both OC and TC settings. However, it is clear that an environment that emphasizes listening and speaking development is mandatory if children are to receive maximum benefit from the device. Cochlear implants have the potential to dramatically improve a deaf child's ability to perceive spoken language and to speak intelligibly. If those two skills are not essential goals within an educational program, it is considered an inappropriate placement for an implanted child. For teaching suggestions related to language development in children using TC, see Robbins (1998a).

Set Both Spontaneous and Structured Language Goals

The tendency is to set goals only for behaviors that the child must demonstrate during structured learning times. Goals for spontaneous use of language define specific communication behaviors that the clinician expects to observe when the child is not in a structured setting, but rather is conversing with the teacher or with a peer. It is important to give parents homework activities that emphasize carryover of language skills learned at school to everyday situations at home.

Comment to Children as Much as You Question

Analyses of language interactions between adults and children with hearing loss reveal an overuse of commands and questions directed at children. Blank and Marquis (1987), in their conversational training program for young children, urge clinicians to recognize the vital importance of comments in conversation. The clinician who makes relevant comments that are at the child's language level provides natural language models to the child, teaches the child about facts ("pumpkins are orange") versus opinions ("pumpkin ice cream is better than vanilla ice cream"), and demonstrates one of the most important functions of language: sharing thoughts and feelings. By their very nature, comments leave a conversational space for communication turn-taking and elicit longer responses than

"Yes-No" or "Wh" questions do. These skills, falling under the rubric of pragmatics, are sometimes mentioned by parents and teachers as being underdeveloped in children with CIs.

Use "Thinking While Listening" Techniques to Interweave Auditory and Language Activities

Auditory and language activities may be interwoven to "double your money" during lessons. Listening and language are not viewed as separate tasks but as interrelated components of communication. The "thinking while listening" approach (Robbins, 1998b) uses many traditional auditory techniques but introduces a twist to make them more meaningful and less predictable.

Monitor Children's Progress in Language

A program should establish milestones for language behaviors that are expected to emerge in children at specific postimplant intervals. Noticeable changes in communication should be seen after 3 months of CI use. In children implanted by 36 months of age, data have been used to establish first-year auditory milestones that are precursors to spoken language proficiency (**Table 13–3**). Extensive post-CI communication benchmarks are also found in McClatchie and Therres (2003). Although children vary in the patterns of development, programs should have pre-established "red flags" for children who are not progressing appropriately. The clinician should keep a watchful eye on how well the chosen methodology works for a given child. If progress is not occurring, the teachers and parents should meet and discuss strategies. Given the research results that show the average implanted child learning 1 year of language in 1 year's time, clinicians and teachers must be concerned about a child whose language progress is significantly slower than this. If limited progress is made after 6 months, something different should be tried. This may mean a host of different things for different children, but the goal is to explore other avenues for accelerating language learning.

Clinicians should record the positive changes occurring in a child's language by using videotaping, testing, or spontaneous language sampling. It is helpful to document instances in which the child repeats something he has overheard in conversation, uses a new word without being directly taught it, or re-auditorizes by "thinking aloud" with language to problem-solve. All of these suggest that the forces of generalization and incidental learning are actively present in the child with a cochlear implant.

Early Intervention (Birth to Age 3) in "Natural Environments"

Implantation within the first months or years of life provides the baby with auditory access to the world at a point in development that is relatively close to that experienced by the normal-hearing infant. This, theoretically, could prevent the effects of developmental asynchrony and the often-seen gap between chronological age and language age observed in children with profound hearing loss.

We approach intervention with implanted babies with the assumption that a significant part of their language will be acquired incidentally, via natural interactions with their parents in a reinforcing environment, overhearing of conversations not spoken directly to them, and in playtime with other children. When working with implanted infants and toddlers who have no additional handicaps, the therapist's job is largely one of *facilitation* rather than *rehabilitation* of language. This facilitation is not conducted haphazardly, however, but with a purposeful, goal-oriented approach. The notion of "natural environments" for CI children has been misinterpreted to mean therapy that always occurs in the child's home. In fact, children with CIs, whose intervention focus is highly auditory, often should receive intervention in a clinic setting for the following reasons: (1) the clinician must be able to control the auditory environment during intervention, an unattainable task in many homes; (2) equipment (karaoke machine, piano, doorbell) that is essential for intervention is impractical or impossible to transport; (3) only a small number of clinicians are trained to work with this population and time spent traveling results in fewer children having access to a specialized therapist; and (4) a "natural environment" for babies is wherever their parents are, not a specific physical location. That being said, intervention should always be directed at helping parents facilitate communication in everyday settings, as outlined by Estabrooks (1998), Robbins (2003a), Rossi (2003), and Sindrey (2002).

Special Populations of Children with Cochlear Implants

As the criteria for implantation have expanded broadly over the past decade, more children with special needs are receiving these devices and require special considerations. Three such populations are multiply disabled deaf children (MD/D), children exposed to multiple languages, and children with auditory neuropathy/dyssynchrony (AN/AD).

Children with Multiple Disabilities

It has been estimated that ~40% of deaf children have one or more additional disabilities (Parrish & Roush, 2004). In the Colorado statewide population of deaf children ages birth to 3 years (Yoshinaga-Itano et al, 1998), between 41% and 47% were reported to have one or more additional disabilities. It is possible that the number of MD/D children is increasing, due largely to higher rates of premature babies from the neonatal intensive care unit (NICU) who survive but are left with significant impairments. Recent studies (Donaldson et al, 2004; Holt and Kirk, 2005; Waltzman et al, 2000) suggest that many MD/D children show benefit from the cochlear implant, although progress is delayed relative to that of typical deaf children. The severity of the delay is typically consistent with the severity of the additional disability. Not every child with MD/D benefits from a CI.

Some clinical guidelines when working with the MD/D population include the following. Evaluate each child individually in the CI candidacy phase. The team should consider what environmental, cognitive, and social value a CI might have for the child, even if the benefit is less than expected. The team also should consider the cost to the family and child if the implant does not enhance the child's quality of life. Exploring parental expectations is critical.

Determine to what degree the child makes use of the sensory information he already has. To the extent that the child uses touch, taste, vision, and other sensory systems to figure out the world, this bodes well for his ability to utilize auditory information from the implant.

For a significantly disabled child, consider a trial diagnostic period with a tactile aid to determine if the child will accept wearing a device and can make associations between sensory input and meaning. Post-CI, evaluate the progress of CI children with severe disabilities in comparison to themselves and from the standpoint of improved quality of life.

A team approach for the MD/D child is essential. Learn from and educate the other specialists working with the child. They have expertise in areas that can be of great value to the implant clinician. Often, other specialists' knowledge of the benefit of auditory input is limited, and they require modeling to see how to incorporate listening and speaking into developmental activities. In addition, implant teams should not consider implanting MD/D children until the team gains experience with a large number of typically developing deaf children.

Multilingual (ML) and English as a Second Language (ESL) Families

Children exposed to multiple spoken languages fall into one of two subgroups, ML or ESL, that require very different clinical management techniques. The ML group is made up of families in which parents are fluent in both English and another language. Children from such homes who have implants are exposed to fluent and sophisticated models of two languages and often attend schools, social events, and houses of worship where the second language is spoken fluently. Recent studies have yielded encouraging outcomes in both languages for children in this subgroup (Robbins et al, 2004a; Waltzman et al, 2003). It should be noted that the children in these studies were all implanted early (usually before age 2), and had excellent speech perception scores and no other significant disabilities (**Fig. 13–4**).

The high language proficiency of CI children from ML families is also related to two important factors: the rich and complex models of language provided by fluent speakers and the ability of ML parents to navigate the medical and educational systems, serving as informed advocates for their children. These factors are not present in the second group of CI children, those from ESL families. The clinical management of children from ESL families, therefore, is more complex and requires a concerted effort on the part of the CI team. It is widely acknowledged that a parent's English-language proficiency by itself is not considered a

Bilingual Subjects Language
Standard Scores

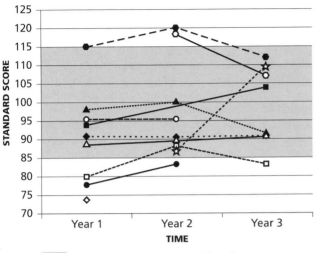

Average range for normal-hearing

Figure 13–4 Individual standard scores on the Oral and Written Language Scales or Reynell Developmental Language Scales representing first-language proficiency in 12 early-deafened, bilingual children wearing the Nucleus cochlear implant. Mean standard score = 100; standard deviation (SD) = 15. The shaded area represents performance within the average range for normal-hearing children. Data points for the same child across 2 or 3 years are connected by a line; single data points without a line indicate a child who was tested at one interval.

selection criterion for a deaf child. On the other hand, family support is still considered an essential component of successful implantation for ESL children, as it is for any CI candidate. As always, the CI team must ensure that the family has appropriate expectations from the implant, can secure the child's full-time use of the device, is comfortable with and able to troubleshoot the equipment, and can learn home carryover of speech, auditory, and language goals. In fact, the latter is absolutely essential for ESL families. For parents with limited English ability, an interpreter ideally should be available during clinic visits. At minimum, an interpreter must be present during preimplant candidacy discussions to ensure that the family has reasonable understanding of and expectations for the implant and to translate parent questions and concerns posed to clinicians. The team should also advise the family members that they play the most important role in their child's success with the implant and must learn language stimulation techniques to use at home *in their first language*. Parents who speak limited English should not be advised to speak English to their deaf child, as the parents will be unable to provide rich, natural, and intelligible models of language in English (Sussman & Lopez-Holzman, 2001). Parent–child therapy time should be spent modeling techniques to the parent using English so that the parents may replicate the techniques in their first language.

Creativity and flexibility are required when dealing with ESL families. Clinicians may administer the Bilingual Family Interview (BIFI) (Robbins, 2004b). The interview

yields information about comprehension, expression, and reading proficiency in English and in the second language for each adult living in the home, which may include extended family members. If ESL parents have a better understanding of written than spoken English, or have family members who read English, clinicians should provide written notes from meetings and therapy sessions. To contact ESL families by telephone, clinics may subscribe to a real-time interpreter service, such as AT&T Language Line. Families may have cultural customs and taboos related to communication to which clinicians should be sensitive. At the same time, the needs of their deaf child may require flexibility on the part of the parents. If the clinician's suggestions are contrary to cultural norms, such as the mother using a strong speaking voice or the child seeking direct eye contact, the clinician may explain their importance at the earliest stages of language use, noting that, once a solid foundation for language is established, the child will have the skills to adapt to these customs.

Coaching Techniques for ESL Families. For ESL families that do not use English with their child, much value can still come out of communication intervention sessions. The clinician's job in such cases is to conduct a language lesson that could be replicated easily in the home [see Rossi (2003) and Bader (2001) for suggestions] with clear modeling of one or two important techniques the parents should use when interacting with their child in their native tongue. These include a strong but natural speaking voice, eye contact, acoustic highlighting techniques, calling the child's name to get his attention, staying at ear level, ensuring a quiet environment, providing additional cues for comprehension, and so on. The clinician models in English, then invites the parents to do the same procedure in their language. Without knowing the second language, the clinician still is able to observe the parents' interaction style and to give feedback. Compliments and praise transcend language barriers and ESL parents need encouragement and validation for their efforts. The John Tracy Clinic (www.jtc.org) offers a correspondence course to families in numerous foreign languages at no charge. Some ESL families have considered the correspondence lessons to be their lifeline because of direct communication in their own language.

Clinicians may model nursery rhymes, songs, finger plays, and children's dances (such as "Ring Around the Rosie" or "Hokey Pokey") in English, and then invite the parents to do the same in their language. Songs and dances are part of the cultural heritage of families and are replete with salient suprasegmental cues. Children from ESL families are at a disadvantage for learning, partially because their parents are less able to advocate for them in English within the educational and health care systems. It is appropriate to encourage ESL parents to learn English, even if they do not speak it at home, as a tool to advocate on behalf of their child.

The management of children from multilanguage backgrounds is challenging but highly rewarding. Even parents who are fluent in English but whose first language is not English report how difficult and unnatural it was to speak English to their child because, as one mother said, "It is not the language of my heart." One can imagine how difficult it would be for limited-English speakers to try to use English with their young child. Communication between a parent and a baby is an intimate and highly emotional exchange and is a central part of how bonding is solidified. Anything that interferes with the naturalness of the exchange may be a hindrance to communication and to parent–child bonding.

Auditory Neuropathy/Dyssynchrony (AN/AD)

Rehabilitation for pediatric auditory neuropathy cases is challenging due to the heterogeneity of this population. One pervasive finding with auditory neuropathy is the poor level of meaningful audition in relation to the degree of hearing loss. While the results of recent studies are promising, a diagnosis of auditory neuropathy is not considered an immediate indicator for cochlear implant referral. Some infants and children diagnosed with auditory neuropathy showed fluctuating auditory responses and significant benefit with conventional amplification (Rance et al, 1999). Therefore, a limited trial period with amplification and monitoring of the stability of audiological thresholds is recommended before cochlear implantation. Postimplant benefits in these children are encouraging and, therefore, an implant should be considered after appropriate hearing aid use and parent counseling.

It has been estimated that about half of all children with AN/AD have global neurological impairments, necessitating an approach similar to that taken with other multiply disabled/deaf children. The CI team must consider whether the child is likely to utilize the signal from the implant. For children with AN/AD who do not have additional neurologic impairments, a therapist experienced with pediatric deafness is essential for informing the CI team about the child's functional communication relative to hearing loss. Because of the nature of this disorder, an audiogram may not be the best indicator of hearing aid benefit.

Some special considerations for the language development of children with AN/AD include the following. Prior to CI, consider emphasis on visual supports for many (not all) children with AN/AD. Progress in a strictly auditory approach is frequently slow but accelerates when visual cues (e.g., speech reading, cues, signs) are used as supplements.

Age-at-implantation effects are similar for this group as for other children. Those AN/AD children who do need a CI will perform better if implanted before a large gap develops between chronological and language age.

Whereas aiding a contralateral ear with residual hearing is desirable in children with CI, it may not be for some children with AN/AD who report that the hearing aid "just makes me hear noise."

Candidacy questions are more pertinent to whether the child performs as would be expected based on his residual hearing, rather than on the audiogram. For this reason, the experienced clinician is essential in making a team decision (J. Shallop, personal communication).

Early reports suggest that several AN/AD children without global neurologic problems still have clinical "soft signs," which may include somewhat low muscle tone, dyspraxic characteristics, mild dysphagia, slightly delayed fine and gross motor development, clumsiness, and sensory integration problems. Clinical experience has shown that many of these problems are responsive to treatment and eventually resolve over time. A vigilant approach, however, is needed with this population, including frequent developmental checks and referral to other therapists because these soft signs can slow language progress.

A range of language benefit has been reported in children with AN/AD who receive a CI, including a number who perform in the superior range. It has been hypothesized that high performers reflect a group with good neural survival and enough usable preimplant hearing to establish a foundation for symbolic communication.

◆ Conclusion

We have defined the urgent problem facing many profoundly deaf children: the struggle to achieve full competence in language. Much has been learned over the past decade about language development in children with cochlear implants but much remains to be learned. The evidence that is available thus far confirms that cochlear implants provide enormous benefit for the development of language in children. Future directions for research include identifying the factors that account for the wide variability in language benefit across implanted children, charting the time course of language skill development postimplant, and more clearly delineating the aspects of linguistic development enhanced by the cochlear implant. In this new science of pediatric cochlear implantation, the roles of both clinician and researcher are vital and interdependent. Neither stands alone. Many of the directions researchers have followed have been based on leads provided by clinicians working with this population. Likewise, clinicians must modify their teaching techniques and expectations in an ongoing way to accommodate the new information revealed in research studies with implanted children. Such a partnership bodes well for the continued progress in helping all children with cochlear implants to fully master the language of their family, their community, and their world.

References

Bader J. (2001). Top Ten Strategies for Parents: Video and Manuals. Washington, DC: AG Bell

Blamey PJ, Sarant J, Paatsch L, et al. (2001). Relationships among speech perception, production, language, hearing loss and age in children with impaired hearing. J Speech Lang Hear Res 44:264–285

Blank M, Marquis MA. (1987). Directing Discourse. Tucson: Communication Skill Builders

Bollard PM, Chute PM, Popp AC, Parisier S. (1999). Specific language growth in young children using the CLARION cochlear implant. Ann Otol Rhinol Laryngol Suppl 177:119–123

Boothroyd A. (1982). Hearing Impairments in Young Children. Englewood Cliffs, NJ: Prentice-Hall

Boothroyd A, Eran O. (1994). Auditory speech perception capacity of child implant users expressed as equivalent hearing loss. Volta Review 96:151–168

Boothroyd A, Geers AE, Moog JS. (1991). Practical implications of cochlear implants in children. Ear Hear 12(4 suppl):81S–89S

Boothroyd-Turner D, Boothroyd A. (1998). Characteristics and attainment of congenitally deaf children with cochlear implants. Paper presented at the AG Bell Convention, June 30, Little Rock, AR

Carney AE, Moeller MP. (1998). Treatment efficacy: hearing loss in children. J Speech Lang Hear Res 41:S61–S84

Connor CM, Hieber S, Arts HA, Zwolen TA. (2000). Speech, vocabulary and the education of children using cochlear implants: oral or total communication? J Speech Lang Hear Res 43:1185–1204

Connor CM, Zwolan TA. (2004). Examining multiple sources of influence on the reading comprehension skills of children who use cochlear implants. J Speech Lang Hear Res 47:509–526

Curtiss S. (1989). Issues in language acquisition relevant to cochlear implants in young children. In: Owens E, Kessler D, eds. Cochlear Implants in Young Deaf Children. Boston: Little, Brown

Davis JM. (1974). Performance of young hearing-impaired children on a test of basic concepts. J Speech Hear Res 17:342–351

Dawson PW, Blamey PJ, Dettman SJ, Barker EJ, Clark GM. (1995). A clinical report on receptive vocabulary skills in cochlear implant users. Ear Hear 16:287–294

Donaldson AI, Heavner KS, Zwolan TA. (2004). Measuring progress in children with autism spectrum disorder who have cochlear implants. Arch Otolaryngol Head Neck Surg 130:666–671

Eisenberg LS, Kirk KI, Martinez AS, Ying EA, Miyamoto RT. (2004). Communication abilities of children with aided residual hearing: comparison with cochlear implant users. Arch Otolaryngol Head Neck Surg 2004;130:563–569

Estabrooks W. (1998). Cochlear Implants for Kids. Washington, DC: AG Bell

Froehlinger VJ. (1981). Into the mainstream of education. Washington, DC: AG Bell

Geers A. (2004). Speech, language and reading skills after early cochlear implantation. Arch Otolaryngol Head Neck Surg 130:634–638

Geers A, Moog J. (1994). Spoken language results: vocabulary, syntax and communication. Volta Review 96:131–150

Geers A, Nicholas J, Sedey AL. (2003). Language skills of children with early cochlear implantation. Ear Hear 24:46S–58S

Goffman L, Leonard J. (2000). Growth of language skills in preschool children with specific language impairment: Implications for assessment and intervention. Am J Speech-Lang Pathol 9:151–161

Hammes DM, Novak MA, Rotz LA, Willis A, Edmondson DM, Thomas JF. (2002). Early identification and cochlear implantation: critical factors for spoken language development. Ann Otol Rhinol Laryngol Suppl 189:74–78

Head J. (1983). Skills + knowledge + x-factors = effective speech teaching. In: Hochberg I, Levitt H, Osberger MJ, eds. Speech of the Hearing Impaired. Baltimore: University Park Press

Holt J, Traxler C, Allen I. (1997). Interpreting the Scores: A User's Guide to 9th Edition Stanford Achievement Test for Educators of Deaf and Hard-of-Hearing Students. Gallaudet Research Institute Technical Report 97-1. Washington, DC: Gallaudet University

Holt R, Kirk KI. (2005). Speech and language development in cognitively delayed children with cochlear implants. Ear Hear 26:132–148

Houston DM, Ying E, Pisoni DB, Kirk KI. (2003). Development of pre-word-learning skills in infants with cochlear implants. Volta Review 2003;103:303–326

Johnson D, Toms-Bronowski S, Pittleman S. (1982). Vocabulary development. Volta Review 84:11–24

Kane MO, Schopmeyer B, Mellon N, Wong N, Niparko JK. (2004). Communication and subsequent language acquisition in children with cochlear implants. Arch Otolaryngol Head Neck Surg 130:619–623

Kirk KI, Miyamoto RT, Lento CL, Ying E, O'Neill T, Fears B. (2002). Effects of age at implantation in young children. Ann Otol Rhinol Laryngol Suppl 189:69–73

Kishon-Rabin L, Taitelbaum R, Elichai O, Maimon D, Debyiat D, Chazan N. (2001). Developmental aspects of the IT-MAIS in normal-hearing babies. Isr J Speech Hear 23:12–22

Kral A, Hartmann R, Tillein J, Held S, Klinke R. (2000). Congenital auditory deprivation reduces syntactic activity within the auditory cortex in a layer-specific manner. Cereb Cortex 10:714–726

Kretschmer R, Kreschmer L. (1994). Discourse and hearing impairment. In: Ripich D, Creaghead N, eds. School Discourse Problems, pp. 263–296. San Diego: Singular

Levitt H, McGarr NS, Geffner D. (1987). Development of Language and Communication Skills in Hearing-Impaired Children. ASHA Monograph No. 26. Rockville, MD: ASHA

Locke J. (1993). The Child's Path to Spoken Language. Cambridge, MA: Harvard University Press

McClatchie A, Therres MK. (2003). Auditory Speech & Language (AuSpLan). Washington, DC: AG Bell

Miyamoto RT, Houston DM, Kirk KI, Perdew AE, Svirsky MA. (2003). Language development in deaf infants following cochlear implantation. Acta Otolaryngol 123:241–244

Miyamoto RT, Svirsky MA, Robbins AM. (1997). Enhancement of expressive language in prelingually deaf children with cochlear implants. Acta Otolaryngol 117:154–157

Moeller MP, McConkey AJ. (1984). Language intervention with preschool deaf children: a cognitive/linguistic approach. In: Perkins W, ed. Current Therapy of Communication Disorders, Hearing Disorders, pp. 11–26. New York: Thieme-Stratton

Moeller MP, McConkey AJ, Osberger MJ. (1983). Evaluation of the communicative skills of hearing-impaired children. Audiology 8(8):113–127

Mohr PE, Feldman JJ, Dunbar JL, et al. (2000). The societal cost of severe to profound hearing loss in the United States. Int J Technol Assess Health Care 16:1120–1135

Moog J, Geers A. (1985). EPIC: a program to accelerate academic progress in profoundly hearing-impaired children. The Volta Review 87:259–277

Nikolopoulos T, Dyar D, Archbold S, O'Donoghue G. (2004). Development of spoken language grammar following cochlear implantation in prelingually deaf children. Arch Otolaryngol Head Neck Surg 130:629–633

Osberger MJ. (1986). Language and learning skills of hearing-impaired students. Summary and implications for research and educational management. ASHA Monogr 23:92–98

Parrish R, Roush J. (2004). When hearing loss occur with other disabilities. Volta Voices 11:20–21

Ponton CW, Eggermont JJ. (2001). Of kittens and kids: altered cortical maturation following profound deafness and cochlear implant use. Audiol Neurootol 6:363–380

Power DJ, Quigley SP. (1973). Deaf children's acquisition of the passive voice. J Speech Hear Res 16:5–11

Rance G, Beer DE, Cone-Wesson B, et al. (1999). Clinical findings for a group of infants and young children with auditory neuropathy. Ear Hear 20:238–252

Rice M, Wexler K, Hershberger S. (1998). Tense over time: The longitudinal course of tense acquisition in children with specific language impairment. J Speech Lang Hear Res 41:1412–1430

Robbins AM. (1998a). Lesson plan for Lilly. In: Estabrooks W, ed. Cochlear Implants for Kids. Washington, DC: AG Bell

Robbins AM. (1998b). Sneaking language into auditory activities: the thinking while listening approach. In: Loud and Clear Newsletter. Sylmar, CA: Advanced Bionics

Robbins AM. (2000). Rehabilitation after cochlear implantation. In: Niparko J, ed. Cochlear Implants Principles and Practices. Philadelphia: Lippincott Williams & Wilkins

Robbins AM. (2003a). Communication intervention for infants and toddlers with CIs. Topics in Language Disorders 23:16–33

Robbins AM. (2003b). Language development in children with cochlear implants. In: Cochlear Implant Research: Present and Future. Proceedings from the tenth annual NIH research symposium, SHHH convention, June 29, 2003, Atlanta, Georgia

Robbins AM. (2005). Clinical Red Flags for Slow Progress in Children with Cochlear Implants. Loud & Clear Newsletter, Issue 1. Valencia, CA: Advanced Bionics Corporation

Robbins AM, Green J, Waltzman SB. (2004a). Bilingual oral language proficiency in children with cochlear implants. Arch Otolaryngol Head Neck Surg 130:644–647

Robbins AM, Green J, Waltzman SB. (2004b). Bilingual spoken language proficiency of children with cochlear implants. Paper presented at 8th International CI Conference, Indianapolis, IN, May 12

Robbins AM, Kirk KI. (1996). Speech perception assessment and performance in pediatric cochlear implant users. Semin Hear 17:353–369

Robbins AM, Koch DB, Osberger MJ, Zimmerman-Phillips SZ, Kishon-Rabin L. (2004). Effect of age at cochlear implantation on auditory skill development in infants and toddlers. Arch Otolaryngol Head Neck Surg 130:570–574

Robbins AM, Svirsky MA, Kirk KI. (1997). Children with implants can speak, but can they communicate? Otolaryngol Head Neck Surg 117(pt 1):155–160

Robbins AM, Svirsky MA, Miyamoto RT. (2000). Aspects of linguistic development affected by cochlear implants. In: Waltzman SB, Cohen N, eds. Cochlear Implants. New York: Thieme

Rossi K. (2003). Learn to Talk around the Clock. Washington, DC: AG Bell

Sharma A, Dorman M, Spahr AJ. (2002). A sensitive period for the development of the central auditory system in children with cochlear implants: implications for age of implantation. Ear Hear 23:532–539

Sindrey D. (2002). Listening Games for Littles. London, Ontario: WordPlay Publications

Spencer LJ, Barker BA, Tomblin JB. (2003). Exploring the language and literacy outcomes of pediatric cochlear implant users. Ear Hear 24:236–247

Sussman K, Lopez-Holzman G. (2001). Bilingualism: Addressing cultural needs in the classroom. Volta Voices 8:11–16

Svirsky MA, Robbins AM, Kirk KI, Pisoni DB, Miyamoto RT. (2000). Language development in profoundly deaf children with cochlear implants. Psychol Sci 11:153–158

Svirsky MA, Teoh SW, Neuburger H. (2004). Development of language and speech perception in congenitally, profoundly deaf children as a function of age at CI. Audiol Neurootol 9:224–233

Tomblin JB, Spencer L, Flock S, Tyler R, Gantz B. (1999). A comparison of language achievement in children with cochlear implants and children using hearing aids. J Speech Lang Hear Res 42:497–511

Waltzman SB, Robbins AM, Green JE, Cohen NL. (2003). Second oral language capabilities in children with cochlear implants. Otol Neurotol 24:757–763

Waltzman SB, Scalchunes V, Cohen N. (2000). Performance of multiply handicapped children using cochlear implants. Am J Otol 21:329–335

Yoshinaga-Itano C, Sedey AL, Coulter D, Mehl A. (1998). Language of early- and later-identified children with hearing loss. Pediatrics 102:1161–1171

Yoshinaga-Itano C, Stredler Brown A, Beams D. (2004). Evidence-based programming for infants and young children with hearing loss. Paper commissioned for Consensus Conference, Effective Interventions for Infants and Young Children with Hearing Loss, Washington, DC, September 10–12

Zimmerman-Phillips S, Osberger MJ, Robbins AM. (2001). Infant-Toddler Meaningful Auditory Integration Scale. Sylmar, CA: Advanced Bionics

14

Speech Production by People with Cochlear Implants

Steven B. Chin and

Mario A. Svirsky

The study of speech production by cochlear implant (CI) users is important on both clinical and theoretical grounds. It is important clinically because, although CIs are by design primarily aids to the perception of speech, they are also an important aid in the development of speech production and oral language in children with congenital or prelingual deafness. Theoretically, however, cochlear implantation also sheds light on the intricate relationship between speech perception and speech production in mature language systems.[1] This chapter discusses studies of pediatric and adult CI users separately. For children, we discuss research on intelligibility, on phonology, and on acoustic and physiologic characteristics of speech. Postlingually deafened adults typically have high intelligibility and intact phonological systems, so we discuss mostly acoustic and physiologic studies in adults.

◆ Speech Production in Children with Cochlear Implants

Clinical trials in children of the Nucleus 22-channel implant (Cochlear Corporation, Sydney, Australia) were initiated in 1986, and this device was approved for use in children by the U.S. Food and Drug Administration in 1990. Most research on speech production in children began during the clinical trial period. To address issues of device efficacy, most studies were comparisons of speech production either at different intervals (e.g., before implantation and after implantation) or in different clinical populations (e.g., CI users and hearing aid users). As the efficacy of cochlear

implantation became established, researchers undertook comparisons of speech production in subpopulations of CI users (e.g., oral communication users and total communication users). Most recently, increased expectations of cochlear implantation benefits have given rise to comparisons of speech production in children with CIs and children with normal hearing.

Intelligibility

Intelligibility refers to the recoverability of a speaker's linguistic message, differing from articulatory or phonological measures in that some aspect of meaning is involved. In cochlear implantation research, units of intelligibility range in size from morphemes to whole sentences. Intelligibility is most often measured with rating scales or write-down (transcription) procedures. Most studies of young CI users have employed write-down procedures, which are considered to have more face validity than rating tasks[2] and less sensitivity to vocal qualities, which may contaminate rating scale responses.[3] Materials for transcription procedures include those by McGarr,[4] Monsen,[5] and Osberger et al[6]; rating scales include the one in Allen et al.[7]

Several studies have compared the speech intelligibility of profoundly deaf children before and after implantation. Tobey et al[8] examined the speech intelligibility of children with CIs, using sentences developed by McGarr.[4] Recordings were transcribed by graduate students; scoring reflected the number of keywords correctly transcribed. Results indicated that speech intelligibility was significantly higher after implantation than before. Similar results were reported by Tobey and Hasenstab[9] and Dawson et al.[10] Similar to the before/after comparisons, Mondain et al[11] examined the effect of increased device use on intelligibility in 16 French children. Mean percent correct scores did increase as length of device use increased.

Osberger et al[12] compared speech intelligibility in pediatric users of single-channel CIs, multichannel CIs, and tactile aids, with users of hearing aids serving as controls. Materials were sentences from Monsen[5] or similar sentences. Children's productions were transcribed by naive listeners. Children with early-onset deafness (before age 4) who received a CI before age 10 had the highest intelligibility scores, whereas children who did not receive a CI until after age 10 had the lowest scores. Osberger et al[13] reported that the intelligibility of CI users began to exceed that of hearing aid users with thresholds at 100 to 110 dB hearing level (HL) after 2.5 years of device use. Studies such as Osberger et al[12] included participants using older strategies such as Multipeak (MPEAK). A later study by Svirsky et al,[14] in which all participants used either the Spectral Peak (SPEAK) or continuous interleaved sampling (CIS) strategy, showed that after 1.5 to 2.5 years of implant use, the speech intelligibility of CI users was similar to that of hearing aid users with pure tone averages (PTAs) of 90 to 100 dB HL. Chin et al[15] examined speech intelligibility in children with CIs and children with normal hearing. Children with normal hearing achieved ceiling levels around the age of 4 years, but a similar peak was not observed for the children with CIs, who were significantly less intelligible than children with normal hearing when controlling both for chronological age and length of auditory experience.

Studies examining relationships between overall intelligibility and other communicative skills include O'Donoghue et al,[16] who assessed speech perception and intelligibility using rating scales. Results indicated strong correlations between intelligibility at 5 years after implantation and earlier speech perception, indicating that speech intelligibility might be predictable by measures of earlier speech perception. Svirsky[17] also found significant and positive correlations between intelligibility and speech perception. Chin et al[18] examined relationships among intelligibility, contrast production, and contrast perception in 20 children with CIs. There were significant overall correlations, but individual feature scores for contrast perception were not correlated with the corresponding production features, and only some perception and production feature scores were correlated with overall intelligibility.

Phonology

Although overall speech intelligibility has high face validity as a measure of communicative ability, much of the research on speech production in children who use CIs has examined such phonological properties as consonants, vowels, and suprasegmentals. Several studies have examined the effects of both cochlear implantation itself and continued use of a CI on phonological properties. Kirk and Hill-Brown[19] appeared just 5 years after commencement of clinical trials of the House/3M (St. Paul, MN) single-channel implant in children. This work examined both segmental (e.g., consonants) and nonsegmental (e.g., vocal duration) properties

in both imitative and spontaneous speech production (based on Ling[20]). Studies reported by Tobey et al[8] and Tobey and Hasenstab[9] also used evaluation procedures from Ling. Results from all three studies showed general improvement trends from before implantation to after implantation. Tobey et al[21] examined production of place, voicing, and manner distinctions as a function of age, with results indicating a significant effect of age on the production of all manner categories.

Studies comparing the effects of different sensory aids on phonological characteristics include that of Tobey et al,[22] which compared speech in users of CIs, hearing aids, and tactile aids. Kirk et al[23] compared feature production in consonant vowel (CV) syllables in CI users and hearing aid users, Ertmer et al[24] examined longitudinal changes in imitative vowel and diphthong production in CI users and tactile aid users, and Sehgal et al[25] examined imitative consonant feature production in CI users and tactile aid users. These studies tended to show greater benefits of CIs over other sensory aids, except hearing aids worn by users with the most residual hearing.

Case studies examining phonological characteristics include Chin and Pisoni,[26] which examined consonant and vowel inventories, syllable structure and phonotactic constraints, and sound correspondences in one child at ~2 years after receiving a CI. Consonant production data from a single child were reported in Ertmer and Mellon,[27] and vowel data from the same child were reported in Ertmer.[28] In addition to individual children, researchers have also focused on individual aspects of phonology. A common one is the inventory of sound segments. The development of consonant and vowel inventories for children with CIs in English-speaking environments was examined by Blamey et al,[29] Serry and Blamey,[30] and Serry et al.[31] Chin[32] examined consonant inventories in children who had used CIs for at least 5 years, comparing inventories of oral communication users with those of total communication users. Dillon et al[33] examined consonant productions in a nonword imitation task. Peng et al[34] examined the inventories of syllable-initial consonants in Mandarin-speaking children with CIs, finding relatively low mastery levels for these children. Consonant clusters were examined as early as Kirk and Hill-Brown[19] in children with single-channel implants; later investigations include those by Chin and Finnegan[35] and Chin.[36] Preliminary work on intonation was reported in O'Halpin,[37] and Carter et al[38] reported results concerning stress placement and number of syllables on a nonword imitation task. Two studies on tone production, one with children in the People's Republic of China[39] and the other in Taiwan,[40] have both indicated deficits in this aspect of phonology for most of the children studied.

Acoustics and Physiology

Researchers have also studied the acoustic and physiologic characteristics of the speech of children who use CIs. Voice onset time (VOT) was examined in Fourakis et al[41] and Tobey et al.[42] Vowel formants (particularly F2) were investigated in Murchison and Tobey,[43] Svirsky and Tobey,[44] Tobey et al,[8] Economou et al,[45] Tobey,[1] and Ertmer.[28] Svirsky et al[46] examined oral-nasal balance, and Higgins et al[47] and Jones et al[48] investigated intraoral pressure.

Recent studies have examined multiple acoustic and physiologic parameters. Uchanski and Geers[49] compared VOT, F2 frequency, spectral moments, nasality, and durations in children with CIs and children with normal hearing. For most of the implant users, most acoustic characteristics had values within the range for children with normal hearing. Higgins et al[50] examined intraoral air pressure, phonatory air flow, electroglottagraph cycle width, fundamental frequency, and intensity, and Higgins et al[51] examined jaw opening, F1, F2, nasal air flow, voice onset time, voicing duration, and intraoral air pressure. Higgins et al[52] examined intraoral air pressure, nasal and phonatory air flow, voice onset time, and fundamental frequency in children with CIs, both longitudinally and in comparison to children with normal hearing.

◆ Speech Production in Adults with Cochlear Implants

In this section we discuss the changes in speech production in postlingually deafened adults after receiving a CI. These changes are more subtle that those observed in prelingually deaf children, who must rely on the auditory information provided by the implant while they learn the sounds and phonological system of their language. Typically, adults who become profoundly to totally deaf after acquiring language do not show major deterioration in their ability to produce speech sounds or to speak intelligibly,[53] suggesting that the role of hearing in speech production is more limited in adults than in children. In fact, from the mid-1980s to the early 1990s there was spirited discussion in the literature about whether adventitious deafness caused disordered speech at all. Goehl and Kaufman[54] examined the speech of five adventitiously deafened adults and concluded that, in spite of the "popular clinical prediction," speech does not deteriorate as a consequence of adventitious deafness. They concluded that "routine recommendations for speech conservation [in postlingually deafened adults] are probably unwarranted." However, this study was forcefully questioned by Zimmermann and Collins,[55] who said it suffered from "logical and methodological flaws" and that following its recommendations "may have adverse clinical effects." The Zimmermann and Collins letter even questioned the editorial policies of the journal that published the article, eliciting a reply from the editor explaining the peer-review procedures of the *Journal of Speech and Hearing Disorders*. Cowie et al[56] also questioned the Goehl and Kaufmann study, pointing to evidence that adventitious deafness "does sometimes affect speech, and the effects may be of more than theoretical significance." Years later, a study by Leder and Spitzer[57] found several abnormalities in the speech of adventitiously deaf subjects. Goehl[58] acknowledged that Leder and Spitzer's study as well as Lane and Webster's[59] showed reliable differences between the speech of the adventitiously deaf and that of the normal hearing, but said that these differences did not rise to the level of "clinically significant disorders." Leder and Spitzer's forceful counter-reply ended by saying that Goehl

et al's "inaccurate and unfounded conclusions cannot be left unchallenged or accepted in the literature." Once again, the polemic included commentary from the journal's editorial board (in this case, *Ear and Hearing*), speculating about possible reasons for the strong disagreement.

The study of the influence of hearing on adult speech production is of interest not only for the clinically related reasons discussed above, but also for theoretical reasons. The effect of prolonged postlingual deafness and that of restored hearing on speech production may provide important information to constrain theories of motor control for speech production. This topic cannot be easily investigated with animal models because speech production is a uniquely human capability (although studies of birdsong may provide important insights). From a basic scientific point of view, postlingually deafened adult users of CIs provide an interesting paradigm for exploring the role of hearing in adult speech production. An excellent example of a careful and comprehensive theory of speech motor control, based in part on data from postlingually deaf CI users, can be found in Perkell et al.[60] The goal of the following section is more modest: we discuss some of the literature on changes in the acoustics and physiology of adult speech production that are associated with the use of a CI. In addition to their theoretical interest, these studies help determine the effectiveness of CIs in adults, as it relates to their speech production.

Acoustics

The role of hearing as an input for the neural mechanisms that control speech production remains controversial. Results obtained with normal-hearing listeners led some researchers to propose that speech production may be controlled by auditory feedback.[61] This hypothesis received indirect support from early studies with the Lombard effect, an increase in vocal effort in the presence of background noise (see Lane and Tranel[62] for a review), and from delayed auditory feedback, in which speakers become disfluent when they hear their own speech delayed by ~200 milliseconds.[61] However, later studies argued against an active role for audition in the moment-to-moment control of speech production, at least at the level of individual phonemes. For example, Borden[63] argued that auditory information about many English phonemes is received too late for the central nervous system to be able to correct ongoing phonemic speech gestures. Most investigators have proposed that auditory feedback serves to calibrate other systems that control speech on a moment-to-moment basis.[64,65]

Interest in this issue motivated several studies of the acoustics of speech production in postlingually deafened adults with CIs. Perkell et al[66] studied vowel production in four recipients of the Ineraid CI (Richards Medical Co., Memphis, TN) before implantation and at regular intervals after implantation. The measured parameters included F1, F2, F0, sound pressure level (SPL), duration and "harmonic difference," a correlate of voice breathiness. Overall trends toward normative values in several parameters were found, but this result was not universal and it was complicated by

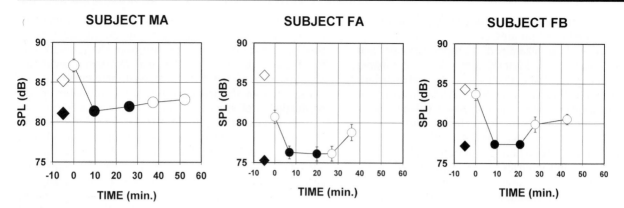

Figure 14–1 Average sound pressure level (SPL) values (circles) averaged across 10 repetitions of six vowels. Filled circles indicate values obtained with the speech processor on, and unfilled circles are the values obtained with the processor off. The first "off" value was obtained after 24 hours of sound deprivation. Filled and unfilled diamonds on the vertical axis indicate postactivation and preactivation values (data from Perkell et al[66]). Error bars are the average of the six standard errors of the mean (one for each vowel). Thus, error bars represent the variability associated with a single vowel and do not include the effect of variability due to cross-vowel differences.

lack of perceptual benefit in one subject, and by earlier deafening in two other subjects. An important result in this study (which parallels the study of nasalance by Svirsky et al[46,67]; see above) is that because speakers respond differently to deafening, their responses to processor activation also differ. Subjects with parameter values that exceed the upper normative boundary may show a decrease after processor activation; subjects with parameters below the lower normative boundary may show an increase after processor activation. Another important result relates to the interactions among measured parameters. The authors studied not only the longitudinal changes in each parameter, but also the correlations between different parameters for each subject. A large degree of interdependency was found among different parameters, some of which may have been due to mechanical interactions among different articulatory adjustments. For example, an increase in speaking rate results in shorter phoneme duration, and the shorter duration may be associated with formant frequency changes because the speaker may not have enough time to reach a steady-state target.

In the Perkell et al[66] study, most longitudinal changes could be attributed to changes in the average settings of speaking rate, F0, and SPL, in conjunction with the general pattern of relationships among parameters. However, the authors also pointed out that some observed F2 realignment may be attributable to the reception of spectral cues, rather than to the average settings of rate, F0, and SPL. A more recent longitudinal study of vowel production by postlingually deafened adult CI users was conducted by Langereis et al.[68] Recordings of 11 Dutch vowels in /hVt/ context were obtained preimplant, and 3 and 12 months postimplant with the processor on and off. They observed an increase in F1 and F2 range when the processor was on, a result that was more marked for some subjects with relatively small formant ranges preimplantation. In addition, vowel formants were closer to normative values 12 months postimplant. One interesting contribution of this study was the measurement of vowel "clustering," defined as the ratio of between-vowel variance of F1 and F2 frequency and the within-vowel variance of three tokens of the same vowel. More clustering was found 12 months postimplant than at the other measurement intervals, suggesting increased ability to produce contrasts between vowels.

Svirsky et al[69] studied three subjects in the Perkell et al[66] study, using an "on-off" paradigm. In each block of the experiment, subjects produced 10 randomized repetitions of six vowels within a carrier sentence. There were five blocks: after 24 hours of auditory deprivation (i.e., the speech processor was turned off); immediately after turning the speech processor on; after at least 10 minutes of having the processor on; immediately after turning the processor off; and at least 10 minutes after the speech processor was turned off. In other words, the testing sequence was off-on-on-off-off. The same six acoustic parameters used in the Perkell et al[66] study were measured in this on-off study. Results for SPL (one of the six parameters) are shown in **Fig. 14–1**. The symbols represent SPL values, averaged across all six vowels, for each individual at each testing block. The figure displays several trends observed in the study, not only for SPL but for the other acoustic parameters. First, there were very significant differences between blocks, particularly when speech processor status changed (i.e., on to off or off to on). Second, these changes were generally (but not always) consistent with the longitudinal changes observed in the Perkell et al study. Finally, changes were generally faster and more pronounced when the speech processor was turned on than when it was turned off. This is a desirable feature in any system that requires calibration to improve its operation, and in the speech production system in particular; when auditory input is withdrawn, it takes time for the acoustic output parameters to drift from their ideal values, but return to the desired range is rapid once the input is restored. How quickly does this happen? This is difficult to assess, due to normal variability in speech production. However, Svirsky et al[69] observed that SPL changes seemed to occur within the first few utterances after turning on the speech processor.

The on-off experimental protocol had been used in a previous study of the speech of multichannel CI users,[70] which investigated the influence of auditory information on speech production, and it was focused on vowel production. The first experiment contrasted vowel formant frequencies produced without auditory stimulation (implant processor off) to those produced with auditory stimulation provided by a Nucleus-22 device (processor on). Significant shifts in second formant frequencies were observed for intermediate vowels (such as those in the words *head* and *hid*) produced without auditory stimulation; however, no significant shifts were observed for the point vowels. Higher first formant frequencies occurred in five of eight vowels when the processor was turned on versus off. Taken together, results from this first experiment suggest that auditory information may play a role in the production of intermediate vowels. Point vowels, on the other hand, may be accurately produced with the help of orosensory (tactile and proprioceptive) feedback or with the use of quantal properties of the speech production system.[71] A second experiment contrasted productions of the word *head* under three conditions: processor on, processor off, and single channel. This third condition was introduced as a control, to obtain speech samples with auditory feedback, but using a signal that carried no spectral information and that was useless for the purpose of calibrating or correcting inappropriately produced formant values. This experiment revealed significant shifts in second formant frequencies between utterances produced in the "on" condition and the other conditions. No significant differences in second formant frequencies were observed between the single-channel and off conditions. These data suggest that auditory stimulation plays a role in vowel production (at least for some vowels, in some speakers), and that the formant frequencies produced by a speaker may be dependent on the type of information delivered by the implant.

Other studies have shown intriguing relations between vowel production and the vowel system of the speaker's language, as well as between a speaker's production of vowel contrasts and the speaker's ability to perceive them. Perkell et al[72] found an interesting cross-language difference in the productive vowel spaces of English- and Spanish-speaking CI users who had used their devices for at least a year. They measured the average vowel spacing (AVS, average intervowel distance in the F1-F2 plane) with the speech processor turned on and off. Vowel distinctiveness (as measured by AVS) was enhanced in the English speakers when the speech processor was turned on, but this did not happen with the Spanish speakers. The authors speculated that vowel production is governed by the competing demands of intelligibility for the listener and economy of effort for the speaker. Speakers may need to produce vowels more distinctly from one another in a language with a relatively crowded space like English, and the information provided by the CI may be necessary to achieve maximum distinctiveness. In contrast, Spanish has a relatively uncrowded vowel space with only five vowels, and vowel production can be more variable without compromising intelligibility. Vick et al[73] studied eight postlingually deaf adults before and after cochlear implantation. Speakers who produced vowels with reduced contrast prior to implant and who were able to perceive those contrasts

postimplant were found to have enhanced production contrasts postimplant in many cases. This result suggests that postimplant changes in vowel production are driven by listeners' ability to hear spectral abnormalities in their own speech. This self-hearing may allow speakers to adjust their articulatory routines to ensure adequate perceptual contrast for listeners.

The effect on speech production of the auditory signal provided by a CI is not limited to vowel acoustics. Matthies et al[74] studied the potential influence of auditory information in the production of /s/ and /ʃ/ by four postlingually deafened adults with four-channel Ineraid CIs (University of Utah, Logan, UT). Analyses of the spectra of the sibilant sounds were compared for speech obtained prior to implant activation, after early implant use, and after 6 months of use. In addition, the electrical output delivered by the Ineraid device (measured at each of the four electrodes) was analyzed with pre- and postactivation speech samples to explore whether the speech production changes were potentially audible to the cochlear-implant user. Results indicated that subjects who showed abnormally low or incorrect contrast between /s/ and /ʃ/ preactivation, and who received significant auditory benefit from their implants were able to increase the distinctiveness of their productions of the two speech sounds. In a follow-up study,[75] the articulator positions of a subject with an Ineraid CI were measured with an electromagnetic midsagittal articulometer (EMMA) system with and without auditory feedback available to the subject via his implant. Acoustic analysis of sibilant productions included specific measures of their spectral properties as well as the F3 formant amplitude. More general postural characteristics of the utterances, such as speech rate and sound level, were measured as well. The shape and central tendency of /ʃ/ was related to tongue blade position, but changes in the spectral contrast between /s/ and /ʃ/ were not related to changes in the more general postural variables of rate and sound level. These findings suggest that auditory feedback provided by the CI allows postlingually deafened adults to monitor their speech and maintain phonemic contrast between /s/ and /ʃ/, and that this is a true effect rather than a by-product of changes in postural variables.

Cochlear implantation affects not only the characteristics of segment production, but also the suprasegmental characteristics of speech. Langereis et al[76] found that the range over which F0 changed while reading a standard text (the "F0 sway") was reduced postimplant for most subjects who had inappropriately large F0 sway preimplant. Consistent with the Langereis et al results, Lane et al[77] found that three out of four postlingually deafened adults in their study reduced the variability of their F0 and SPL contours after implantation. The one subject who did not change significantly was the one with least contour variability preimplant. In an interestingly complementary part of this study, Lane et al also tested a subject whose hearing had been severely reduced following surgery to remove an auditory neuroma. This subject was tested before and after surgery. It was found that the variability of her SPL and F0 contours increased after her hearing loss, in complementary fashion to the results observed in CI users.

Are these changes in speech acoustics accompanied by changes in intelligibility? A study of postlingually deaf adults before activation of their speech processors and at 6 months and 1 year after activation showed improvement in vowel intelligibility for seven of the eight subjects and in consonant intelligibility for six of the eight.[78] Another study of 20 postlingually deaf adults found that the vowels they produced were more intelligible 12 months postimplant than prior to implantation.[79] Individual differences in vowel intelligibility were closely related to the vowel's first and second formant frequencies.

In summary, cochlear implantation has been shown to have a beneficial effect on the production of speech, including both segmental and suprasegmental aspects, by postlingually deafened adults. In addition, the study of speech production in this population has proven to be an exciting new paradigm to help fine-tune current theories about the link between speech perception and speech production in mature speakers.

Physiology

Given that several acoustic aspects of speech were found to be abnormal in postlingually deaf adults and that the use of a CI tended to have a normalizing influence, it is not surprising that several studies of the physiologic parameters that underlie speech production reached conclusions similar to those in the acoustic studies. In this section we review longitudinal and on-off studies of speech breathing, speech aerodynamics, and nasal balance by postlingually deafened adults with CIs (the kinematic study by Matthies et al[75] was discussed in the previous section because it had a strong acoustic component, but it may also be considered a physiologic study).

Speech breathing is known to be severely disordered in congenitally deaf speakers.[80,81] They tend to expend excessive amounts of air, and to start their sentences with lung volumes well below normal. Both of these factors force them to encroach on respiratory reserve volume to produce sentences, working against inspiratory recoil forces. These abnormal speech breathing patterns are accompanied by voices characterized as "breathy" or "harsh," and by low levels of intelligibility. Lane et al[82] measured lung volume during speech production on three postlingually deafened adults before and after they received CIs. Preimplant, one subject had abnormally high levels of average airflow and the other two subjects had abnormally low levels. Postimplant, all values changed toward the normative range: the high one decreased and the low ones increased. The subject with high airflow was the only one who used respiratory reserve volume preimplant, reflecting inappropriate control of speech breathing. However, this behavior was normalized postimplant, as the subject took advantage of his newfound economy of air expenditure. In summary, this study showed that abnormalities in speech breathing are not restricted to the prelingually deaf, and that cochlear implantation can have a beneficial effect in the control of speech breathing. The authors suggested that some of the acoustic changes that take place postimplantation may be mediated by the normalization of breath-stream mechanisms. In addition, they pointed out that inappropriate laryngeal valving was a prime suspect in the search for explanations of improper speech breathing.

This explanation finds support in a study by Leeper et al,[83] who observed changes in laryngeal resistance (among several other speech aerodynamics changes) in five adventitiously deafened adults who used the Nucleus-22 CI. The hypothesis about a link between laryngeal valving and airflow also found support in the close relation between average airflow and an acoustic measure of breathiness observed by Svirsky et al[69] in on-off studies and by Perkell et al[66] and Lane et al[84] in longitudinal studies. Lane et al found that most postlingually deaf speakers who received prosthetic hearing reduced their sound level (SPL), and tended to normalize their speech breathing parameters. More specifically, their air expenditure moved toward normative values, and their respiratory limbs terminated closer to functional residual capacity. The authors attributed these results to changes in respiratory and glottal posture aimed at reducing SPL and economizing effort.

As indicated above, the abnormalities in the speech of postlingually deafened adults are subtle, much less extensive than those observed in prelingually deafened speakers. For example, a study of nasal balance[85] found that 18 out of the 21 postlingually deaf CI users who were tested had preimplant values within the normal range. However, nasalance for some of the individuals with high preimplant values changed toward the normative values.

◆ Conclusion

A substantial body of literature, part of which has been discussed here, shows that cochlear implantation has a beneficial effect on speech production. This effect is rather pronounced in the case of prelingually deaf children, many of whom develop intelligible speech with the help of the implant. This newfound ability to speak in a manner that can be understood by naive listeners has its foundation in the development of a phonological system, and is expressed in acoustic and physiologic measures as well as in longitudinal and on-off experiments. The changes in speech production by postlingually deafened adults when they receive an auditory signal from their CIs are more subtle than those observed in children, but they are no less significant from a theoretical and a practical standpoint. The literature that studies these adult speakers has provided, and will continue to provide, important insights into the workings of normal speech production and the relation between what we hear and how we speak.

Acknowledgments

We dedicate this chapter to the memory of our colleague Maureen B. Higgins. This work is supported by grants to Indiana University from the National Institutes of Health, R01DC005594, R01DC000423, and R01DC003937.

References

1. Tobey EA. Speech production. In: Tyler R, ed. Cochlear Implants: Audiological Foundations. San Diego CA: Singular, 1993:257–316

2. Metz DE, Schiavetti N, Sitler RW. Toward an objective description of the dependent and independent variables associated with intelligibility assessments of hearing-impaired adults. In: Subtelny JD, ed. Speech Assessment and Speech Improvement for the Hearing Impaired. Washington, DC: Alexander Graham Bell Association, 1980:72–81

3. Samar VJ, Metz DE. Criterion validity of speech intelligibility rating-scale procedures for the hearing impaired population. J Speech Hear Res 1988;31:307–316

4. McGarr NS. The intelligibility of deaf speech to experienced and inexperienced listeners. J Speech Hear Res 1983;26:451–458

5. Monsen RB. The oral speech intelligibility of hearing-impaired talkers. J Speech Hear Disord 1983;48:286–296

6. Osberger MJ, Robbins AM, Todd SL, Riley AI. Speech intelligibility of children with cochlear implants. Volta Review 1994;96:169–180

7. Allen C, Nikolopoulos TP, Dyar D, O'Donoghue GM. Reliability of a rating scale for measuring speech intelligibility after cochlear implantation. Otol Neurotol 2001;22:631–633

8. Tobey EA, Angelette S, Murchison C, et al. Speech production performance in children with multichannel cochlear implants. Am J Otol 1991;12(suppl):165–173

9. Tobey EA, Hasenstab S. Effects of a Nucleus multichannel cochlear implant upon speech production in children. Ear Hear 1991;12(suppl):48S–54S

10. Dawson PW, Blamey PJ, Dettman SJ, et al. A clinical report on speech production of cochlear implant users. Ear Hear 1995;16:551–561

11. Mondain M, Sillon M, Vieu A, et al. Speech perception skills and speech production intelligibility in French children with prelingual deafness and cochlear implants. Arch Otolaryngol Head Neck Surg 1997;123:181–184

12. Osberger MJ, Maso M, Sam LK. Speech intelligibility of children with cochlear implants, tactile aids, or hearing aids. J Speech Hear Res 1993;36:186–203

13. Osberger MJ, Robbins AM, Todd SL, Riley AI, Miyamoto RT. Speech production skills of children with multichannel cochlear implants. In: Hochmair-Desoyer IJ, Hochmair ES, eds. Advances in Cochlear Implants. Vienna: Manz, 1994:503–508

14. Svirsky MA, Sloan RB, Caldwell M, Miyamoto RT. Speech intelligibility of prelingually deaf children with multichannel cochlear implants. Ann Otol Rhinol Laryngol Suppl 2000;185(12 pt 2):123–125

15. Chin SB, Tsai PL, Gao S. Connected speech intelligibility of children with cochlear implants and children with normal hearing. Am J Speech Lang Pathol 2003;12:440–451

16. O'Donoghue GM, Nikolopoulos TP, Archbold SM, Tait M. Cochlear implants in young children: the relationship between speech perception and speech intelligibility. Ear Hear 1999;20:419–425

17. Svirsky MA. Speech intelligibility of pediatric cochlear implant users and hearing aid users. In: Waltzman SB, Cohen NL, eds. Cochlear Implants. New York: Thieme, 2000:312–314

18. Chin SB, Finnegan KR, Chung BA. Relationships among types of speech intelligibility in pediatric users of cochlear implants. J Commun Disord 2001;34:187–205

19. Kirk KI, Hill-Brown C. Speech and language results in children with a cochlear implant. Ear Hear 1985;6(suppl):36S–47S

20. Ling D. Speech and the Hearing Impaired Child: Theory and Practice. Washington, DC: Alexander Graham Bell Association, 1976

21. Tobey EA, Pancamo S, Staller SJ, Brimacombe JA, Beiter AL. Consonant production in children receiving a multichannel cochlear implant. Ear Hear 1991;12:23–31

22. Tobey E, Geers A, Brenner C. Speech production results: speech feature acquisition. Volta Review 1994;96:109–129

23. Kirk KI, Diefendorf E, Riley A, Osberger MJ. Consonant production by children with multichannel cochlear implants or hearing aids. Adv Otorhinolaryngol 1995;50:154–159

24. Ertmer DJ, Kirk KI, Sehgal ST, Riley AI, Osberger MJ. A comparison of vowel production by children with multichannel cochlear implants or tactile aids: Perceptual evidence. Ear Hear 1997;18:307–315

25. Sehgal ST, Kirk KI, Svirsky M, Ertmer DJ, Osberger MJ. Imitative consonant feature production by children with multichannel sensory aids. Ear Hear 1998;19:72–84

26. Chin SB, Pisoni DB. A phonological system at 2 years after cochlear implantation. Clin Linguist Phon 2000;14:53–73

27. Ertmer DJ, Mellon JA. Beginning to talk at 20 months: Early vocal development in a young cochlear implant recipient. J Speech Lang Hear Res 2001;44:192–206

28. Ertmer DJ. Emergence of a vowel system in a young cochlear implant recipient. J Speech Lang Hear Res 2001;44:803–813

29. Blamey PJ, Barry JG, Jacq P. Phonetic inventory development in young cochlear implant users 6 years postoperation. J Speech Lang Hear Res 2001;44:73–79

30. Serry TA, Blamey PJ. A 4-year investigation into phonetic inventory development in young cochlear implant users. J Speech Lang Hear Res 1999;42:141–154

31. Serry T, Blamey P, Grogan M. Phoneme acquisition in the first 4 years of implant use. Am J Otol 1997;18(suppl):S122–S124

32. Chin SB. Children's consonant inventories after extended cochlear implant use. J Speech Lang Hear Res 2003;46:849–862

33. Dillon C, Pisoni DB, Cleary M, Carter AK. Nonword imitation by children with cochlear implants: consonant analyses. Arch Otolaryngol Head Neck Surg 2004;130:587–591

34. Peng S-C, Weiss AL, Cheung H, Lin Y-S. Consonant production and language skills in Mandarin-speaking children with cochlear implants. Arch Otolaryngol Head Neck Surg 2004;130:592–597

35. Chin SB, Finnegan KR. Consonant cluster production by pediatric users of cochlear implants. Volta Review 2002;102:145–156

36. Chin SB. Realization of complex onsets by pediatric users of cochlear implants. Clin Linguist Phon, in press

37. O'Halpin R. Intonation issues in the speech of hearing impaired children: analysis, transcription and remediation. Clin Linguist Phon 2001;15:529–550

38. Carter AK, Dillon CM, Pisoni DB. Imitation of nonwords by hearing impaired children with cochlear implants: Suprasegmental analyses. Clin Linguist Phon 2002;16:619–638

39. Xu L, Li Y, Hao J, Chen X, Xue SA, Han D. Tone production in Mandarin-speaking children with cochlear implants: a preliminary study. Acta Otolaryngol 2004;124:363–367

40. Peng S-C, Tomblin JB, Cheung H, Lin Y-S, Wang LS. Perception and production of Mandarin tones in prelingually deaf children with cochlear implants. Ear Hear 2004;25:251–264

41. Fourakis M, Geers AE, Tobey EA. Voice onset time constraints in the speech of profoundly hearing impaired children. J Acoust Soc Am 1994;95(5 pt 2):3012

42. Tobey E, Uziel A, Vieu A, et al. Acoustic characteristics of consonant production in French children with cochlear implants. Presented at IIIrd International Congress on Cochlear Implants, Paris, France, 1995

43. Murchison C, Tobey E. Rapid changes in speech production with and without auditory stimulation. In: Proceedings of the Second Annual Southeastern Allied Health Research Symposium. New Orleans: Louisiana State University Medical Center, 1989:260–268

44. Svirsky MA, Tobey EA. Effect of different types of auditory stimulation on vowel formant frequencies in multichannel cochlear implant users. J Acoust Soc Am 1991;89:2895–2904

45. Economou A, Tartter VC, Chute PM, Hellman SA. Speech changes following reimplantation from a single-channel to a multichannel cochlear implant. J Acoust Soc Am 1992;92:1310–1323

46. Svirsky MA, Jones D, Osberger MJ, Miyamoto RT. The effect of auditory feedback on the control of oral-nasal balance by pediatric cochlear implant users. Ear Hear 1998;19:385–393

47. Higgins MB, Carney AE, McCleary E, Rogers S. Negative intraoral air pressures of deaf children with cochlear implants: physiology, phonology, and treatment. J Speech Hear Res 1996;39:957–967

48. Jones DL, Gao S, Svirsky MA. The effect of short-term auditory deprivation on the control of intraoral pressure in pediatric cochlear implant users. J Speech Lang Hear Res 2003;46:658–669

49. Uchanski RM, Geers AE. Acoustic characteristics of the speech of young cochlear implant users: A comparison with normal-hearing age mates. Ear Hear 2003;24:90S–105S

50. Higgins MB, McCleary EA, Schulte L. Altered phonatory physiology with short-term deactivation of children's cochlear implants. Ear Hear 1999;20:426–438

51. Higgins MB, McCleary EA, Schulte L. Articulatory changes with short-term deprivation of the cochlear implants of two prelingually deafened children. Ear Hear 2001;22:29–45

52. Higgins MB, McCleary EA, Carney AE, Schulte L. Longitudinal changes in children's speech and voice physiology after cochlear implantation. Ear Hear 2003;24:48–70

53. Cowie R, Douglas-Cowie E, Kerr AG. A study of speech deterioration in post-lingually deafened adults. J Laryngol Otol 1982;96:101–112

54. Goehl H, Kaufman D. Do the effects of adventitious deafness include disordered speech? J Speech Hear Disord 1984;49:58–64

55. Zimmermann GN, Collins MJ. The speech of the adventitiously deaf and auditory information: a response to Goehl and Kaufman. J Speech Hear Disord 1985;50:220–223

56. Cowie R, Douglas-Cowie E, Stewart P. A response to Goehl and Kaufman (1984). J Speech Hear Disord 1986;51:183–185

57. Leder SB, Spitzer JB. A perceptual evaluation of the speech of adventitiously deaf adult males. Ear Hear 1990;11:169–175

58. Goehl H. Is disordered speech production a consequence of adventitious deafness? A comment to Leder and Spitzer. Ear Hear 1993;14:217–218

59. Lane H, Webster J. Speech deterioration in postlingually deafened adults. J Acoust Soc Am 1991;89:859–866

60. Perkell JS, Guenther FH, Lane H, et al. A theory of speech motor control and supporting data from speakers with normal hearing and with profound hearing loss. Journal of Phonetics 2000;28:233–272

61. Fairbanks G. Selected vocal effects of delayed auditory feedback. J Speech Hear Res 1955;20:333–345

62. Lane H, Tranel B. The Lombard sign and the role of hearing in speech. J Speech Hear Res 1971;14:677–709

63. Borden GJ. An interpretation of research on feedback interruption in speech. Brain Lang 1979;7:307–319

64. Zimmermann G, Rettaliata P. Articulatory patterns of an adventitiously deaf speaker: implications for the role of auditory information in speech production. J Speech Hear Res 1981;24:169–178

65. Cowie R, Douglas-Cowie E. Speech production in profound postlingual deafness. In: Luttman ME, Haggard MP, eds. Hearing Science and Hearing Disorders. New York: Academic Press, 1983:183–231

66. Perkell J, Lane H, Svirsky M, Webster J. Speech of cochlear implant patients: A longitudinal study of vowel production. J Acoust Soc Am 1992;91:2961–2978

67. Svirsky MA, Jones D, Osberger MJ. Control of oral-nasal balance by pediatric cochlear implant patients, with and without auditory feedback. Sixth Symposium on Cochlear Implants in Children, Miami, FL, 1996

68. Langereis MC, Bosman AJ, van Olphen AF, Smoorenburg GF. Changes in vowel quality in post-lingually deafened cochlear implant users. Audiology 1997;36:279–297

69. Svirsky MA, Lane H, Perkell JS, Wozniak J. Effects of short-term auditory deprivation on speech production in adult cochlear implant users. J Acoust Soc Am 1992;92:1284–1300

70. Svirsky MA, Tobey EA. Effect of different types of auditory stimulation on vowel formant frequencies in multichannel cochlear implant users. J Acoust Soc Am 1991;89:2895–2904

71. Stevens KN. The quantal nature of speech: evidence from articulatory-acoustic data. In: Denes PB, David EE Jr, eds. Human Communication, A Unified View. New York: McGraw-Hill, 1972:51–66

72. Perkell J, Numa W, Vick J, Lane H, Balkany T, Gould J. Language-specific hearing-related changes in vowel spaces: a preliminary study of English- and Spanish-speaking cochlear implant users. Ear Hear 2001;22:461–470

73. Vick JC, Lane H, Perkell JS, Matthies ML, Gould J, Zandipour M. Covariation of cochlear implant users' perception and production of vowel contrasts and their identification by listeners with normal hearing. J Speech Lang Hear Res 2001;44:1257–1267

74. Matthies ML, Svirsky MA, Lane HL, Perkell JS. A preliminary study of the effects of cochlear implants on the production of sibilants. J Acoust Soc Am 1994;96:1367–1373

75. Matthies ML, Svirsky MA, Perkell JS, Lane HL. Acoustic and articulatory measures of sibilant production with and without auditory feedback from a cochlear implant. J Speech Hear Res 1996;39:936–946

76. Langereis MC, Bosman JJ, van Olphen AF, Smoorenburg GG. Effect of cochlear implantation on voice fundamental frequency in post-lingually deafened adults. Audiology 1998;37:219–230

77. Lane H, Wozniak J, Matthies ML, et al. Changes in sound pressure and fundamental frequency contours following changes in hearing status. J Acoust Soc Am 1997;101:2244–2252

78. Gould J, Lane H, Vick J, Perkell JS, Matthies ML, Zandipour M. Changes in speech intelligibility of postlingually deaf adults after cochlear implantation. Ear Hear 2001;22:453–460

79. Langereis MC, Bosman AJ, van Olphen AF, Smoorenburg GF. Intelligibility of vowels produced by post-lingually deafened cochlear implant users. Audiology 1999;38:206–224

80. Hixon TJ. Kinematics of the chest wall during speech production: volume displacements of the rib cage, abdomen, and lung. J Speech Hear Res 1973;16:78–115

81. Forner LL, Hixon TJ. Respiratory kinematics in profoundly hearing-impaired speakers. J Speech Hear Res 1977;20:373–408

82. Lane H, Perkell J, Svirsky M, Webster J. Changes in speech breathing following cochlear implant in postlingually deafened adults. J Speech Hear Res 1991;34:526–533

83. Leeper HA, Gagne JP, Parnes LS, Vidas S. Aerodynamic assessment of the speech of adults undergoing multichannel cochlear implantation. Ann Otol Rhinol Laryngol 1993;102(4 pt 1):294–302

84. Lane H, Perkell J, Wozniak J, et al. The effect of changes in hearing status on speech sound level and speech breather: a study conducted with cochlear implant users and NF-2 patients. J Acoust Soc Am 1998;104:3059–3069

85. Langereis MC, Dejonckere PH, van Olphen AF, Smoorenburg GF. Effect of cochlear implantation on nasality in post-lingually deafened adults. Folia Phoniatr Logop 1997;49:308–314

15

Interventional Approaches and Educational Options in the United States for People with Cochlear Implants

Rosemarie Drous

Over the past 30 years, there has been a dramatic shift in both intervention and educational options available to deaf and hard of hearing children in the United States. Certainly one of the major influences has been cochlear implantation, approved for children with hearing losses as young as 1 year of age. Some implant centers are also implanting children younger than one in the presence of minimal auditory benefit with amplification. Mandated newborn hearing screenings, with the stated goal of the hearing impaired infant enrolled in an intervention program by 6 months of age, as well as Individuals with Disabilities Education Act (IDEA), which supports free appropriate public education (FAPE) and least restrictive environment (LRE), are equal and accompanying influences.

Historically, deaf education has been influenced by the technology of the time, and attempts to use hearing for spoken language development. In the United States, Dr. Max Goldstein advocated for the acoustic method in 1939 (Pollack et al, 1997). This auditory training method encouraged the use of audition to stimulate for speech perception without visual or tactile support. In the 1940s and 1950s, Hudgins at the Clarke School for the Deaf in Massachusetts began working with group amplification systems and demonstrated the ability of even profoundly deaf children to use some auditory information. In the 1950s and 1960s, the auditory global method was introduced with an emphasis on listening, speech reading, and using amplification as early as possible. This method also supported the role of parents in the habilitation process and more natural language learning versus the analytic approaches used previously.

Beginning in the 1950s, professionals in the field of audiology, speech pathology, and education of the deaf

(e.g., Doreen Pollack, Helen Beebe, and Daniel Ling) began to discuss the use of amplified residual hearing as the primary means for hearing impaired children to learn spoken language. The discussion extended from training the ears to the impact of auditory learning on the cortical functioning of the brain. The goal was to create an early and lasting auditory imprint by following the typical developmental learning patterns of normally hearing children.

During the 1970s, total communication became the predominant methodology in public deaf education programs. Auditory oral and auditory verbal methods continued to be available, but was generally a private versus a public option. In the late 1980s cochlear implants were introduced for children. With that came a gradual reemergence of auditory-based intervention and education, particularly for children from birth through early elementary age.

The decade beginning in 2000 has seen a steady increase in the numbers of children mainstreamed (Sorkin et al, 2004) as well as receiving early and intensive auditory, speech, and spoken language services. The goal of these early intensive services is to prepare children to learn, if possible, alongside their typically hearing peers in mainstream education. With the ever-changing technology of implants, and the ability to identify children with hearing losses at birth, it would be reasonable to expect the numbers of children who have early access to audition for learning to increase. Accompanying that will be the anticipated increased numbers of children who are a part of regular education.

This chapter reviews communication and educational options available to families of children with cochlear implants; the research demonstrating the impact of cochlear implants on auditory, speech, and language outcomes in educational programs; educational law and its influence on professionals and institutions responsible for developing educational plans for deaf or hard-of-hearing children; and the method to determine appropriate educational placement and services.

◆ Early Intervention and the Law

Three of every 1000 babies born in the United States each year have a profound hearing loss. Given this statistic, ~33 infants are diagnosed daily with a hearing impairment. Another two or three of 1000 babies are born with mild to severe hearing losses (Johnson et al, 1993). The educational cost for not identifying children early is estimated at $420,000, with a lifetime cost of approximately $1 million per individual. From a cost-benefit perspective, the impact of early identification and early auditory access and language development cannot be overstated (Francis et al, 1999).

According to the Centers for Disease Control and Prevention, as of 2004, newborn hearing screening is mandated in 37 states. Early Detection and Hearing Intervention (EDHI) programs have the following stated goals:

1. Screening an infant before 1 month of age
2. Audiologic management, including the use of amplification, by 3 months of age for those children with a hearing loss
3. Entry into an early intervention program by 6 months of age

Early intervention programs have been in existence since 1986. Congress established the Program for Infants and Toddlers with Disabilities (Part C of IDEA), a federal grant program with the following functions:

1. Enhance the development of infants and toddlers with disabilities
2. Reduce educational costs by minimizing the need for special education through early intervention
3. Minimize the likelihood of institutionalization, and maximize independent living
4. Enhance the capacity of families to meet their child's needs

An understanding of the implications of Part C of IDEA benefits professionals whose charge it is to guide and counsel families as they enter the early intervention system. As previously stated, cochlear implants are approved for children as young as 1 year of age and younger if appropriate. If we are giving infants auditory access to spoken language with cochlear implants during this critical period for learning, a primary goal of early intervention is to maximize the auditory potential for the development of competent oral communication. With earlier implant there is the potential for the stages of auditory, speech, and oral language development of the hearing impaired infant to closely approximate that of his typically hearing peer, given appropriate interventions, and family support.

Of greatest significance is wording in the law that recognizes the family members' role as decision makers regarding how their infant or toddler will communicate. Given that the majority of hearing impaired children are born into families whose parents are typically hearing, recognition of the viability of spoken language as a communication option for deaf or hard-of-hearing infants warrants attention. With an early emphasis on spoken language development due to available hearing technology, the other immediate and obvious mandate of early intervention (i.e., reduce institutionalization) is the potential shift to community-based programs for greater numbers of deaf and hard-of-hearing children as they age out of early intervention.

◆ Communication Therapy Options in the United States

Auditory-Verbal (Unisensory) Method

The emphasis is on audition as the primary means for learning to process spoken language. Principles of the approach (Pollack et al, 1997) include:

1. Early detection of hearing impairment, with an emphasis on newborn hearing screening
2. Appropriate medical and audiologic management to ensure that amplification or a cochlear implant allow for maximum access to spoken language
3. Parents and caregivers are viewed as the primary models for spoken language development, and remain as active participants throughout the child's intervention and education.
4. Integrating audition into the personality of the child so that listening is viewed as meaningful and primary for learning and functioning in the mainstream of society
5. Auditory verbal development is grounded in one-on-one teaching that includes the therapist and parent caregiver. Hearing-impaired children are not grouped together for learning.
6. Development of an auditory feedback loop so that the child monitors not only his own speech but also the speech of others
7. Communication follows typical developmental patterns to promote listening, speech, language, and cognition in natural communicative exchanges.
8. Ongoing assessment of the child's development; auditory verbal therapy is diagnostic in nature and supports ongoing analysis of the child's progress
9. Integration into regular education as much as possible to allow for typical speech, language, and auditory models, as well as a typical curriculum that supports age-appropriate academic and social learning

The hallmark of auditory verbal therapy is its emphasis on listening for the development of spoken language. Speech reading and other visual supports are not used, except to bridge the child to maximum use of audition if necessary. Children are taken through the normal developmental process of speech and language learning without the traditional didactic teaching seen in some schools for oral deaf or hard-of-hearing students. Natural learning in the context of meaningful experiences is highlighted, particularly in the early years. The family is viewed as instrumental in the developmental process, and parents are guided and supported in their role as the "first teachers" of their children. The therapist serves to model techniques, goals, and objectives that the family can carry out in the home environment. School placement, beginning in the nursery school years, is with children who are typically hearing, and often reflects the culture of the family and the community in which the family resides.

Auditory-Oral Method

The emphasis is on spoken language development through the use of appropriate-fit amplification or a cochlear implant, and individual and small group learning with hearing-impaired peers. Auditory oral programming varies in its defining characteristics, from advocacy for early mainstreaming using one-on-one teaching and small group instruction, to full-time programming with other hearing-impaired children. As a result of early diagnosis and cochlear implants, there is a growing emphasis on auditory-oral early intervention and preschool education to prepare the child for entry into regular education during the elementary years. The Alexander Graham Bell Association (1998) has published *Components of a Quality Auditory Oral Program*, which has a checklist with the specifics of an appropriate program using this approach for hearing-impaired children.

Cued-Speech Method

Cued Speech supports spoken language learning through eight visual cues that distinguish consonant phonemes, using four different placements near the mouth to distinguish vowels. These cues are used while speaking to make the ambiguous components of spoken language visual, particularly those that look similar on the lips such as [b], [p], and [m]. Spoken language is the goal with integration into mainstream education. Use of amplification or a cochlear implant is supported by available visual cues and speech reading. The parents must use the cuing system whenever they communicate with the child, and work toward proficiency in the use of cues while speaking.

Total-Communication Method

Total communication uses a combination of sign language in English word order, speech, and audition to develop language. Speech, speech reading, sign language, natural gestures, print, and hearing are used in this approach. Children are grouped according to their age and diagnosis as they enter the preschool years. This approach believes that children will respond to the sensory modality (i.e., hearing, vision, touch), which facilitates their learning at any given time, and parents learn signing to provide consistent modeling of this multisensory approach at home. Signing and speaking (i.e., simultaneous communication) is the general expectation within a total communication approach; however, that can vary from program to program.

American Sign Language/English as a Second Language (ASL/ESL): Bilingual/Bicultural Method

This approach uses manual language that is distinctly different from spoken language in grammar and syntax. It is the accepted language of the deaf community and is found generally in schools for the deaf in the United States. English is learned as a second language, using print and increased fluency in American Sign Language as a primary avenue to spoken word order and grammar. The emphasis is on a manually encoded language system that allows for early communication. Audition and spoken language are not emphasized when using American Sign Language. Access to appropriate language models fluent in the language of sign is critical. Parents of hearing-impaired children must be able to communicate in the chosen language. Not only is it important for the child to be immersed in the language and culture of the deaf, but it is equally or perhaps more critical that the family members immerse themselves in American Sign Language.

◆ Cochlear Implant Research Supporting Auditory-Based Learning

In a study completed at Central Institute for the Deaf (Geers et al, 2003), 181 8- and 9-year-old children were evaluated over a 4-year period. These children were from 33 different states and five Canadian provinces. All of the children were diagnosed with deafness prior to the age of 3, implanted by 5 years of age, and had used their implants for more than 3 years. The study consistently demonstrated significantly higher outcomes on all tested measures for implanted children in educational environments where listening and speaking are the expectation. In addition, educational placement changed as the children developed auditory, speech, and language skills. Initially, the children were evenly split relative to auditory oral and total communication educational placement. Significantly, the implanted children tended to shift toward public education in mainstream classes as auditory, speech, and spoken language skills improved. Of those children, speech perception 4 to 6 years postimplant averaged 50% open set using listening alone, and almost 80% with combined auditory and lip-reading cues. Intelligibility of speech was also greatly improved, from 60% for the unschooled listener to 80% intelligibility for half of the evaluated children when compared with their typically hearing peers. Children who were enrolled in auditory oral programs where the emphasis is on listening and speaking for communication were better able to use the information provided by the implant to understand speech, and demonstrated improved speech intelligibility. Over half the population studied produced English syntax comparable to their same-age hearing peers.

It appeared that use of a manually coded sign system did not translate to oral syntactical development. In this study, all performance measures were significantly higher for children in auditory oral settings.

In a study completed by Svirsky et al (2000), 70 children with cochlear implants were assessed ~4 months before receiving their cochlear implants, and 6, 12, 18, 24, and 30 months after implantation. The purpose of the study was to determine the English language abilities of children with cochlear implants. Their scores were compared with the language age they might obtain as a function of chronological age, residual hearing, and communication mode. Children who received cochlear implants had a mean rate of language development similar to that of children with normal hearing, and greater than that of deaf children who were not implanted. There was a relationship between better speech perception scores and more normal oral language development. Children who were oral communicators versus children using total communication demonstrated this effect to a greater degree. Overall, children with high speech perception were developing oral language skills based on the auditory input of the cochlear implant. In a study by Kirk et al (2002), the oral communication early-implanted children demonstrated spoken word recognition improving at a faster rate, and the oral communication children made more rapid gains in communication abilities than did the children who used total communication. Finally, in a study completed by Osberger et al (2002), age at implantation, educational setting, and communication mode influenced speech perception performance with a cochlear implant. Children from oral educational backgrounds demonstrated more benefit than did those from total communication programs. Individual variance in performance remains regardless of the educational option; however, generally speaking, as a group, children in auditory-oral programs are demonstrating better auditory, speech, and language skills, which translate to greater academic performance and the ability to learn in regular education settings.

◆ Auditory Development and the Implanted Child

Regardless of the communication and educational option, the stages of listening as established by Erber (1982) from detection to comprehension are the foundation for developing the ability to use audition meaningfully, and learning spoken language. For children who are not in programs where spoken language is the only expectation, the practitioner must be vigilant in ensuring appropriate integration of this developmental process. The typical expectation is at least a year's progress in a year's time relative to auditory, speech, and language development. For those children who are not meeting that minimal expectation, assessment must begin to determine the appropriateness of the intervention and the educational setting, as well as determine if there are other possible contributing influences, such as level of family involvement and other learning issues.

Hierarchy of Listening Skills from Detection to Comprehension (Adapted from Erber, 1982)

Detection

The ability to respond to the presence or absence of sound: the child learns to respond to sound, pay attention to sound, and not respond when there is no sound.

- Selective attention to sound
- Searches for and localizes sound
- Conditioned response to sound
- Spontaneous awareness of sound

Discrimination

The ability to perceive similarities and differences between two or more speech stimuli: the child learns to attend to differences among sounds, or to respond differently to different sounds.

Identification

The ability to label by repeating, pointing to, or writing the speech stimulus heard.

Suprasegmentals

- Prosodic features of speech (duration, pitch, loudness, rhythm, stress, intonation)
- Recognition of a man's, a woman's, and a child's voice
- Learning to Listen Sounds

Segmentals

- Learning to Listen Sounds
- Words varying in number of syllables
- One-syllable words varying in vowel and consonant content
- Stereotypic messages (familiar expressions and directions)
- Words in which the consonants are identical and the vowels differ
- Words in which the vowels are identical and the consonants differ in manner and place of articulation, and in voicing
- Words in which the vowels are identical and the consonants differ only in manner of articulation
- Words in which the vowels are identical and the consonants differ only in voicing

Comprehension

The ability to understand the meaning of speech by answering questions, following instruction, paraphrasing, or participating in conversation. The child's responses must be qualitatively different from the stimuli presented.

Auditory Sequencing

- Familiar expressions
- Follow single directions
- Follow classroom directions
- Sequence 2, 3, and 4 critical elements
- Sequence 5 directions
- Sequence multielement directions

Auditory/Cognitive Skills in Structured Listening Set

- Sequence series of multielement directions
- Identify based on related descriptors
- Sequence 3, 4, and 5 events
- Recall 5 details of an event, story, or lesson
- Understand main idea of a lesson or complex story

Auditory/Cognitive Skills in Conversation

- Answer questions requiring comprehension of the main idea of a short conversation
- Paraphrase remarks of another
- Offer spontaneous remarks

Auditory learning encompasses both receptive and expressive spoken language development, as well as speech perception and production. No skill is taught in isolation, hence listening, speech, and spoken language develop simultaneously. Learning is viewed from a typical developmental perspective in the early years. Progression should parallel that of the implanted child's same-age hearing peers, realizing that the older the age of the implanted child with limited oral experience, the more systematic and intensive the approach to speech and language learning.

◆ Education for Deaf/Hard-of-Hearing Students in the United States

Transition from Early Intervention to School (Preschool and Older)

Families are enrolled in early intervention programs under Part C of IDEA transition to Part B, Children with Disabilities (3 to 21 years) at or around age 3. The focus shifts from family-centered to child-centered programming. Local education agencies assume responsibility under the state Department of Education. An individual education plan (IEP) is developed based on multidisciplinary assessment, and is influenced by the stated communication option. This legal document is critical for establishing not only the appropriate placement but also the approach. Hearing-impaired preschoolers are placed in a continuum of educational settings, from typical nursery schools alongside their same-age hearing peers to self-contained groupings as part of a program for hearing-impaired children, some with the option for inclusion with typically hearing children or part-time placement in regular educational settings. Another alternative is placement in noncategorical groupings with children with various diagnoses. For the child with additional handicapping conditions, placement in a program that specializes in other diagnoses may be considered. Children who are not placed in specialized programs for hearing-impaired children generally require support services from a teacher of the deaf and speech pathologist familiar with cochlear implants.

Determining Placement and Services

Critical to placement decisions and the development of either the individual family service plan (IFSP) in early intervention or the individual education plan (IEP) after age 3 is assessment that reflects an understanding of cochlear implants and their impact on speech perception, production, and language development. These assessments define how effectively the child is using audition for learning. As a result of these assessments, recommendations are made for appropriate acoustic learning environments that allow for auditory access to the curriculum, as well as an ongoing focus on auditory, speech, and spoken language development. They serve as the guide in developing goals and objectives for the child in his new educational program, as well as providing baseline information about the present level of performance to gauge the rate of progress. Rate of progress is especially important as we look at children who will be or are educated alongside their same-age typically hearing peers because not all children enter the mainstream with the same listening and linguistic abilities as their hearing peers. The child's ability to close that gap with appropriate services, as well as the depth of that gap, is invaluable information.

Clearly, assessment must be completed by professionals not only familiar with the hearing-impaired population and strategies to elicit the desired response, but also familiar with auditory learning and cochlear implants. Interpretation of test results should include knowledge of other children with similar pre- and postimplant histories. Tests normed on normal-hearing children are an integral part of the assessment battery. Because the cochlear implant is an auditory prosthesis, with spoken language being one of the expected outcomes, test measurements must be compared with those of normal-hearing children in addition to those of implanted peers. With the swing toward educational placement on a continuum toward mainstreaming, standardized tests normed on hearing children provide the educational team with comparative data.

Speech and language assessments are only a part of a battery of tests administered that assist in determining appropriate placement for the student with a cochlear implant. Other assessments include, but are not limited to, audiology, psychoeducational, and a functional look (i.e., classroom observation) at the student by a teacher of the deaf or other qualified professional in the learning environment. Functional evaluations provide additional information about auditory, speech, and language in the environment in which the student is learning, and how those skills are impacting on academic and social development.

Functional Observations

Classroom observation provides information about how the child is integrating auditory learning in his everyday learning activities as compared with test results. That information assists the classroom teacher by providing strategies to teach the implanted child, as well as promoting an understanding of why the child responds differently in various auditory learning situations.

Continuum of Auditory Skill Development

Easy	*Difficult*
Look and listen	Listen alone
Close	Distance
Quiet	Noise
Nonverbal response	Verbal response
Closed set	Open set
Suprasegmentals	Segmentals
Gross contrasts	Minimal contrasts
Context bound	Contextually limited

Ying E. (1990). Speech and language assessment: communication evaluation. In: Ross M, ed. Hearing-Impaired Children in the Mainstream. Parkton, Maryland: York Press; 45-60. Used with permission.

Questions to answer when observing a child:

• When does the child use audition to receive information? Pair auditory cues with visual cues? How dependent is the child on visual cues?

• What is the impact of distance and noise on attention and listening?

• Is the child's response to verbal requests and instruction appropriate? Is there only a nonverbal response required, or a verbal?

• Does the student have the ability to use a range of auditory skills in the classroom, from use of suprasegmental information to segmentals?

• Can the child listen to new information without contextual supports? How much contextual support is needed?

Information about how a child listens in controlled environments, such as one-on-one teaching, is not sufficient to develop individual educational plans. Ultimately, the goal for a child with a cochlear implant is to compare the results on standardized measures with auditory, speech, and language function in the environment in which the implanted child is learning. Because we know that the acoustic signal degrades as distance and noise increase, and because linguistic demands increase, the natural learning environment of the home and classroom offer challenges to auditory learning that cannot be assessed solely in controlled situations.

The course of the child's learning experience in school changes significantly throughout the day: listening during seated instruction is uniquely different from participating in small group discussion that is rapid-fire in pace. There are times during the day when language is familiar, such as directions or review of previous material. Unfamiliar language, such as the language of math, may require different strategies for access. In addition to providing teaching strategies to maximize listening and speaking, classroom observation also can lead to a discussion about alternative placements if the child is not appropriately challenged, or lead to changes in the written goals and objectives to maximize auditory learning.

Classroom observations usually consist of discussion of the acoustic environment, teacher style, peer interaction, the implanted child's skills, and the support team (Talbot, 2000). Considerations for auditory learning on an IEP generally start with adaptations to the acoustic environment. Classrooms are notoriously noisy environments for any child to listen and learn. For a child with a cochlear implant, a room that has not been managed acoustically poses an obstacle to *access*, a keyword in disability law. In 1957, J. E. J. John addressed the issue of noisy classrooms by stating the following: "One of the main tasks of those who are responsible for the education of most deaf children is to help them to get maximum benefit from the use of hearing aids, and this task does not end when a child has been given an aid and switched it on.... It is a sad fact that in a great number of schools little or nothing is done about room acoustics; in such conditions, hearing aids cannot be used efficiently" (Crandall and Smaldino, 2001).

Substitute cochlear implant for hearing aid in the above quote. Noise in a classroom that has not been acoustically treated minimizes the implanted child's ability to be an active learner. Acoustic treatments for a classroom could include acoustic tiling, carpeting, and soft porous materials for the walls. The most effective management, however, is the use of an frequency modulated (FM) system, either sound field or personal. FM systems increase the intensity of the speaker's voice in the child's ear in response to noise, distance, and issues of reverberation in a classroom. Bilateral implantation is also being seriously considered to address the issue of noise and localization, two key listening issues in a classroom.

Determination of the appropriateness of an FM system is based on assessment by an audiologist. There is a growing demand for educational audiologists to be included in the implanted child's IEP given the increased numbers of children in regular education. The Educational Audiology Association (1994) has published *Minimum Competencies for Educational Audiologists*, and extended that to include a description of the educational audiologist working with implanted students. Presently the responsibility for monitoring cochlear implants and assistive listening devices in regular education falls to the teacher of the deaf or other related service providers such as a speech pathologist, although schools for the deaf and larger public and private programs established for hearing-impaired children generally have the advantage of there being an educational audiologist on staff.

Beyond academic performance, one of the key components of a functional observation is the implanted child's level of peer interactions. Social learning plays a critical role in the communication, as well as social emotional development of the child. The quality of the implanted child's interactions with his peers, as well as a fellow student's ability to provide appropriate auditory, speech, and spoken language models, influences questions of placement and the extent of intervention necessary to facilitate that interaction.

Areas to include in a written report of an observation is a student's ability to participate in classroom discussion; to attend during various learning activities; his level of dependence on additional cues, such as visual supports; use of clarification skills to get missed information or make oneself clear; and academic, speech, and language standing relative to his peers in class.

◆ The Relationship Between the Implant Center and the School

It is important to remember that early intervention programs and school districts may have limited or no experience with a hearing-impaired child, particularly a child with a cochlear implant. When a child is placed in an early intervention or educational program, it is imperative that the cochlear implant team has the personnel to respond to not only the needs of the child but also the needs of the school responsible for implementing the goals and objectives of the IEP. Members of the cochlear implant team can act as a resource, attend planning meetings, offer in-service training, and advocate for appropriate programming, services, and assistive listening devices for the implanted child. Regardless of the expertise of the educational program, ongoing communication between the school and implant center is critical, particularly relative to questions about device programming, cochlear implant equipment, and use of FM systems, or consultation regarding the child's progress in auditory, speech, and language development, academic standing, additional teaching strategies to employ, or questions of additional learning issues.

Implant centers also play a critical role in assisting programs to bridge children from visual learning to auditory-based learning. Generally, children who are in total communication programs do not have the same expectation to use audition throughout the course of the day if a visual representation of language is consistently available. The challenge when looking at educational placement is to rethink opportunities for auditory learning for those implanted children. The goal is to move the child along the continuum of auditory, speech and language development while supporting his academic learning visually. This is particularly true for those children who are implanted later, and have an established visual communication system. At the start, this could include using detection of sound to expect the student to be alert to his name, when set to listen, or the use of suprasegmental contours for vocabulary learning. Auditory learning must be integrated, consistently and systematically, into the academic and social curriculum.

For the later-implanted student or adult who has learned visually, teaching strategies employed must recognize the listener's interest level. Listening to associated sounds is not a meaningful exercise for a teenager; listening to music may be more motivating to develop the ability to listen and possibly recognize familiar songs through audition. Also practice with conversation using rehearsed scripts of familiar routines to the implant user, as well as tracking, which requires verbatim repetition of what was heard, are useful transition exercises. Both an analytic and synthetic approach is of value, combining listening to sounds of speech individually, for example, with listening to those same sounds in running speech. The key is to start at the implanted student's auditory and motivational level, bridging him with known visual cues such as speech reading to an auditory emphasis.

Another category of implanted student is the child with multiple handicaps. Given the myriad needs of these children, teaming with educational programs plays an important role in integrating auditory skills with the global goals of the child. It is estimated that ~40% of children with the diagnosis of deafness have other learning issues (Luterman, 2004). Those additional learning issues could include learning disabilities, mild to profound cognitive issues, attention deficit disorders, and developmental spectrum disorders, such as Asperger's syndrome or pervasive developmental disorder (PDD), or children with global developmental challenges, such as a diagnosis of CHARGE syndrome (coloboma of the eye, heart anomaly, atresia choanae, retardation, and genital and ear anomalies).

Obviously, learning to use audition is influenced by other handicapping conditions impacting on the hearing-impaired child. The decision regarding placement and communication intervention strategies requires input from a multidisciplinary team. In addition, function must be seriously considered for generalized learning. Using audition meaningfully may require many more opportunities for experiential learning, and a longer time frame for integration of those skills. Placement often cannot be solely based on the child's hearing loss given the need for professionals with experience in such fields as oral motor development, special education, and adaptive physical and occupational therapy.

The parameters that define educational placement and services are as individual as the child. *Deaf children are more variable as a population than hearing children. When we apply a common label such as deafness to children, there is an implicit invitation to regard them as somehow more alike than is the norm* (Wood et al, 1986). Placement and the process of learning are never static but rather are dependent on the progress of the student's auditory, speech, and language abilities, in addition to considerations of other variables, such as additional disabilities. Decisions about communication approaches and educational placement must also consider the family's preferred option. Any placement and subsequent development of educational goals and objectives must address the acoustic environment, the ability of the program and service providers to maximize listening and speaking (including but not limited to the teacher of the deaf, speech pathologist, and educational audiologist), the availability of appropriate peer models for oral communication, the integration of the family as key members of the team, annual communication evaluations to assess response to the strategies of intervention and educational programming, and coordination with the implant center to assist in developing appropriate MAPs (a 'listening program' stored in the memory of the speech processor) for the implanted child, as well as the implant team functioning as a resource regarding the overall educational management of the implanted child.

◆ Conclusion

A cochlear implant is an auditory prosthesis and with time will become increasingly more sophisticated. Yet to know the impact of earlier implantation on the auditory processes of the brain, such as auditory memory and sequencing. With increasingly sophisticated technology and programming strategies, ongoing medical research, and greater collaboration across disciplines to avoid a myopic view of the child, we may see changes in future outcome studies relative to performance.

Deaf education, one could reasonably expect, accompanied by educational law and the impact of identifying hearing loss in infants, may also continue to make a dramatic shift from a self-contained model as more and more implanted children enter public mainstream education. There is no argument that cochlear implants have made a difference in the auditory, speech, and spoken language outcome of hearing-impaired children and adults. Research now is moving toward questions of higher order processing as a result of oral language development. Language-related performance in such areas as reading and writing is of great interest as is the influence of implants on the social and emotional development of implanted children who are in increasing numbers learning alongside their typically hearing peers.

For families of hearing-impaired children, ensuring equal access to information about choices in communication and educational options, as well as implant technology, falls to the practitioners in the field of deaf education and related fields. The mandate is to be prepared professionally to respond to the expectations presented as technology opens the door for greater auditory access, and the potential for spoken language development in addition to the child's own innate abilities. At present, educational placement in the United States, beginning in early intervention, remains as varied as the population of implanted children. The range of professional training and experience relative to auditory learning and spoken language development is equally variable.

References

Alexander Graham Bell Association for the Deaf and Hard of Hearing. (1998). Components of a Quality Auditory Oral Program (booklet). Washington, D.C.: Alexander Graham Bell Association for the Deaf

Centers for Disease Control and Prevention. National Center for Birth Defects and Developmental Disabilities, Early Hearing Detection and Intervention Program. http://www.cde.gov/ncbddd/ehdi/default.htm

Crandall CC, Smaldino JJ. (2001). Classroom acoustics: understanding barriers to learning, monograph. Alexander Graham Bell Association for the Deaf and Hard of Hearing. Volta Review 101, p.1

Educational Audiology Association. (1994). Minimum Competencies for Educational Audiologists (handout) – 800.460.7322

Erber N. (1982). Auditory Training. Washington, DC: A. G. Bell Association for the Deaf

Francis HW, Koch ME, Wyatt R, Niparko JK. (1999). Trends in educational placement and cost-benefit considerations in children with cochlear implants. Arch Otolaryngol Head Neck Surg 125:499–505

Geers AE, Kirk KI. (2003). Background and educational characteristics of prelingually deaf children implanted by five years of age. Ear and Hearing, 24(1):2S–14S (Geers, Ann and Brenner, Chris)

Johnson JL, Mauk GW, Takekawa KM, Simon PR, Sia CC, Blackwell PM. (1993). Implementing a statewide system of services for infants and toddlers with hearing disabilities. Semin Hear 14:105–119

Kirk KI, Miyamoto RT, Lento CL, Ying E, O'Neill T, Fears B. (2002). Effects of age at implantation in young children. Ann Otol Rhinol Laryngol Suppl 189:69–73

Luterman D. (2004). Counseling families of children with hearing loss and special needs. Multiple challenges-multiple solutions: children with hearing loss and special needs. Volta Review 104:215–220

Osberger MJ, Zimmerman-Phillips S, Koch DB. (2002). Cochlear implant candidacy and performance trends in children. Ann Otol Rhinol Laryngol Suppl 189:62–65

Pollack D, Goldberg D, Caleffe-Schenk N. (1997). Educational Audiology for the Limited Hearing Infant and Preschooler. Springfield, IL: Charles C. Thomas

Sorkin DL, Zwolan TA. (2004). Trends in educational services for children with cochlear implants. Int Congr Ser 1273:417–421 (reprinted by 0531-5131/2004 Elsevier B.V.)

Svirsky MA, Robbins AM, Kirk KI, Pisoni DB, Miyamoto RT. (2000). Language development in profoundly deaf children with cochlear implants. Psychol Sci 11:153–158

Talbot P. (2000). Classroom Observation and Evaluation (handout) Washington, D.C.: Alexander Graham Bell Association for the Deaf

Wood D, Wood H, Griffiths A, Howarth I. (1986). Teaching and Talking to Deaf Children. New York: John Wiley

Ying E. (1990). Speech and language assessment: communication evaluation. In: Ross M, ed. Hearing-Impaired Children in the Mainstream. Parkton, Maryland: York Press; 45–60

16

Cochlear Implantation and Deaf Education: Conflict or Collaboration?

Sue M. Archbold

By 2004 there were ~40,000 children under the age of 16 worldwide who had received implants (personal communication with the three major manufacturers) and, indeed, in the United Kingdom, the majority of profoundly deaf children now have a cochlear implant. This rapid growth over the past 10 years means that in many educational settings, in many countries, profoundly deaf children with implants outnumber those with hearing aids. For parents, the reality is now that cochlear implantation is a very real choice, and one that may be made earlier than ever. With the advent of newborn hearing screening in many areas in the world, although patchy in places, parents now have the diagnosis of deafness earlier, and are making choices on behalf of their children earlier, and often when still undergoing adjustments to the child's deafness. It may be that at this vulnerable time, cochlear implantation may be seen as a "fix" for deafness rather than as an extremely efficient form of amplification. Even at an early stage after diagnosis, parents have major concerns about the future education of their deaf child, and it is more important than ever that the educational implications of cochlear implantation are fully discussed and that parents are informed of their options as fully as possible by fact rather than rhetoric.

This chapter discusses the historical context of deaf education and the controversies, the current practice of cochlear implantation, the current research into educational outcomes from implantation, the emerging challenges, and the ways in which we can ensure the best possible service provision for this growing group of deaf children. Individual education plans (IEPs), which are common for deaf children and for those with implants, should be based on up-to-date knowledge of the educational implications of implantation.

The issues discussed here are relevant throughout the world, where the same topics are debated by parents and those charged with the education of deaf children, in whatever context.

◆ The Context of Education for the Deaf

Deaf education has a long history of debate about what comprises good practice. The impact of deafness on the acquisition of language, taken for granted with hearing children, has a key influence on the practice of deaf education. Rather than being concerned largely with the acquisition of skills such as literacy and numeracy, of knowledge, and of social skills, deaf education has to take account of the acquisition of language, and how this is best achieved without normal hearing. A review of good practice in deaf education in the United Kingdom (Powers et al, 1999) found commonality in views of helping deaf children maximize their potential, and their right to language, literacy, and communication, but found strong differences in the ways in which these were best achieved.

Organizations and educational services differ to varying degrees about where and how deaf children should be educated to achieve these educational goals. These questions of educational placement and communication approach and the comparative effectiveness of different choices, have long been the subject of debate, but, to observers, the debates often seemed fueled by rhetoric rather than reality, and with a lack of evidence or objectivity. Indeed a literature review of deaf education in the United Kingdom (Powers et al, 1998) found little evidence in favor of one environment and education management over another.

Within this already controversial area, the rapid growth of cochlear implantation in children has added another dimension to the debate, and indeed evidence on outcomes after implantation and the influence of education is mixed, too. Parents, faced with yet another decision about the management of their deaf child, now routinely have another choice: that of implantation. Do they have the information on which to base these choices?

Deaf children were traditionally educated in schools for the deaf, often residential, and often in remote areas involving travel some distance from home. Large schools for the deaf were established in many countries in the 19th century, and children were taught according to the prevailing philosophies in those establishments. In the second half of the 20th century, increasing numbers of children with disabilities have been educated in mainstream schools with support, and teachers of the deaf led the way in promoting the movement toward mainstream placement of children with disabilities. Units, or special classes, were established in mainstream schools, staffed by teachers of the deaf, particularly in the United Kingdom, and since the 1970s more and more deaf children have been placed full-time in to mainstream schools with varying levels of support. For deaf children, the development of more effective hearing aids and the provision of frequency modulated (FM) systems have given them the possibility of greater use of audition to facilitate participation in mainstream education. The availability of cochlear implants is now moving this trend forward again.

There is a worldwide trend to educate all children with disabilities in the same mainstream class with their age peers, and increasingly in their local schools, with specialist support being provided in the class (Chute et al, 1996; Powers, 1996a). This movement responded to the growing awareness of the rights of those with disabilities, and the parallel demands by many minority groups for inclusion in the mainstream of society. For deaf children, it has led to the closure of some specialist schools for the deaf, which may be seen by the deaf community as a threat to their culture. Schools for the deaf have traditionally been centers where deaf culture and language have been transmitted, and where there has been a center of expertise in deaf education. With more children in mainstream, a reduction in special schools may mean greater difficulty in providing specialist support to deaf children, and greater difficulty in accessing those working with them in the mainstream for continuing professional development.

To summarize, the options for educational placement are as follows:

- A school for the deaf (residential or day)
- A unit or resource base in mainstream school (with varying degrees of integration)
- Mainstream school (with varying degrees of support in quality and quantity)

These situations are not mutually exclusive, but overlap to a large degree, with wide variations in practice, particularly in the degree of support. This makes comparisons about educational independence in varying educational settings complex, and hence comparing the effectiveness of different educational settings complex. Koch et al (1997) produced a useful matrix of educational resource use, illustrating the continuum of support; for example, a child in the mainstream with full-time support in class may in fact have less educational independence than a child in a class of 10 in a special school.

In addition to the debate about the relative value of different types of educational placement and levels of support, the debate as to which communication approach is most effective for deaf children continues. Traditionally there have been two extreme views: those of the oralists, who hold that all deaf children should communicate by spoken language alone, and those of the manualists, who hold that all deaf children should communicate by the language of the deaf, sign language. Although the oral view was held strongly in the 19th and the first half of the 20th centuries, it was challenged by reports of poor linguistic and educational attainments and speech intelligibility of deaf children, and by the increasing voice of the deaf community, wanting recognition of its own language and culture. In response, signed methods of communication were increasingly introduced to educational systems in many countries. This frequently took the form of total, or simultaneous, communication, where spoken language is used with signed support. In the 1980s there was the growth of interest in the use of sign bilingualism, using the language of the deaf community and the hearing community. However, as sign languages have their own grammar, it is not possible to use the two languages simultaneously, and transition to the written form of the hearing language (whatever it is) may be difficult. In the United States, the abbreviation "bi-bi" is often used, to denote bilingual and bicultural approaches.

Although terminology may vary, communication approaches may be grouped into three broad categories:

- Oral/aural alone
- Those using speech and sign simultaneously
- Bilingualism (Lynas, 1994)

The degree of dominance of one approach over another varies from country to country and from area to area in each country. For example, bilingualism is particularly strong in Scandinavia, where sign language has long been recognized as an official language. Within and across each category are subcategories, such as auditory verbal approaches, or structured oralism, complicating comparisons between categories. As with comparisons of the effectiveness of the different types of education placement that are available, the comparisons of the effectiveness of communication approaches on the attainments of deaf children are also inconclusive, for similar reasons (Powers et al, 1998). In the field of cochlear implantation, research into the comparative effectiveness of different modes of communication on progress after implantation has also often been inconclusive (Thoutenhoofd et al, 2005).

In this already changing and challenging area of deaf education, the advent of implantation has brought another dimension to the debates. It is worth noting that in the

United Kingdom in 1989, the first child received a multi-channel cochlear implant system, and the first bilingual educational service for deaf children was established, with rather different levels of funding.

The Development of Pediatric Cochlear Implantation

Although there has been a global increase in the numbers of children receiving implants worldwide, the trend has not been consistent across countries, and there has not been equity of access to the new technology, regardless of the state of a country's economy (O'Donoghue, 2004). Factors that have been observed to influence the availability of cochlear implantation for young children include the following:

- Development of child-appropriate technology
- Parental pressure
- Pressure from the deaf community
- Educational issues, including prevailing policies
- Evidence of outcomes
- Financial constraints
- Individual endeavors (Archbold, 2003)

Some of these factors moved implantation forward, whereas others delayed progress. It may be that "individual endeavors" is the strongest category of influence; for example, a country in Europe at the present time with one of the greatest incidences of childhood implantation is Croatia, largely due to the efforts of one particular individual. However, although pediatric implantation has moved ahead rapidly in terms of global numbers, it has not always been appreciated that the decision often made by parents on behalf of their child will have communication, language, and educational implications, and that the education system in which their child is placed is also likely to have an influence on outcomes from implantation.

The interaction between implantation and the education of the deaf has not yet been resolved: which influences the other? In efforts to utilize education as an outcome from implantation it may be that the influence of deaf education itself on implantation has not been sufficiently researched, nor have the most effective ways of educating the varied children who receive implants yet been identified. Ever more demanding groups of children are receiving implants, who require educational involvement in their long-term care:

- Very young deaf infants, following newborn hearing screening and earlier diagnosis
- Teenagers choosing implantation for themselves
- Children with very complex additional needs
- Those with more residual hearing, wearing a hearing aid and an implant
- Those with bilateral implants
- Deaf children of deaf parents

The research endeavors that have taken place into outcomes from cochlear implantation have identified influences such as age at implantation and duration of use, but have yet to identify more than 40 to 60% of the variance in outcomes for children with implants (Spencer and Marschark, 2003). It may be that some of the reasons for some of this variance lie in this difficult to assess area of educational management.

◆ Cochlear Implantation and Deaf Education

Surveys of implant professionals (Archbold & Robinson, 1997) and parents of children with implants (Archbold et al, 2002a; Hasenstab et al, 1997; Sorkin & Zwolan, 2004) found concerns about the education of children after implantation. In the questionnaire survey of parents by Sorkin and Zwolan, 30% of parents had experienced difficulty in obtaining the educational services they felt their child needed, and went on to describe the need for training about implantation, and for cochlear implant staff to be involved. In the qualitative study by Archbold et al, the links between the cochlear implant center and the local educational services was one of the major issues to arise spontaneously from parents. It is clear that cochlear implantation has brought together the medical and educational worlds in ways not previously envisaged, and requires professionals from different backgrounds to work together more closely than before. Educators, medical professionals, and audiologists may have different priorities following implantation: for the audiologist and the medical professional, the safety of the procedure and the changing of hearing thresholds may be the major goal, whereas for a teacher, the development of language, of literacy skills may be more important (Thoutenhoofd et al, 2005). The involvement of the child's local educator in the implantation process may pose difficulties for a clinic-based implant team, organized on a medical model (Nevins and Chute, 1996); the child's local educator may not be involved in the decision to implant or in the process itself, but may be left with the responsibilities for the long-term management of the child (Geers and Moog, 1995) and of the outcomes from implantation. It would not be surprising if many teachers felt under threat by the development of implantation, and uncertain of their role in the care of these children. It does seem clear that parents want a strong working link between the implant center and the educational system, wherever their child is educated; how this is managed is crucial to the sustained long-term management of children with implants.

A survey of implant centers in Europe (Archbold and Robinson, 1997) found that, in the centers' view, 25% of their children were in inappropriate educational settings; these were specialist educational settings where there was little emphasis on the use of audition, and mainstream education with insufficient specialist support. Although implant teams acknowledged the importance of the educational support of the child following implantation, there was no clear consensus as to what this support should be, and there was a wide variation in practice. With the recent results of the survey by Sorkin and Zwolan (2004) in the United States, there is little reason to suppose that the situation has changed overall. Other surveys of both teachers and parents reveal similar findings: Archbold et al (1998) found that teachers of the deaf in the United Kingdom emphasized the need for flexibility of both educational placement and communication mode, had difficulty with the diverse advice they received, and wanted more training. For Geers and Moog (1995), the implications for teachers of the deaf had impact on time, training, and money: time and training in managing an implant system, with the consequent financial implications and the need for long-term support. Dryden (1997) found that the conflicts for teachers were in reconciling the needs of children with implants with the needs of the others in their care; the other major conflict was that of resolving the balance of oral and signed input after implantation. She recommended that implant centers produced guidelines for teachers on the management of children with implants; this has been now done in many countries, and a wide range of resource materials is now available. However, a recent survey by Most et al (2004) reported that there was still a need for professional training.

Earlier, mention was made of the importance parents place on the liaison between the implant center and educational services (Archbold et al, 2002a) and of the finding of Sorkin and Zwolan (2004) that a significant proportion of parents felt that their child had inappropriate or no support. Hasenstab et al (1997) found that 30% of parents paid for additional services. The authors summarized the situation by quoting one parent: "If I had one wish for all implanted kids and their families, it would be to have excellent services locally. Services are usually available and even funded but too often woefully poor or inappropriate." It seems that the situation had not improved in the United States in the intervening 7 years, and are unlikely to have improved elsewhere. In those 7 years there had been a great deal of work on rehabilitation materials for children with implants from a variety of sources, and many implant centers provided rehabilitation services. Why does the situation seem not to have improved?

◆ Conflicts Between Cochlear Implant Centers and Educational Services

Public services worldwide are under tremendous pressure to provide and improve their services as measured against specified targets. For implant centers, in medical contexts, and teachers, in educational services, these pressures may produce further tensions in meeting different goals. For teachers, providing educational services in societies with changing expectations and demands, the advent of cochlear implantation has brought fresh challenges and responsibilities. Although there is evidence on the efficacy of implantation in terms of improved auditory perception and hence speech perception and production (Thoutenhoofd et al, 2005), there remains wide variation in outcome, and the delays in deaf children's language continue to be a challenge for educators (Spencer & Marschark, 2003).

Although cochlear implant centers continue to be based in medical environments, and teachers and classroom support are provided in educational institutions, there remain several potential conflicts; how they are resolved is vital for the secure future of current child implant users. For educators, the perceived conflicts are as follows:

- Inequity in the time and money it takes to teach children with and children without implants
- Inconsistency of input, expectations, and goals among implant centers, parents, and educational services
- Pressure on educator's time to acquire new and changing knowledge
- Responsibility for the day-to-day management of rapidly changing, complex technology
- Pressure on educators' financial budgets for training, spare parts for the implant systems to be used in school
- Demands on educators to be responsible for ongoing support for children with implants, often without advice or support from an implant center
- Pressure on educators to be responsible for outcomes from implantation for implant teams, which may not be the priority of the educator
- Managing the changing needs of children following implantation: changes in placement and in communication mode, requiring flexibility of management
- Confusion over roles and responsibilities

With growing numbers of children receiving cochlear implants, it is timely to look anew at the ways of managing them; their needs may not be so very different from those of hearing aid users, and they should be brought into the mainstream of deaf education, which may not necessarily be mainstream education itself! What are their educational needs? In common with other deaf children, they require the following opportunities:

- To acquire communication and language skills
- To develop their cognitive potential
- To access a curriculum appropriate for their stage of development
- To develop their personal self-esteem and to develop age-appropriate social skills

To utilize the implant system fully in these educational goals, they also require the following:

- An optimally working implant system at all times
- Good acoustic conditions to promote the development of listening within the learning environment
- High expectations of high-frequency speech information

For children with implants, the use of the implant system to its optimum is dependent on the combined skills and expertise of the implant center and educators responsible for the child. The implant center is likely to retain the specialist knowledge about implant systems and their management, and the educators are likely to know the child and the learning situation best. How can this responsibility be shared?

◆ Implant Centers and Educational Services: Sharing the Care?

With adult implantation, models of rehabilitation after implantation were developed that were largely clinic-based, which was essential for adults who were unlikely to have other sources of support. With the advent of childhood implantation, these models continued, with clinic-based rehabilitation after implantation being common. However, as the need to provide long-term care for children with implants became apparent, several service models developed to address these issues (Chute et al, 1996; Cowan, 1997; Robbins, 2000). Cowan identified three forms of pediatric rehabilitation:

- Solely in implant clinics
- Specialized educational settings or schools, incorporating or liaising with an implant center
- Outreach programs from implant centers

These models have been described over the years: Bertram (1996) and Sillon et al (1996) described two clinic-based rehabilitation services, and an innovative model of service delivery has been discussed by Muller et al (1996), who describe the development of a complete implant support system. This established cooperation between school and clinic, with shared personnel and facilities. Nevins (1991) and Archbold (2003) describe the educational liaison model in which educational consultants from the implant center visit the child's own educational setting to liaise with educators directly, the aims being:

- To provide direct contact between implant center and home and school
- To ensure that the implant system is managed appropriately at all times
- To ensure that ongoing support is appropriate
- To provide training for teachers of the deaf in cochlear implantation
- To monitor the child's progress in real-life settings

Working with the local educators may well be the most time- and cost-effective way of working in the long term (Chute et al, 1996). Passing on the skills to those in daily contact with the child may serve several purposes:

- Supporting the use of the implant in appropriate children
- Extending the skills of the local educators in the management of children with implants
- Anticipating and smoothing out possible areas of conflict between the implant center and the educators, ensuring consistency of care
- Promoting cooperation between implant clinic and educators

In the United States, the international group Network of Educators of Children with Cochlear Implants (NECCI) (Nevins and Chute, 1996) has long been established and continues to work with educators supporting children with implants, and in the United Kingdom, the teachers of the deaf employed by implant teams meet as a group, ICTOD (Implant Center Teachers of the Deaf), to ensure consistency of practice. They have developed guidelines for good practice, published by Royal National Institute for the Deaf (RNID) (2003). Educational liaison is seen as essential, but must be based on ongoing professional development. Cochlear implant centers and companies provide a great deal of training for the many professionals working with children with cochlear implants; are we sure that we are reaching those who manage the child in the classroom on a daily basis? With more children in mainstream it is more difficult to target those supporting individual children, who may not be a teacher of the deaf, and who may be difficult to reach for training. In the United Kingdom, the Ear Foundation provides ongoing training for a range of professionals, but particularly for teachers working with deaf children with implants on a daily basis. These courses cover up-to-date criteria and processes, and the management of a range of deaf children, from those implanted as infants, to the different needs of teenagers. One of the greatest demands is for training for classroom assistants who provide individual support for deaf children in mainstream classes but who may have no training. The aim of such continuing professional development is to provide an informed infrastructure for the children wherever they live, and to ensure that they have local technical support and appropriate expectations wherever they attend school; 20% of delegates attending the courses do so from outside the United Kingdom, indicating a demand for such training. Educational services are changing in response to the demands of cochlear implantation, but there is little evidence that they are changing as a whole sufficiently to develop the potential we now know is possible for children with implants, in light of the lengthier experience we now have. Conferences of groups of teachers of the deaf around the world often do not feature the needs of those with implants, who now form a significant group of profoundly deaf children. Do teachers of the deaf know what the educational implications of cochlear implantation are for the children in their care?

◆ Educational Outcomes from Cochlear Implantation

The major decisions parents face about the education of their deaf child are those of educational placement and communication mode. The other major educational issue for them is that of educational outcomes. What are the known influences of cochlear implantation in these areas? Research on the progress of deaf children has long been regarded as complex, owing to the number of confounding factors. Any group of deaf children is heterogeneous, and for children with cochlear implants there are additional variables to be considered: age at implantation, duration of deafness, and processing strategies used, among others. Implant professionals are, rightly, asked to provide detailed outcomes, but the complexities of the variables influencing progress make the drawing of robust conclusions difficult. However, funders of health care provision, which includes cochlear implantation, are asking more sophisticated questions about outcomes, including educational ones, and these outcomes are heavily reliant on input from teachers. Increasing accountability in both educational and health care fields demands that we address these issues.

First, educational placement has been of particular interest in considering the outcome of pediatric cochlear implantation, as it has been used in studies of cost-benefit (Cowan, 1997; Francis et al, 1999; O'Neill, 2000; Schulze-Gattermann et al, 2002; Summerfield et al, 1997). It must be recognized from the outset that placement decisions may be influenced by political influences and availability as much as by the assessed needs of the child; this is true within and across countries. However, the current evidence shows that significantly more children with cochlear implants tend to go to mainstream schools than those with hearing aids. Both Chute and Nevins (1994) and Archbold et al (1998) showed a trend to mainstream provision; Archbold et al found that age at implantation and duration of deafness were significant predictors of educational placement. Archbold et al (2002) compared aged-matched groups (5 to 7 years of age) in the United Kingdom with and without implants; all those implanted were implanted before the age of 5. They found that significantly more of the profoundly deaf with implants were attending mainstream schools and significantly fewer schools for the deaf. However, the conclusions still remain tentative: these were young children, and secondary or high school education remains a challenge. It is necessary to follow up these results as more children, receiving implants as young children, enter secondary education and we have the numbers to carry out such studies. However, Fortnum et al (2002) reached a similar conclusion in a UK study of 757 children with cochlear implants. Another large, US-based study reported by Geers and Brenner (2003) found that children tended to move from private and special school settings to mainstream provision after implantation; the evaluations were performed 4 to 7 years after implantation on children who were implanted before the age of 5. Daya et al (2000) also report a trend to mainstream placement.

However, the real educational outcomes are those of educational attainment; Powers (1996b) suggested that investigating educational outcomes is crucial in any discussion of the value of educational placement. Some reports claim that the educational attainments of those deaf children in mainstream schools are higher than those in special schools for the deaf. Such conclusions are confounded by the "chicken and egg" factor: it may be that those placed in mainstream schools have greater potential than those placed in special schools, and this was the very valid reason for the placement decision. Claims that mainstreamed children attain higher educational attainments than those in special schools may not take into account all the factors.

Although it is hoped that increased spoken language abilities will improve the literacy levels of profoundly deaf children, little work has been undertaken to look at attainments following implantation (Spencer and Marschark, 2003; Thoutenhoofd et al, 2005). A major UK study undertaken by Summerfield (2004) and Fortnum et al (2002) also looked at attainments of the children with cochlear implants and those with hearing aids. When educational attainment was estimated by teachers as a composite of abilities in reading, writing, and arithmetic, and compared with hearing loss, as hearing loss increases, attainments decrease for those with hearing aids, but is roughly constant for children with implants—for those with hearing losses over 100 dB. The children in this study were those implanted later than the current candidates and were implanted with earlier devices than those currently used; it may well be that these outcomes prove conservative in the long run.

Geers (2003) also reported on outcomes in reading skill development, an area where deaf children have a long history of very delayed development. Although finding a wide variation, Geers found in a group of 181 8- and 9-year-olds that early implantation was associated with a more normal rate of reading development. Spencer et al (1997) also reported improved reading scores for children with implants, but Wauters et al (2002) found no difference in reading skills in those who had implants. Clearly there have not yet been enough children with long-term usage of up-to-date devices to make reliable conclusions; however, the growing evidence is that early implantation in particular is linked with improved linguistic outcomes and hence educational attainments, such as reading.

In addition to looking at educational attainments of children with implants, we need to consider the psychosocial perspective of placing a deaf child in a mainstream school. Children remain deaf after implantation, and even a mild, unilateral loss can affect a child's classroom performance (Most, 2004). Chute et al (2004) also reported children with implants having difficulties in areas of classroom management and behaviors, when compared with their hearing peers. Many consider that education solely with hearing children deprives them of their need for a peer group and to learn about issues of deaf culture. There is a need to ensure that educational placement decisions are made with regard to the needs of the child, rather than political issues. The checklist devised by Chute and Nevins (1996), and the Screening Instrument for Targeting Educational Risks (SIFTER), devised by Anderson (1989) are useful in ensuring that these decisions be made with an element of objectivity by classroom observation rather than for political or economic reasons.

Whatever the complexities of the issue of educational placement for children following implantation, there does seem to be some early evidence that children who receive implants when young tend to go to mainstream schools, compared with conventionally hearing-aided children, and fewer to schools for the deaf, with implications for the organizations of educational services. What of the evidence of the influence of cochlear implantation on the decisions with regard to the communication mode used with profoundly deaf children? Again, we are faced with the question of which comes first, the choice of communication mode, or the evidence of its effectiveness. The evidence is mixed, but where there is a difference it is in favor of oral settings.

Most studies of the influence of communication mode on outcomes after implantation do not make clear whether the communication mode was assessed prior to implant, or whether the communication mode was that of the child or the parent or teacher. In total, or simultaneous, communication settings, the comparative balance of oral and signed communication is always difficult to assess, as is the quality of the communication being offered the deaf child. Some of these issues may account for the lack of definitive outcomes. The studies are also often confounded by a lack of clarity in terminology, using spoken language to equate with speech perception, for example.

In early studies, McConkey Robbins (McConkey Robbins et al, 1997) and Connor et al (2000) showed little or no difference in outcomes from those in oral or total communication settings. Tait et al (2000) reported that it was the quality of the early communication of children and caregivers, rather than modality, that influenced progress after implantation. In a study looking at language progress, Svirsky et al (2000) found no difference in language levels between those in total communication and those in oral settings. When they looked at only spoken language, there was a difference in favor of those in oral settings; this illustrates the importance of being clear about the use of terminology in these research studies. In tests of speech perception and production it is highly likely that those in oral settings will outperform those in total communication or signed settings; for educational purposes, we must look carefully at language outcomes.

Osberger et al (1998) observed children in oral settings significantly outperforming those in total communication settings. Miyamoto et al (1999) also found significant effects of oral communication mode in tests of speech perception and production. In more recent work, Geers et al (2003) found oral communication strongly linked with speech perception skills and language skills. In the same study, Tobey et al (2003) found oral communication also linked with speech production skills.

Archbold et al (2000) investigated children in oral settings and those using signed approaches, finding that, 3 years after implantation, those in oral settings outperformed those in signed settings on measures of speech perception and production. However, when those who had always been oral communicators were compared with those who had used sign and changed to oral communication 3 years after implantation, there was no significant difference between the two groups. In a further study of 176 children, 5 years after implantation, (Watson et al, 2006), the changes in groups of children after implantation were studied. Changes in communication mode were significantly related to age at implant; in children implanted before the age of 3, 90% were using signing prior to implant, and 5 years after, 83% of the same group were using oral communication. For children implanted young, changes tended to take place in the first 2 years of implant use, and to take place later and over a longer period of time for older implanted children. Clearly it is possible for children to change communication mode after implantation, and it is essential that educational services recognize this and provide services that monitor and facilitate such changes. Those children who had little audition prior to implantation, and therefore used sign communication, may well, as they grow used to improved access to speech via audition through the implant, become able to use spoken language as their main means of communication, of acquisition of language, and of access to the curriculum. They will need

an education system that can provide communication choice and can facilitate the change.

Based on recent reports, it would appear that the majority of children implanted young are developing the ability to use spoken language as their main means of communication and hence for education. What is difficult to determine is to what extent the cochlear implant influences the outcome and to what extent the outcome from cochlear implantation is dependent on the educational support of the child. Research into outcomes from cochlear implantation in young children has only served to confirm what deaf researchers have always known: the relative influences of the many variables are difficult to identify (Wood et al, 1986).

We asked whether cochlear implantation was influencing educational practice, or vice versa. On reviewing the evidence available, the answer would appear to be that each is influencing the other: educational policies and practice may well have influenced the varying levels of practice of implantation in different countries and influenced outcomes, and implantation itself would appear to be influencing decisions of placement, communication mode, and educational attainments themselves. The practices of education and implantation seem to be inextricably linked. How can we move educational services forward so that children with implants receive the best possible long-term care?

◆ The Future of Deaf Education for Children with Cochlear Implants: Addressing the Differences

With the current numbers of children with implants and the continued expansion of implantation in countries where it is well established, most teachers of the deaf will be required to teach a child with an implant at some time in their careers. Implant teams' emphasis on the specialist rehabilitation of children after implantation may have deskilled teachers of the deaf. Has unnecessary mystique built up to support an industry of rehabilitation for children with implants? Are there differences between a child with useful hearing with a hearing aid and one wearing an implant? The major differences that are emerging more clearly are as follows:

- The access to high-frequency hearing is rare in a hearing aid user.
- The complexity of monitoring device functioning
- The complexity of device programming
- The implementation of changes in technology over time
- The management of device and technology difficulties
- The length of time taken for progress—often years not months
- The flexibility of educational support required: placement, levels of support, and communication may change over time
- The medical risks associated with implantation

There are three other major differences emerging as we gain more experience:

1. It may be that implants often work too well. The speech intelligibility of some children may appear normal and such that there appears to be no difficulties for the child, whereas if we explore the child's functioning in everyday life, rather than in the clinic, we may notice the more subtle difficulties experienced by someone with a moderate, rather than a profound, hearing loss. Then the expertise of the teacher of the deaf will be required in subtle ways to monitor and facilitate progress to ensure that the child's linguistic and educational potentials are achieved.

2. There are other children who do not do as well as one might have predicted; a recurring theme in the literature is the variability of outcomes. It is likely that these children have difficulties not identifiable prior to implantation. Once the child has some useful hearing, it may become apparent that the child has a language difficulty, for example, and the major difficulty may no longer be deafness. Cochlear implantation is enabling teachers of the deaf to identify these children for the first time, but we may not know how best to educate them.

3. Another recurring theme in discussions about implantation is the management of those with implants as they grow through adolescence, and maintaining and developing implant use through these challenging times (Beadle, 2004). At this time, implant system malfunctions may appear after several years, and require sensitive handling with the implications that changes in hearing levels may have at a time of demanding education. During adolescence, there are reports of changes in levels and occasional sensations of pain. Again, these need sensitive educational responses to ensure that the necessary changes are made. A child may reach adolescence and question the value of the implant system, as many do with hearing aids, and question the decision made by parents. An adolescent who received an implant early and uses spoken language well, may wish to talk more fully about deaf issues. The issues of adolescent management are unlikely to be best met by implant center staff or by parents; educators may be in the best position to handle these situations, but not in isolation.

For experienced teachers of the deaf, cochlear implantation should not bring major challenges, if there is a commitment to the use of audition in the child's development of communication and language and a link with the child's implanting center. Educational services often provide these services over the years for those with hearing aids; they should be able to do so for those with implants. However, they will require close liaison with the implanting team, and to be enabled to take on these roles. Implant teams need to recognize the local educators as partners, so that, in the long term, the day-to-day responsibilities for managing the implant system and promoting its use on an everyday basis are shifted to the local teacher.

In order for teachers to become experts in the ways in which cochlear implants can offer new opportunities for the children in their care, initial and ongoing training is required. In both the United States and the United Kingdom, there are active training opportunities for teachers to acquire the necessary knowledge and skills. Teachers need to know about the following:

- The differences between cochlear implants and hearing aids
- Appropriate candidature
- Expectations from implantation for different populations
- The fundamentals of an implant system
- The basics of the tuning process
- Monitoring the system functioning and trouble-shooting it
- Monitoring the child's progress

These are some of the everyday knowledge and skills required; however, for them to be put in place and utilized effectively, there may need to be some organizational changes, for both educational services and implant centers. Educational services need to look at the following:

- How they organize their services to provide effective, trained support in the classroom for those in mainstream
- How they provide placement and communication choices as children's needs change
- How they provide appropriate education for those for whom an additional language difficulty may become apparent after implantation
- How they provide support for the implant system in the demanding environment of secondary or high school
- How they implement changes in technology and support them throughout the child's educational life
- How they provide for the psychosocial needs of the children as the children grow to independence

This cannot be done without the expertise of the implant center team and without ongoing professional training—given in the right place and in accessible ways. Increased liaison between implant teams and the child's own educator should ensure consistency of care, optimize the teacher's knowledge about implantation, and be cost effective in the long term. The potential conflicts of discrepancy between rehabilitation implemented by an implant team and the educational goals and the disruption to education by possibly unnecessary visits to an implant center can be minimized and the child's ongoing care ensured by the implementation of an informed infrastructure. As teachers of the deaf become more familiar with the technology and expected range of outcomes, they would be able to be more effective in the assessment period, helping to ensure that appropriate children receive implants, and that all concerned have realistic expectations. Training educators and linking implant center and educational service can take place utilizing the new technologies, providing monitoring, support, and training via video links, and Webcams, ensuring it is available for all.

Those of us working in the field of cochlear implantation have a responsibility not only to those with implants but to deaf children in general. Perhaps the difficult questions that have been asked about outcomes from cochlear implantation, and the interaction among the educational, medical, and scientific field, will benefit all deaf children, in that the

level of provision for all deaf children has been under scrutiny. Then the final conflict, that of the perceived discrepancy of support between those with hearing aids and those with cochlear implants, may be resolved.

References

Anderson K. (1989). Screening Instrument for Targeting Educational Risk (SIFTER). Tampa, FL: Educational Audiology Association

Archbold S, Nikolopoulos T, O'Donoghue G, Lutman M. (1998). Educational placement of children following cochlear implantation. Br J Audiol 32:295–300

Archbold S, Robinson K, Hartley D. (1998). UK teachers of the deaf: working with children with cochlear implants. Br J Teachers of the Deaf 22(2):24–30

Archbold S. (2003). A paediatric cochlear implant programme: current and future challenges. In McCormick B, Archbold S, eds, Cochlear Implants for Young Deaf Children. Second Edition. London: Whurr, 96–134

Archbold S, Nikolopoulos T, O'Donoghue G, Lutman M. (1998). Educational placement of children following cochlear implantation. Br J Audiol 32:295–300

Archbold SM, Lutman ME, Gregory S, O'Neill C, Nikolopoulos TP. (2002a). Parents and their deaf child: their perceptions three years after cochlear implantation. Deafness Education Int 4:12–40

Archbold SM, Nikolopoulos TP, Lutman ME, O'Donoghue GM. (2002b). The educational settings of profoundly deaf children with cochlear implants compared with age-matched peers with hearing aids: implications for management. Int J Audiol 41:157–161

Archbold SM, Nikolpoulos TP, Tait M, O'Donoghue GM, Lutman ME, Gregory S. (2000). Approach to communication, speech perception and intelligibility after paediatric cochlear implantation. Br J Audiol 34:257–264

Archbold S, Robinson K. (1997). A European perspective on pediatric cochlear implantation, rehabilitation services, and their educational implications. Am J Otol 18(6 Suppl):S75–S78

Beadle E. (2004). Supporting teenagers and young people with cochlear implants. Paper presented at 7th European Symposium on Paediatric Cochlear Implantation, Geneva, May

Bertram B. (1996). An integrated rehabilitation concept for cochlear implanted children. In: Allum DJ, ed. Cochlear Implant Rehabilitation in Children and Adults. London: Whurr

Chute PM, Nevins ME. (1994). Educational placement of children with multi-channel implants. European Symposium on Paediatric Cochlear Implantation, Montpellier.

Chute PM, Nevins ME. (1996). Managing educational issues through the process of implantation. In Allum DJ, Ed. Cochlear Implant Rehabilitation in Children and Adults. London: Whurr, pp. 164–218

Chute P, Nevins ME, Parisier SC. (1996). Managing educational issues through the process of implantation. In: Allum DJ, ed. Cochlear Implant Rehabilitation in Children and Adults. London: Whurr

Chute PM, Nevins ME, Parisier SC. (2004). Performance of children with cochlear implants in mainstream elementary school settings. Paper presented at 7th European Symposium on Paediatric Cochlear Implantation, Geneva, May

Connor CM, Hieber S, Arts HA, Zwolan TA. (2000). Speech, vocabulary, and the education of children using cochlear implants: oral or total communication? J Speech Lang Hear Res 43:1185–1204

Cowan RSC. (1997). Socio-economic and educational and management issues. In Clark GM, Cowan RSC, Dowell RC, eds. Cochlear Implantation for Infants and Children Advances, pp. 223–240. San Diego: Singular

Daya H, Ashley A, Papsin BC. (2000). Changes in educational placement and speech perception ability after cochlear implantation in children. J Otolaryngol 29:224–228

Dryden R. (1997). A study of the collaboration between implant professionals and local educators in the rehabilitation of children with cochlear implants. Deaf Educ 21:3–9 (JBATOD)

Fortnum HM, Marshall DH, Bamford JM, Summerfield AQ. (2002). Hearing-impaired children in the UK: education setting and communication approach. Deafness Education Int 4:123–141

Francis HW, Koch ME, Wyatt JR, Niparko JK. (1999). Trends in educational placement and cost-benefit considerations in children with cochlear implants. Arch Otolaryngol Head Neck Surg 125:499–505

Geers A. (2003). Predictors of reading skill development in children with early cochlear implantation. In: Geers A, ed. Cochlear Implants and Education of the Deaf Child. Ear Hear 2003 (suppl)

Geers A, Brenner C. (2003). Background and educational characteristics of prelingually deaf children implanted by 5 years of age. In: Geers A, ed. Cochlear Implants and Education of the Deaf Child. Ear Hear (suppl)

Geers A, Brenner C, Davidson L. (2003). Factors associated with the development of speech perception skills in children implanted by age 5. In: Geers A, ed. Cochlear Implants and Education of the Deaf Child. Ear Hear (suppl)

Geers A, Moog J. (1995). Impact of cochlear implants on the educational setting. In: Uziel A, Mondain M, eds. Cochlear Implants in Children. Basel: Karger

Hasenstab S, VanderArk WD, Kastetter SK. (1997). Parent report of Support Services for their Children using Cochlear Implants. Presented at the Vth International Cochlear Implant Conference, New York, May

Koch ME, Wyatt R, Francis HW, Niparko JK. (1997). A model of educational resource use by children with cochlear implants. Otolaryngol Head Neck Surg 117:174–179

Lynas W. (1994). Education Options in the Education of Deaf Children. London: Whurr

Most T. (2004). The effects of degree and type of hearing loss on children's performance in class. Deafness Education Int 6:154–166

Most T, Weisel A, Ben-Itzhak D. (2004). The effect of knowledge and experience on beliefs and expectations about cochlear implants. Paper presented at 7th European Symposium on Paediatric Cochlear Implantation, Geneva, May

Miyamoto R, Kirk K, Svirsky M, Sehgal S. (1999). Communication skills in paediatric cochlear implant recipients. Acta Otolaryngologica 119:219–224

Muller, R, Allum DJ, Allum JHJ. (1996). A service network of rehabilitation of cochlear implant users. In: Allum DJ, ed. Cochlear Implant Rehabilitation in Children and Adults, 102–118. London: Whurr

Nevins ME, Chute PM. (1996). Children with Cochlear Implants in Educational Settings. San Diego: Singular

Nevins ME, Kretschmer RE, Chute PM, Hellman SA, Parisier SC. (1991). The role of an educational consultant in a paediatric cochlear implant programme. Volta Review 93:197–204

O'Donoghue GM. (2004). Cochlear implant service provision: Are all of Europe's children equal? Paper presented at 7th European Symposium on Paediatric Cochlear Implantation. Geneva, May

Osberger M, Fisher L, Zimmerman-Phillips I, Geier L, Barker M. (1998). Speech recognition performance of older children with cochlear implants. Am Otol 19:2152–2158

O'Neill C, O'Donoghue GM, Archbold SM, Normand C. (2000). A Cost-utility analysis of pediatric cochlear implantation. The Laryngoscope, 110:156–160

Powers S. (1996a). Inclusion is an attitude not a place: Part 2. J Br Assoc Teachers Deaf 20:365–369

Powers S. (1996b). Deaf children's achievements in ordinary schools. J Br Assoc Teachers Deaf. 20:3111–3123

Powers S, Gregory S, Lynas W, et al. (1999). A Review of Good Practice in Deaf Education. London: RNID

Powers S, Gregory S, Thoutenhoofd ED. (1998). The Educational Achievements of Deaf Children, A Literature Review. Research report 65. London: Department of Education and Employment

RNID. (2003). Educational Guidelines Project: working with children with cochlear implants. London: RNID

Robbins AM, Svirsky M, Kirk KI. (1997). Children with implants can speak, but can they communicate? Arch Otolaryngol Head Neck Surg 117:155–160

Robbins AM. (2000). Rehabilitation after cochlear implantation. In: Niparko J, Iler Kirk K, Mellon NK, Robbins AM, Tucci DL, Wilson B, eds, Cochlear Implants: Principle and Practices, pp. 323–360. Philadelphia: Lippincott Williams & Wilkins

Schulze-Gattermann H, Illg A, Schoenermark M, Lenarz T, Lesinski-Shiedat A. (2002). Cost-benefit analysis of paediatric cochlear implantation: the German experience. Otol Neurotol 23:674–681

Sillon M, Vieu A, Pirou JP, et al. (1996). The management of cochlear implanted children. In: Allum DJ, ed. Cochlear Implant Rehabilitation in Children and Adults, pp. 83–101. London: Whurr

Sorkin DL, Zwolan TA. (2004). Trends in educational services for children with cochlear implants. International Congress Series 1273:417–421. New York: Elsevier

Spencer PE, Marschark M. (2003). Cochlear implants: issues and implications. In: Spencer PE, Marschark M, eds. Deaf Studies, Language and Education, pp. 434–450. New York: Oxford University Press

Spencer L, Tomblin JB, Gantz BJ. (1997). Reading skills in children with multi-channel cochlear implant experience. Volta Review 99:193–202

Summerfield AQ. (2004). Current issues in cochlear implantation. National Cochlear Implant Users Association Newsletter, Summer

Summerfield AQ, Marshall DH, Archbold SM. (1997). Cost-effectiveness considerations in paediatric cochlear implantation. Am J Otol 18:S166–S168

Svirsky M, Robbins A, Kirk K, Pisoni D, Miyamoto R. (2000). Language development in profoundly deaf children with cochlear implants. Psychological Science 11:153–158.

Tait M, Lutman ME, Robinson K. (2000). Preimplant measures of preverbal communication behaviour as predictors of cochlear implant outcomes in children. Ear Hear 21:18–24

Thoutenhoofd ED, Archbold SM, Gregory S, Lutman ME, Nikolopoulos TP, Sach TH. (2005). Paediatric Cochlear Implantation: Evaluating Outcomes. London: Whurr

Tobey EA, Altuna D, Gabbert G. (2003). Factors associated with development of speech production skills in children implanted by age 5. In: Geers A, ed. Cochlear Implants and Education of The Deaf Child. Ear Hear (Suppl)

Watson L, Archbold S, Nikolopoulos TP. (2006). Changing communication mode after implantation: by age at implantation. Cochlear Implant International

Wauters LN, van Bom WHJ, Tellings A. (2002). Reading comprehension of deaf students in primary and secondary education. Paper presented at the Society for Scientific Studies of Reading, Chicago

Wood DJ, Wood HA, Griffiths AJ, Howarth CI. (1986). Teaching and Talking with Deaf Children. New York: John Wiley

17

Speech Perception by Adults with Multichannel Cochlear Implants

Michael F. Dorman and
Anthony J. Spahr

This chapter reviews the speech perception abilities of patients fit with the current generation of multichannel cochlear implants. It describes selected acoustic cues for speech perception; reviews errors in phonetic identification made by patients; describes the signal processing strategies that can encode the acoustic cues; reviews the levels of speech recognition achieved by normal-hearing subjects listening to speech processed by the signal processing strategies, focusing on the issue of how many channels of stimulation are necessary to transmit speech in quiet and in noise; describes the performance of average and above-average patients on tests of speech, voice, and music recognition; and compares patient performance with the potential level of performance that could be achieved if all of the information delivered to the electrode array were received by the patient.

◆ The Speech Signal

Division of Information in the Speech Signal

It is convenient to divide information in the speech signal into two categories. In one category is information that exists in the amplitude envelope of the signal. This information could be coded by stimulation delivered to a single electrode. In the other category is information about the identity of a sound that exists in the frequency domain above several hundred Hertz. This information must be coded by the place of stimulation provided by multiple, intracochlear electrodes.

Rosen (1992) divides information in the amplitude envelope into envelope cues, periodicity cues, and fine, temporal-structure cues. As shown in **Fig. 17–1** (top), the very low-frequency envelope (2–50 Hz) of a signal can, but does not always, provide information about the number of word-sized units in the signal. The envelope, in the best case, can also provide information about the number of phoneme-sized elements in the signal (e.g., in "Sam").

As shown in **Fig. 17–2** the envelope of a signal can provide information about the manner of consonant articulation; that is, whether a signal is from the category stop consonant, semivowel, nasal, fricative, affricate, or vowel. In a vowel-consonant-vowel environment stop consonants (e.g., /d/ and /t/) are characterized by a period of silence in the signal. Semivowels and nasals (e.g., /l/ and /m/) are characterized by periodic energy greater than that for a stop but less than that for a vowel. The acoustic signature of fricatives (e.g., /s/ and /f/) is aperiodic energy or "noise." For /s/ and "sh," the level of the noise relative to the accompanying vowel can be 20 dB higher than for /f/ and "th." In this instance, an envelope cue can provide partial information about place of articulation. Affricates (e.g., "ch") are fricatives following a stop consonant and are characterized by a period of silence followed by a brief fricative noise with a rapid onset.

Periodicity cues provide information about the voicing status of a segment and about sentence intonation. As shown in **Fig. 17–2**, the acoustic realization of voice pitch is a series of high-amplitude modulations of the speech waveform. The interval between the peaks specifies the pitch period. Because voice pitch can vary over a large range (e.g., 80 Hz for a deep male voice and 300 Hz for a infant cry), the pitch period can vary, for these examples,

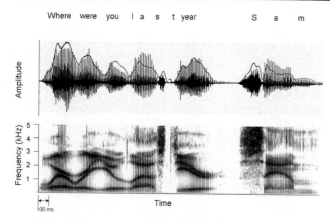

Figure 17–1   Two representations of the sentence, "Where were you last year, Sam?" At the top is the time waveform. The speech envelope is indicated by the solid black line. At the bottom is a spectrogram showing the frequencies that signal each of the phonetic elements in the sentence. Darkness specifies signal intensity.

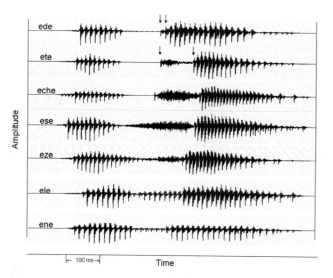

Figure 17–2   Amplitude envelopes for vowel-consonant-vowel syllables. For /ede/ and /ete/ the first arrow indicates the burst and the second arrow indicates the onset of voicing. The interval between arrows is the voice-onset time (VOT).

between 12.5 milliseconds and 3.3 milliseconds. Voiced sounds, such as /d/, /l/, and /n/, are periodic. Voiceless sounds, such as /t/, /s/, and "ch," are noise-excited and aperiodic. The voicing characteristic of stop consonants (e.g., /d/ versus /t/) in syllable-initial position is signaled by distinctive time/amplitude envelopes, related to differences in voice-onset time (VOT) and the presence or absence of aspiration before the onset of the vowel. The voicing status of fricatives is signaled by a different set of cues—the presence or absence of voicing during the production of the fricative noise [compared in **Fig. 17–2**, lines 1 and 2 (/ada/ vs. /ata/) and lines 4 and 5 /asa/ vs. /aza/].

Fine, temporal structure cues, realized as the intervals between the low-amplitude fluctuations and between the high-amplitude voicing pulses in **Fig. 17–2**, could, for implant patients, provide information about signal

frequency, at least in the domain of the first formant of the speech signal (e.g., 300 to 700 Hz for a male voice).

How might time/amplitude cues be useful to cochlear implant patients? Zue (1985) reports that if all the words in a 126,000-word vocabulary are defined in terms of six envelope/periodicity cues (vowel, strong fricative, weak fricative, nasal, semivowel, and stop), then for a given sequence of features only 2.4 words, on average, are possible word candidates. Thus, information in the time/amplitude envelope—information that could be conveyed by stimulation of a single electrode—could allow a listener to significantly restrict a set of possible word candidates.

If the correct word is to be identified from a set of possible word candidates, then information must be available from the frequency domain above several hundred hertz because the cues that specify place of articulation reside in that frequency domain. As shown in the spectrogram (**Fig. 17–1**, bottom) of the utterance, "Where were you last year, Sam?" speech is composed of frequencies that can range from ~300 Hz, the first formant for /u/, to 4 to 5 kHz, the frequencies that signal the presence of "s" in "Sam." The upper range of frequencies in female and children's speech can be, for "s," as high as 7 to 9 kHz.

Fig. 17–1 illustrates that, in the frequency domain, the sounds of speech are characterized by multiple concentrations of energy, or formants. To identify a vowel sound, an implant must be able to resolve, and then specify, where concentrations of energy occur in the frequency domain. The vowel "ou" in "you" is characterized by energy at 301 and 980 Hz. The vowel "a" in "last" has concentrations of energy at 592 and 1357 Hz. In the case of vowel sounds that are very similar, such as the vowels in "bit" and "bet," an implant must be able to resolve, at the level of the input filters, differences in formant frequencies of 100 to 200 Hz. These differences in input frequency must then be encoded by the relative depth, or position, of an electrode in the cochlea, or by the pattern of activity among adjacent electrodes in the cochlea.

Because vocal tract shapes change nearly continuously during the production of speech, frequencies of the speech signal will change from moment to moment. For example, as shown in **Fig. 17–1**, the "y" in "you" is characterized by a falling second formant that changes in frequency over a period of ~135 milliseconds. Other sounds change more quickly; for example, the formant frequencies in "b," "d," and "g" (not shown in **Fig. 17–1**) change over a period of 10 to 30 milliseconds. Thus, an implant must be able to resolve the frequency of multiple formants at a given moment in time and must be able to resolve rapid changes in formant frequencies over time. The duration of changes in formant transitions per se can be a cue to consonant manner as in the case of stops (10- to 30-millisecond duration) vs. semivowels (80- to 120-millisecond duration) (Liberman et al, 1956).

The stop consonant place of articulation is specified by the onset frequency and direction of change of brief, second, and third formant transitions and the frequency of the accompanying brief release burst (Cooper et al, 1952). Release bursts can differ in center frequency by as much as 2 kHz. The perceptual value of release bursts varies greatly with the vowel context in which the stop is articulated.

The acoustic cues for nasal place of articulation reside in the nasal resonance and in the second and third formant transitions that precede the accompanying vowel (Liberman et al, 1954). The different nasal resonances have similar, but not identical, spectra with the most energy concentrated under 400 Hz. The formant transition cues are brief as in the case of stop consonants.

Semivowel—/w r l j/—place of articulation is signaled by changes in the second and third formant transitions (O'Connor et al, 1957). In /r/ vs. /l/ the third formant transition is of special importance. Formant duration is longer for semivowels than for stops.

Fricative place of articulation is specified by both the center frequency of the long-duration fricative noise and by the formant transitions that follow the noise (Harris, 1958). When the noise signatures are very different, as in /s/ and "sh," then formant transitions play a relatively minor role in perception. When noise signatures are similar, as in the case of /f/ and "th," then formant transitions (and amplitude envelope cues) play a major role in perception.

Implications for Signal Processor Design

Signal processors need to be able to encode information in both the envelope and in the frequency domain. If we assume, following Wilson (1997), that pulse rate in a implant signal processor must be four to five times the highest frequency to be transmitted, then pulse rates as low as 250 Hz would preserve envelope information. The relatively large differences in envelope shape across manner categories and stop voicing should make consonant manner of articulation and stop voicing relatively well identified by patients fit with modern cochlear implants.

If temporal fine structure cues in the domain of voice pitch are to be faithfully preserved, then pulse rates of 1 kHz (5×200 Hz) per channel may be necessary. If first formant frequencies are to be encoded by temporal, fine-structure information, then pulse rates of 2500 to 3500 pulses per second (pps) may be necessary.

Providing sufficient coding to resolve place of articulation, especially for minimal pairs such as the vowels in "bit" and "bet" or for stop consonant and nasal place of articulation, could require a large number of input filters and output channels. We should suppose that the more input filters and the more electrodes, the better an implant would function.

◆ Strategies to Transmit Speech via a Cochlear Implant

Rubinstein (see Chapter 4) and Wilson (2000, 2006) provide detailed accounts of current signal processing strategies for cochlear implants. (For other reviews of signal processing strategies see, for example, Brown et al, 2003; Clark, 2000; David et al, 2003; Loizou, 1998, 1999; Wilson, 2000, 2004; Wouters et al, 1998.)

Current strategies to transmit information in the speech signal to an implant patient are variants or combinations of two designs. In one strategy, the n-of-m strategy, the signal is divided into m channels, the n channels with the largest energy are determined, and the electrodes associated with those channels are stimulated. Wilson et al (1988) described this strategy in a generic form for cochlear implants, and it is implemented, or can be implemented, on most modern cochlear implants (Arndt et al, 1999; Kiefer et al, 2001; Lawson et al, 1996; McDermott et al, 1992; Vandali et al, 2000; Ziese et al, 2000). The n-of-m strategy is an excellent way to transmit speech because only the peaks in the spectrum, or the formant frequencies, are transmitted, and as the formant frequencies change so also do the electrodes being stimulated. The change in location of stimulation mimics the normal change in location of spectral peaks along the basilar membrane. Experiments with normal-hearing listeners dating to the late 1940s and early 1950s have shown that speech can be transmitted with a high level of intelligibility if only information about the location of the formant peaks is transmitted (see, for example, the first experiments on the pattern playback speech synthesizer by Cooper et al, 1950, and experiments on peak-picking vocoders by Peterson and Cooper, 1957, as cited in Flanagan, 1972).

The other strategy to transmit speech by means of an implant is to divide the signal into frequency bands or channels and to transmit information about the energy in all of the bands at each processor update cycle. This strategy (and its variants, see Battmer et al, 1999; Firszt, 2004; Kessler, 1999; Koch et al, 2004; Loizou et al, 2003; Osberger and Fisher, 2000; Wilson et al, 1991; Zimmerman-Phillips and Murad, 1999) can be termed a fixed-channel strategy, in contrast to a channel-picking, or n-of-m strategy. Experiments dating to Dudley (1939) have shown that normal-hearing individuals can achieve a high level of speech understanding when speech is transmitted by a relatively small number (7 to 10) of fixed channels (e.g., Halsey and Swaffield, 1948; Hill et al, 1968).

◆ The Potential of n-of-m and Fixed-Channel Signal-Coding Strategies

Several research groups have performed experiments in which speech signals were processed by n-of-m and fixed-channel strategies and were presented to *normal-hearing listeners* for identification. These experiments differed from the earlier experiments cited above (e.g., Halsey and Swaffield, 1948; Hill et al, 1968) in terms of the motivation for the experiments (the earlier experiments were designed to principally investigate sound *quality* for speech transmission systems) and in the details of the implementations of the signal processors (in the recent experiments signal processing has been based on cochlear-implant signal processors, instead of speech transmission systems). The experiments have proved to be useful on at least three grounds. First, by presenting signals acoustically to normal-hearing individuals, we can establish how well implant patients would perform if electrode arrays were able to reproduce, by artificial electrical stimulation, the stimulation produced by acoustic signals. These data can serve as a baseline to assess how near or how far away we are from re-creating, with artificial electrical stimulation, the stimulation provided by acoustic stimulation of the cochlea. Second, experiments with normal-hearing listeners allow factors, normally confounded in implant patients, to be examined in isolation. For example, it is difficult to assess the effects of depth of electrode insertion on speech understanding because in patients with deep insertions there may be no viable neural elements near the electrode, whereas in patients with shallow insertions there may be viable neural elements. Of course, patients differ in many other ways, all of which are uncontrollable in a given experiment. Third, the experiments indicate how many channels are necessary to achieve a high level of speech understanding for both n-of-m and fixed-channel systems, a question that is central to the design of cochlear implants.

Signal Processing

In experiments with fixed-channel processors, signals are first processed through a pre-emphasis filter (e.g., low-pass below 1200 Hz, −6 dB per octave) and then band-passed into m logarithmic frequency bands using, for example, sixth-order Butterworth filters. The envelope of the signal is extracted by full-wave rectification, and low-pass filtering (e.g., second-order Butterworth with a 400-Hz cutoff frequency). Two types of outputs have been used. In some experiments, sinusoids are generated with amplitudes equal to the root-mean-square (rms) energy of the envelopes (computed every 4 milliseconds, for example) and frequencies equal to the center frequencies of the bandpass filters. In other experiments noise bands the width of the input filters are generated. The sinusoids or noise bands are finally summed and presented to listeners at a comfortable level. Signal processing for n-of-m processors is similar, in broad measure, to that for fixed-channel processors. However, instead of outputting the signals in each m channel, an algorithm chooses the n channels with the highest energy and outputs those channels.

Before the data for normal-hearing listeners are described, it is important to note that the normal-hearing listeners in these experiments have had, most generally, only very limited experience listening to signals processed into channels. Thus, the levels of performance obtained by the listeners are a conservative estimate of the levels of performance they might achieve if they had not hours but years of experience with the signals (as do implant patients).

Recognition in Quiet with Fixed-Channel and n-of-m Processors

The number of channels necessary to reach maximum performance varies as a function of test material and signal processing strategy. For fixed-channel processors, Dorman et al (2002b) report that Hearing in Noise Test (HINT) sentences (Nilsson et al, 1994) could be identified with 90% accuracy using four channels of stimulation (see the pioneering study of Shannon et al, 1995; see also Dorman et al, 1997; Friesen et al, 2001). Consonants could be identified with

greater than 90% accuracy with six channels of stimulation, and multitalker vowels required eight channels to reach 90% intelligibility. Dorman et al (2002a) report that between eight and 12 channels of stimulation are necessary to provide 90% intelligibility for monosyllabic words (see also Friesen et al, 2001). These results are reassuringly similar to those reported by researchers using different methods nearly a half century ago (e.g., Halsey and Swaffield, 1948).

For n-of-m processors, Dorman et al (2002a) report that a 3-of-20 processor allowed 90% correct recognition of vowels, consonants, and sentences. Dorman et al (2000) report that a 6-of-20 processor allowed a mean score of 90% correct for monosyllabic words. The results of these experiments are consistent with the much older literature on "peak-picking" channel vocoders (e.g., Peterson and Cooper, 1957) and demonstrate that a very high level of speech intelligibility can be achieved when picking only a small handful of high-amplitude channels from a set of 16 to 20 channels.

Recognition in Noise with Fixed-Channel and n-of-m Processors

The number of channels necessary to reach maximum performance in noise depends on the nature of the test material and the signal-to-noise ratio (Dorman et al, 1998, 2002a; Friesen et al, 2001; Fu et al, 1998). For example, 10 fixed channels allow 70% correct recognition of multitalker vowels at −2 dB signal-to-noise ratio (SNR); allow 70% correct recognition of consonants at +4 dB SNR; and allow 70% correct recognition of HINT sentences at 0 dB SNR (Dorman et al, 2002a). As the signal-to-noise level becomes poorer, the number of channels necessary to reach asymptotic performance increases. Dorman et al (1998) report that at +2 dB SNR, performance on sentences reached asymptote (85% correct) with 12 channels of stimulation. At −2 dB SNR, performance reached asymptote (63% correct) with 20 channels of stimulation. Results with n-of-m processors mirror the results for fixed-channel processors. Increasing the value of both m and n results in better performance (Kendall et al, 1997; Loizou et al, 2000). Dorman et al (2002a) report equal levels of performance (near 70% correct) for a 10 fixed-channel processor and a 9-of-20 processor when sentences were presented at 0 dB SNR.

One of the important findings from the literature reviewed above is that processors that allow scores equal to that of unprocessed speech in quiet do not allow scores equal to unprocessed speech in noise. For example, Fu et al (1998) report that a 16-band processor, which allowed scores similar to those for unprocessed speech in quiet, allowed much poorer scores than unprocessed speech at +12 to 0 dB SNR. Qin and Oxenham (2003) compared the speech reception threshold in noise for unprocessed speech and for speech processed through 4, 8, and 24 channels. Although the 24-channel processor provided near-normal resolution of formant peaks in quiet, the speech reception threshold for speech in noise was as much as 10 dB poorer than for unprocessed speech.

The poor performance of fixed-channel and channel-picking processors in noise can be exacerbated when the noise is a competing speech signal. In most real-world environments, noise changes over time, that is, the noise is temporally modulated. Normal-hearing subjects listening to speech in noise benefit from listening during "dips" in modulated noise (Bacon et al, 1998; Gustafsson and Arlinger, 1994). In contrast, normal-hearing subjects listening to speech coded into as many as 24 channels do not benefit from dips in a temporally modulated masker, especially if the masker is a single talker (Nelson and Jin, 2004; Qin and Oxenham, 2003; Stickney et al, 2004).

Summary

The studies reviewed above suggest that if cochlear implants could provide 12 channels of stimulation, then patients would enjoy near perfect recognition of speech in quiet. As few as four channels would allow a high level of performance for predictable sentences. This observation is critical because most conversations are relentlessly predictable. Predictability, in an important sense, allows the current generation of implants to be very effective for a very large number of patients. To understand a conversation in a level of noise commonly found in the workplace, an implant would need more channels—the number needed depends on the level and type of noise. Even a very large number of channels (e.g., 24) may fail to allow normal recognition of speech when the noise is temporally and spectrally modulated.

◆ Speech Recognition by Adult Cochlear-Implant Patients

In the previous section the potential of signal processing schemes for cochlear implants was documented. In this section the performance of postlingually deafened patients fit with cochlear implants is described.

Fig. 17–3 shows monosyllabic word recognition and sentence recognition for 54 patients fit with an eight-channel cochlear implant. The data are a superset of the data reported by Helms et al (1997) and are replotted from Wilson (2000, 2006). Observations were made of patient performance at 1, 3, 6, 12, and 24 months postfitting. At most measurement intervals word scores ranged from near 0% correct to near 90% correct. Mean scores increased from 37% correct at 1 month to 55% at 12 months. The mean score at 24 months did not differ from the mean score at 12 months. The number of patients with scores greater than 80% correct increased at the 24-month interval. For sentences, average performance was high (69% correct) following 1 month of experience. Performance was constrained by ceiling effects at subsequent test intervals. At 24 months the mean score was 90% correct.

The level of performance shown in **Fig. 17–3** for an implant with eight electrodes appears to be representative of the performance allowed by devices with more electrodes and different processing schemes. Wilson (2006) reports similar mean scores, near 55% correct, on CNC words for patients fit with devices with eight to 16 fixed channels and for a device that employs channel-picking with 20 or more input channels (see David et al, 2003; Koch et al, 2004).

Performance of the "Average" Patient

A common yardstick for performance is the performance of the "average" patient. In **Fig. 17–3**, the average score following 12 to 24 months of implant use was near 55% correct on a test of monosyllabic word recognition. In **Table 17–1**, scores are shown for 20 average patients (mean CNC score = 58% correct) and 21 above-average patients (mean CNC score = 80% correct) on a battery of tests of speech, voice, and music recognition. The data were collected in the context of a comparative study of cochlear implant performance (Spahr and Dorman, 2004). In the average group, 12 patients used a device with a 16-channel, high-rate, continuous interleaved sampling (CIS) processor, and eight used an implant with a lower-rate, 12-channel CIS processor. In the above-average group, 12 patients used a 16-channel CIS processor and nine used a 12-channel CIS processor.

The mean age of the patients in the average group was 58 years. The patients had been profoundly deaf for an average period of 18 years before implantation. Scores on the clearly articulated City University of New York (CUNY) sentences (Boothroyd et al, 1985) were at the ceiling (97% correct) of performance. The sentence data in **Fig. 17–3** show a similar outcome for an unselected set of patients. Thus, the average implant patient, when listening to the average, predictable conversation in quiet, should be able to communicate with relative ease. However, scores from sentences that were spoken by multiple talkers in a more normal, casual speaking style (the AzBio sentences) averaged only 70% correct. This outcome suggests more difficulty understanding speech in quiet than suggested from experiments using the CUNY or HINT sentences. At +10 dB SNR, performance on the CUNY sentences fell to 70% correct. At +10 dB SNR performance on the AzBio sentences fell to 42% correct. At +5 dB SNR, a common level in many work environments, performance on the AzBio sentences was only 27% correct. The difference in performance for casually spoken sentences in quiet and in noise (43%) highlights the difficulty faced by the average implant patient when attempting to understand speech presented against a background of noise.

To assess the recognition of voice pitch/voice quality, subjects were presented with pairs of words produced by the same talker or different talkers. The words in the pairs always differed, for example, "ball" from one talker and "brush" from the other talker. When one talker was male and the other female, patients were highly accurate (mean score = 93% correct) in judgments of same or different speaker. However, when both speakers were the same gender, performance was only slightly better than chance (65% correct).

To assess the recognition of melodies, each subject selected five familiar melodies from a list of 33 melodies. Each melody consisted of 16 equal-duration notes and was synthesized with MIDI software that used samples of a grand piano. The frequencies of the notes ranged from 277

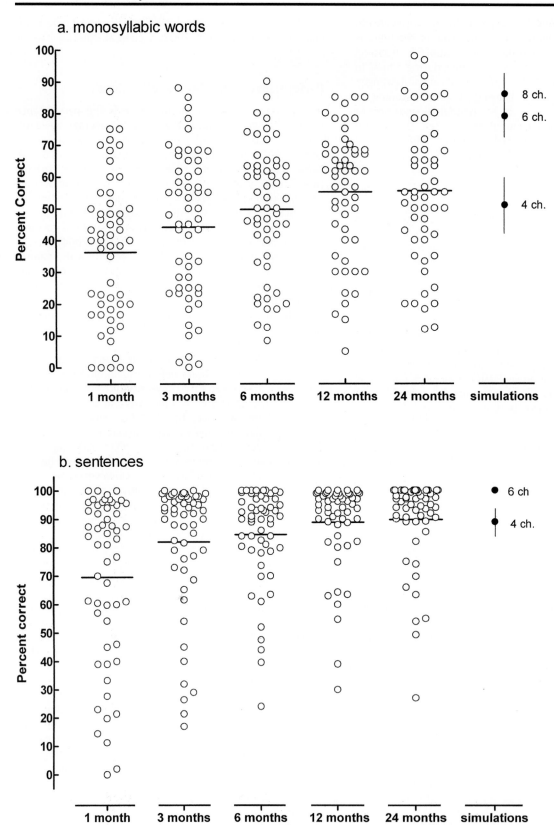

Figure 17-3 Scores on CNC words (top) and sentences (bottom) as a function of time for patients fit with an 8-channel cochlear implant. The data are from Helms et al (1997) and Wilson (2006). Each open circle indicates the performance of one patient. The mean score at each test interval is indicated by a solid line. The performance of normal-hearing subjects listening to similar material processed in the manner of a cochlear implant with 4, 6, or 8 channels is shown at the far right on each x-axis. The data are from Dorman et al (2002a). Standard deviations are shown by vertical lines.

Table 17–1 Average Age, Duration of Deafness, and Scores on Tests of Speech, Voice, and Music Recognition for Patients Who Achieve Average Scores (58% Correct) and Above-Average Scores (80% Correct) on Tests of CNC Word Recognition

	Average	Above-Average
Age	58 (14)	48 (11)
Duration of Deafness	18 (18)	11 (14)
CNC	58 (9)	80 (7)
Consonants	66 (19)	84 (6)
Vowels	58 (18)	72 (17)
CUNY Quiet	97 (3)	99 (2)
AzBio Quiet	70 (16)	90 (7)
CUNY +10	70 (20)	90 (8)
Az Bio +10	42 (20)	72 (14)
Az Bio +5	27 (15)	52 (15)
Voice: Male vs. Female	93 (5)	96 (5)
Voice: Within Gender	65 (6)	70 (6)
Five Melodies	33 (20)	56 (34)

to 622 Hz. The melodies were created without distinctive rhythmic information. Patient performance on this very simple task was very poor (33% correct).

The results from the voice discrimination task and the melody recognition task combine to demonstrate that patients cannot extract low-frequency information from the time waveform with a high degree of fidelity. This is the case even when the pulse rate is sufficiently high to provide good resolution of the time waveform.

The mean score on a 20-item test of consonant recognition (e.g., "a bay," "a day") was 66% correct. The confusion matrix is shown in **Table 17–2**. As should be expected from the discussion of envelope-based cues for speech recognition, manner of articulation was transmitted effectively (81% information transmitted). The error patterns for manner are instructive. For example, the relatively long interval between burst and the onset of voicing for /g/ apparently led to confusion with other sounds that shared a similar place but had a longer low-amplitude aspirated segment (/k/) or a silent interval ("dj"). Confusion between a silent interval and low amplitude aspiration also accounts for the /t k/ and "ch" errors.

The scores for voicing were poorer than for manner. With the exception of the /k/ for /g/ errors noted above, most voicing errors were within the fricative category. Errors

were not symmetrical between voiced and voiceless fricatives; the voicing status of voiced stops was much more likely to be misidentified.

Place of articulation was transmitted with the least effectiveness. Errors on /f/ and "th" were common, as would be expected from the similar noise spectra of the two sounds. In the high, front-vowel environment of /e/, alveolar and velar stops are more similar in terms of formant movement and burst spectra than labial stops. This could account for the better identification of /b p/ than /d t g k/. The very poor identification of nasal place suggests that neither the small differences in low-frequency spectra of the nasal resonances nor the following formant transitions were well received.

The mean score on a computer-synthesized, 16-item test of vowel recognition in "bVt" environment (Dorman et al, 1989) was 58% correct. The confusion matrix and vowel formant frequencies are shown in **Table 17–3** and **Fig. 17–4**. Back vowels (e.g., in "boot") and diphthongs with low, closely spaced F1 and F2 ("bout" and "boat") caused the most difficulty. The diphthongs in "bait" and "bite," characterized by widely spaced formants and extensive formant movement, were among the best-identified signals in the test set. Error responses for all signals were, most generally, vowels one up or one down in the vowel quadrangle (see Valimaa et al, 2002, for a review of vowel and consonant confusion errors for a different language—Finnish).

Performance of the "Better" Patients

As shown in **Table 17–1**, the highest performing patients (CNC mean score = 80% correct) were younger than the average patients (48 years vs. 58 years) and had been deaf for a shorter duration (11 years vs. 18 years). Four aspects of their performance, relative to that of patients in the average group, were notable. First, scores on the CUNY test did not separate patients in the two groups because of a ceiling effect. Second, performance on sentences produced in a casual speaking style in quiet was high (90% correct), demonstrating that the better patients can function at a very high level in a quiet environment even when multiple speakers are not trying to speak clearly and predictably. Third, at an SNR commonly found in the workplace (+5 dB SNR), performance fell to 52% correct. This suggests that even the better patients have difficulty understanding

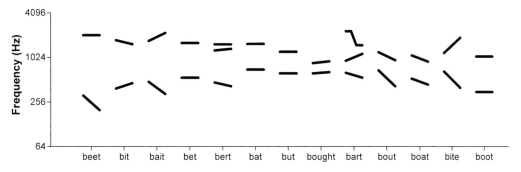

Figure 17–4 Stylized spectrograms of formant frequencies for the vowels in the test set. The vowels were computer synthesized in "bVt" context, e.g., "beet," "bit," "bet," etc. All vowels were of equal duration.

Table 17–2   Consonant Confusion Matrices for Patients with **(A)** Average (58% Correct) and **(B)** Above-Average (80% Correct) CNC Scores

A

	b	d	g	p	t	k	w	r	l	y	m	n	v	z	dj	ch	s	sh	f	th
b	74	12	1	11							1	1								
d	18	64	8	5	1		1			1			1							1
g		4	56	3	3	14	1			2			1	2	13					1
p		1		79	10	4							1	1		1			2	1
t			1	7	49	30							1		3	3		1	1	4
k		1	1	9	16	65							1	1			3			
w				2			63	13	16	3	2		1							
r							4	93					2	1						
l							6	19	72	1	1		1							
y	1	1	1	1	1	1	1	3		58			8	17	1					3
m		2	1				1		7	2	62	23	2							
n		2	1				1		4		29	61	1				1			
v	7	4		1	1		1	1	2		2	2	57	2		1			6	13
z													6	76	1	3	9	2		3
dj				6	2									2	87		1			1
ch			3	8	11					2			1	1	5	56	1	6	1	5
s		1											1	1	3		69	7	14	4
sh																9	15	73	2	1
f													5	2		4	7	8	67	6
th	2		1	2	1								14	6	1		7	1	27	38

B

	b	d	g	p	t	k	w	r	l	y	m	n	th	v	z	dj	ch	s	sh	f
b	92	8																		
d	3	90	6										1							
g		4	77		2	10			1				1	1	2	2				
p				93	4	3														
t				2	81	12							2			1	1	1		
k				3	16	77														
w			5				84			5					3	4				
r							4	96												
l							2	10	87			1								
y			5							84	5				3	4				
m	3								4		64	30								
n									2		19	79								
th													46	20	6		2			25
v	7							1	1	1			15	72						3
z									1					1	97		1			
dj																100				
ch				4	5											3	88	1		
s													1	2				97		
sh															5			3	92	
f													6	4				2		89

Darker lines encompass manner categories. Within the stop, fricative, and affricate manner categories, voicing categories are setoff by shading. The consonants were produced by a single male speaker in /eCe/ ("a bay," "a day," etc.) context. Key to symbols: "y" as in "yellow"; "th" as in "thin"; "dj" as in "jello."

speech in a noisy work environment. Fourth, performance on the tests of within-gender speaker recognition and melody recognition, although superior to that of the patients in the average group, was still poor.

The relatively few errors on the test of consonant identification (**Table 17–2B**) were predominantly "place" errors. As was the case for the group of average performers, /f/ versus "th" and /m/ versus /n/ were troublesome. There were very few errors on manner and only one common error on voicing. Errors on the test of vowel identification (**Table 17–3B**) were similar to those committed by patients in the average group. Back vowels and diphthongs with low, closely spaced formants remained difficult to identify.

One patient fit with a 16-channel, high-rate CIS processor and a modiolar-hugging electrode array achieved a score of 100% correct on the test of CNC word identification and must be considered one of the highest performing patients in the world. For that reason, his scores on other tests are of interest. On the difficult AzBio sentences, he scored 98% correct—a score within the range of performance of normal-hearing listeners tested with unprocessed AzBio sentences. On tests of vowel and consonant identification he

Table 17–3   Vowel Confusion Matrices for Patients with **(A)** Average CNC Scores (Correct Responses are Set Off by Shading), and **(B)** for Patients with Above Average CNC Scores

A

	beet	bit	bait	bet	Bert	bat	but	bought	Bart	bout	boat	bite	boot
beet	71	9	17	1		2							
bit	6	60	3	19	2	7			1	1			1
bait	17	4	62	8	1	4			2		1		
bet		26	2	53	1	13			1	2	1		1
Bert		1			76	1	6	2	5	2	2		5
bat	1	1	2	21	1	63	10			1			
but		1		5	3	15	52	8	4	8	1	2	1
bought					1	1	11	73	2	5	6		1
Bart				5		6	26		54	3	4		2
bout					1		4	3	5	30	52		5
boat			1	8	1	1	13	12	6		51		7
bite		4	5	9	4	5	1		3			69	
boot		1			12		7	15	8	5	17		35

B

	beet	bit	bait	bet	Bert	bat	but	bought	Bart	bout	boat	bite	boot
beet	88	4	9										
bit		79	10	6	1		2						3
bait	7	6	84	1	2								1
bet		20	5	65	1	7							
Bert					90			2			2	2	3
bat		1		20	1	73	4						
but		1		2	2	9	76	2	2	3		4	
bought				2		5	10	79	1	2	1		
Bart					1	1	19		77	1	1		
bout					1	1	3	2		56	35		2
boat				4		1	8	9	9		61		9
bite			3		1					4	3	88	
boot					28	1	2				19		48

scored 97% correct and 94% correct, respectively. Normal-hearing subjects listening to unprocessed speech score 99% correct on these tests. At +10 dB SNR he scored 90% correct on the AzBio sentences; at +5 dB SNR he scored 77% correct. Normal-hearing subjects listening to unprocessed speech score 99% correct on these tests. His scores were relatively poor on tests of within-gender voice identification (72% correct) and melody identification (48% correct). These scores suggest that even the very best patients do not receive a high-fidelity representation of low-frequency information.

Estimating the Number of Functional Channels of Stimulation

The data reviewed in the sections above were collected from patients fit with devices with 8 to 16 electrode contacts. A central issue in the field of implant design is how many functional channels are derived from that number of electrical contacts. One way to estimate the number is to compare the performance of normal-hearing subjects listening to acoustic simulations with the performance of patients fit with cochlear implants (see, for example, Dorman and Loizou, 1998; Friesen et al, 2001; Fu and Shannon, 1999). That comparison is made in **Fig. 17–3** for monosyllabic words and sentences. On the test of monosyllabic word recognition, the average score after 24 months of experience

was no better than that achieved by normal-hearing subjects listening to four channels of stimulation. The better patients received the equivalent of six or eight channels of stimulation. Only two patients with scores near 100% correct received the equivalent of more than eight channels of stimulation. This result parallels the results of experiments in which electrodes were selectively turned off in arrays with as many as 20 electrodes. Performance with four to seven active electrodes was as good as performance with 20 active electrodes (e.g., Fishman et al, 1997; Friesen et al, 2001; Wilson, 1997). Both results demonstrate that implant patients do not extract the full amount of information available in the stimulation patterns delivered to the electrode array.

Conclusion and Speculation

The statistically average, postlingually-deafened patient can, in a quiet environment, understand carefully articulated, conversational speech with a very high degree of accuracy. This ability allows the average patient to use that most necessary modern toy, the cell phone. However, in many common environments speech understanding remains relatively poor. In a quiet environment, only about three quarters of the words in sentences that are spoken casually by multiple talkers are recognized. Speech understanding is poor in any environment with background noise.

The statistically above-average patient enjoys near perfect speech understanding in quiet, even when sentences are spoken in a conversational style and when multiple takers speak in turn. In modest amounts of noise, performance falls and is relatively poor at a SNR ratio found in busy work environments.

In terms of processor design, how might we make speech more understandable for patients? One obvious answer is to make each physical channel a functional channel. The evidence reviewed in this chapter suggests that if patients were to receive all of the information coded into 12 to 20 channels—the number of electrodes in current devices— then the average patient would achieve near-perfect recognition of CNC words and would achieve high, but not normal, scores on tests of speech perception in noise. It is generally supposed that the difference between physical and functional channels is caused by current spread or interaction at the level of the spiral ganglion or by overlap in the representation of these patterns at more central locations in the auditory pathway. To date, no method of altering current fields, other than ensuring that the fields are not on at the same time (Wilson et al, 1991), has provided a significant improvement in speech understanding.

Another way to create higher levels of speech understanding is to improve the transmission of low-frequency information. For patients with very high scores on tests of word and sentence identification, we have documented poor reception of: (1) voice pitch/voice quality; (2) low- frequency, closely spaced formants; (3) the low-frequency nasal resonance; (4) voicing for fricatives; and (5) simple, low-frequency note sequences, that is, melodies. It has been suggested that the poor coding of pitch is a major factor in the poor recognition of speech when speech is presented against a background of other speech (e.g., Qin and Oxenham, 2003; Nelson and Jin, 2004; Turner et al, 2004). Rubinstein (see Chapter 4) suggests that the use of a high rate, "conditioning" pulse train may create: (1) an environment in which neurons can be coaxed to fire in a more stochastic pattern and (2) an environment in which low-frequency information in the temporal fine structure is better coded. However, even if temporal fine structure were well coded, Oxenham et al (2004) suggest that the temporal information would have to be delivered to the correct "place" in order for frequency to be resolved with normal fidelity. As the authors note, "it will be extremely challenging to recreate the complex pattern of activity produced within each cycle of the cochlear traveling wave, should the neural code be based on spatiotemporal excitation patterns." Given this pessimistic view, we should hope that near-normal fidelity of low-frequency information will suffice for the perception of speech in noise.

Another way to improve the reception of low-frequency information by implant patients is to implant electrode arrays into patients with low-frequency acoustic hearing to 500 Hz (Kiefer et al, 2005; Lawson et al, 2000; von Ilberg et al, 1999; see also Chapter 19). Patients who hear by a combination of electric and acoustic stimulation (EAS) commonly achieve higher levels of speech understanding in noise than when hearing by electric stimulation alone. For some patients the improvement in speech understanding can be as large as 70 percentage points (Kiefer et al, 2005). Given this outcome, the best solution to the problem of providing detailed low-frequency information to an implant patient may be to let the acoustically driven auditory system code the information. If acoustic hearing can be reliably preserved following implant surgery, then the large and growing population of aging individuals with relatively good low-frequency acoustic sensitivity but poor high-frequency sensitivity may be the most successful users of cochlear implants.

Acknowledgment

The writing of this chapter was supported by National Institute on Deafness and Other Communication Disorders (NIDCD) grant RO1-DC-000654–14.

References

Arndt P, Staller S, Arcaroli J, Hines A, Ebinger K. (1999). Within-subjects comparison of advanced coding strategies in the Nucleus 24 cochlear implant. Technical report. Englewood, CO: Cochlear Corporation

Bacon S, Opie J, Montoya D. (1998). The effects of hearing loss and noise masking on the masking release for speech in temporally complex backgrounds. J Speech Lang Hear Res 41:549–563

Battmer RD, Zilberman Y, Haake P, Lenarz T. (1999). Simultaneous analog stimulation (SAS)–continuous interleaved sampler (CIS) pilot comparison study in Europe. Ann Otol Rhinol Laryngol Suppl 177:69–73

Boothroyd A, Hanin L, Hnath T. (1985). A Sentence Test of Speech Perception: Reliability, Set Equivalence and Short-Term Learning. Internal Report RCI 10. New York: City University of New York

Brown CJ, Geers A, Herrmann B, Iler-Kirk K, Tomblin JB, Waltzman S. (2003). Cochlear implants. Technical Report. American Speech-Language-Hearing Association. ASHA Suppl. 24:1–35

Clark GM. (2000). The cochlear implant: a search for answers. Cochlear Implants Int 1:1–15

Cooper F, Delattre P, Liberman A, Borst J, Gerstman L. (1952). Some experiments on the perception of synthetic speech sounds. J Acoust Soc Am 24:597–606

Cooper F, Liberman A, Borst J. (1950). Preliminary studies of speech produced by a pattern playback. J Acoust Soc Am 22:678

David E, Ostroff JM, Shipp D, et al. (2003). Speech coding strategies and revised cochlear implant candidacy: an analysis of post-implant performance. Otol Neurotol 24:228–233

Dorman MF, Dankowski K, Smith L, McCandless G. (1989). Identification of synthetic vowels by patients using the Symbion multichannel cochlear implant. Ear Hear 10:40–43

Dorman MF, Loizou P. (1998). The identification of consonants and vowels by cochlear-implant patients using a 6-channel CIS processor and by normal-hearing subjects using simulations of processors with 2–9 channels. Ear Hear 19:162–166

Dorman MF, Loizou PC, Fitzke J, Tu Z. (1998). The recognition of sentences in noise by normal-hearing listeners using simulation of cochlear-implant signal processors with 6–20 channels. J Acoust Soc Am 104:3583–3585

Dorman M, Loizou P, Fitzke J, Tu Z. (2000). The recognition of NU-6 words by cochlear-implant patients and by normal-hearing subjects listening to NU-6 words processed in the manner of CIS and SPEAK strategies. Ann Otol Rhinol Laryngol 109:64–66

Dorman MF, Loizou P, Rainey D. (1997). Speech intelligibility as a function of the number of channels of stimulation for signal processors using sine-wave and noise-band outputs. J Acoust Soc Am 102:2403–2411

Dorman MF, Loizou PC, Spahr AJ, Maloff E. (2002a). A comparison of the speech understanding provided by acoustic models of fixed-channel and channel-picking signal processors for cochlear implants. J Speech Lang Hear Res 45:783–788

Dorman MF, Loizou PC, Spahr AJ, Maloff E. (2002b). Factors that allow a high level of speech understanding by patients fit with cochlear implants. Am J Audiol 11:119–123

Dudley H. (1939). Remaking speech. J Acoust Soc Am 11:169–177

Flanagan J. (1972). Speech Analysis, Synthesis and Perception, 2nd ed., pp.329–331. New York: Springer-Verlag

Firszt JB. (2004). HiResolution Sound Processing. Technical report. Sylmar, CA: Advanced Bionics Corporation http://www.cochlearimplant.com/printables/HiRes-WhtPpr.pdf

Fishman K, Shannon R, Slattery W. (1997). Speech recognition as a function of the number of electrodes used in the SPEAK cochlear implant speech processor. J Speech Lang Hear Res 40:1201–1215

Friesen LM, Shannon RV, Baskent D, Wang X. (2001). Speech recognition in noise as a function of the number of spectral channels: comparison of acoustic hearing and cochlear implants. J Acoust Soc Am 110:1150–1163

Fu Q-J, Shannon R. (1999). Recognition of spectrally degraded and frequency shifted vowels in acoustic and electric hearing. J Acoust Soc Am 105:1889–1900

Fu Q-J, Shannon R, Wang X. (1998). Effects of noise and spectral resolution on vowel and consonant recognition: Acoustic and electric hearing. J Acoust Soc Am 104:3586–3596

Gustafsson H, Arlinger S. (1994). Masking of speech by amplitude-modulated noise. J Acoust Soc Am 95:518–529

Halsey R, Swaffield J. (1948). Analysis-synthesis telephony, with special reference to the vocoder. Institute of Electrical Engineers (London) 95(pt III):391–411

Harris K. (1958). Cues for the discrimination of American English fricatives in spoken syllables. Lang Speech 1:1–7

Helms J, Muller J, Schon F, et al. (1997). Evaluation of Performance with the COMBI 40 cochlear implant in adults: a multicentric clinical study. ORL J Otorhinolaryngol Relat Spec 59:23–35

Hill JJ, McRae PP, McClellan RP. (1968). Speech recognition as a function of channel capacity in a discrete set of channels. J Acoust Soc Am 44:13–18

Kendall M, Summerfield A, Chambers J. (1997). Digital signal-processing simulation of the Spectra-22™ speech processor. Manuscript from the MRC Institute of Hearing Research, Nottingham, UK

Kessler DK. (1999). The CLARION multi-strategy cochlear implant. Ann Otol Rhinol Laryngol Suppl 177:8–16

Kiefer J, Hohl S, Sturzebecher E, Pfennigdorff T, Gstoettner W. (2001). Comparison of speech recognition with different speech coding strategies (SPEAK, CIS, and ACE) and their relationship to telemetric measures of compound action potentials in the nucleus CI 24M cochlear implant system. Audiology 40:32–42

Kiefer J, Pok M, Adunka O, et al. (2005). Combined electric and acoustic stimulation (EAS) of the auditory system – Results of a clinical study. Audiol Neurootol 10:134–144

Koch DB, Osberger MJ, Segel P, Kessler DK. (2004). HiResolution and conventional sound processing in the HiResolution Bionic Ear: using appropriate outcome measures to assess speech-recognition ability. Audiol Neurootol 9:214–223

Lawson D, Wilson B, Wolford B, Brill S, Schatzer R. (2000). Speech processors for auditory prostheses. Eighth quarterly progress report. NIH project N01-DC-8-2105. Bethesda, MD: Neural Prosthesis Program, National Institutes of Health, http://www.rti.org/capr/caprqprs.htm)

Lawson DT, Wilson BS, Zerbi M, Finley C. (1996). Speech processors for auditory prostheses: 22 electrode percutaneous study—results for the first five subjects. Third quarterly progress report. NIH project NO1-DC-5-2103. Bethesda, MD: Neural Prosthesis Program, National Institutes of Health, http://www.rti.org/capr/caprqprs.htm

Liberman AM, Delattre PC, Cooper FS, Gerstman LJ. (1954). The role of consonant-vowel transitions in the perception of the stop and nasal consonants. Psych Mono 68:

Liberman AM, Delattre PC, Gerstman LJ, Cooper FS. (1956). Tempo of frequency change as a cue for distinguishing classes of speech sounds. J Exp Psychol 52:127–137

Loizou PC. (1998). Mimicking the human ear: An overview of signal processing strategies for cochlear prostheses. IEEE Sig Proc Mag 15:101–130

Loizou PC. (1999). Signal-processing techniques for cochlear implants. IEEE Eng Med Biol Mag 18:34–46

Loizou P, Dorman MF, Tu Z, Fitzke J. (2000). The recognition of sentences in noise by normal-hearing listeners using simulations of SPEAK-type cochlear-implant signal-processors. Ann Otol Rhinol Laryngol Suppl 185:67–68

Loizou P, Stickney G, Mishra L, Assmann P. (2003). Comparison of speech processing strategies used in the Clarion implant processor. Ear Hear 24:12–19

McDermott HJ, McKay CM, Vandali AE. (1992). A new portable sound processor for the University of Melbourne/Nucleus Limited multielectrode cochlear implant. J Acoust Soc Am 91:3367–3391

Nelson PB, Jin SH. (2004). Factors affecting speech understanding in gated interference: cochlear implant users and normal-hearing listeners. J Acoust Soc Am 115:2286–2294

Nilsson M, Soli S, Sullivan J. (1994). Development of the Hearing in Noise Test for the measurement of speech reception thresholds in quiet and noise. J Acoust Soc Am 95:1085–1099

O'Connor J, Gerstman L, Liberman A, Delattre P, Cooper F. (1957). Acoustic cues for the perception of initial /wjrl/ in English. Word 13:24–43

Osberger MJ, Fisher L. (2000). New directions in speech processing: Patient performance with simultaneous analog stimulation. Ann Otol Rhinol Laryngol Suppl 185:70–73

Oxenham A, Bernstein J, Penagos H. (2004). Correct tonotopic representation is necessary for complex pitch perception. Proc Natl Acad Sci USA 101:1421–1425

Peterson G, Cooper F. (1957). Peakpicker: a bandwidth compression device. J Acoust Soc Am 29:777(A)

Qin MK, Oxenham AJ. (2003). Effects of simulated cochlear-implant processing on speech reception in fluctuating maskers. J Acoust Soc Am 114:446–454

Rosen S. (1992). Temporal information in speech and its relevance for cochlear implants. Philos Trans R Soc Lond [B] Biol Sci 336:333–367

Shannon R, Zeng F-G, Kamath V, Wygonski J, Ekelid M. (1995). Speech recognition with primarily temporal cues. Science 270: 303–304

Spahr A, Dorman M. (2004). Performance of subjects fit with the Advanced Bionics CII and Nucleus 3G cochlear implant devices. Arch Otolaryngol Head Neck Surg 130:624–628

Stickney G, Zeng F-G, Litovsky R, Assmann P. (2004). Cochlear implant speech recognition with speech maskers. J Acoust Soc Am 116: 1081–1091

Turner CW, Gantz BJ, Vidal C, Behrens A, Henry BA. (2004). Speech recognition in noise for cochlear implant listeners: Benefits of residual acoustic hearing. J Acoust Soc Am 115:1729–1735

Valimaa TT, Maatta TK, Lopponen HJ, Sorri MJ. (2002). Phoneme recognition and confusions with multichannel cochlear implants: vowels. J Speech Lang Hear Res 45:1039–1054

Vandali AE, Whitford LA, Plant KL, Clark GM. (2000). Speech perception as a function of electrical stimulation rate: using the Nucleus 24 cochlear implant system. Ear Hear 21:608–624

Von Ilberg C, Kiefer J, Tillein J, et al. (1999). Electric-acoustic stimulation of the auditory system. ORL J Otorhinolaryngol Relat Spec 61:334–340

Wilson B. (1997). The future of cochlear implants. Br J Audiol 31: 205–225

Wilson BS. (2000). Strategies for representing speech information with cochlear implants. In: Niparko J, Kirk K, Mellon N, Robbins A, Tucci D, Wilson B, eds. Cochlear Implants: Principles and Practices, pp. 129–170. Philadelphia: Lippincott Williams & Wilkins

Wilson B. (2004). Engineering design of cochlear implant systems. In: Zeng F-G, Popper AN, Fay RR, eds. Auditory Prostheses: Cochlear Implants and Beyond, pp. 14–52. New York: Springer-Verlag

Wilson B. (2006). Speech Processing Strategies. In: Cooper H, Craddock L, eds. Cochlear Implants: A Practical Guide, 2nd ed., pp. 21–69, London: Whurr

Wilson BS, Finley CC, Farmer JC Jr, et al. (1988). Comparative studies of speech processing strategies for cochlear implants. Laryngoscope 98:1069–1077

Wilson BS, Finley CC, Lawson DT, Wolford RD, Eddington DK, Rabinowitz WM. (1991). Better speech recognition with cochlear implants. Nature 352:236–238

Wouters J, Geurts L, Peeters S, Vanden Berghe J, van Wieringen A. (1998). Developments in speech processing for cochlear implants. Acta Otorhinolaryngol Belg 52:129–132

Ziese M, Stutzel A, von Specht H, et al. (2000). Speech understanding with the CIS and the n-of-m strategy in the MED-EL COMBI 40+ system. ORL J Otorhinolaryngol Relat Spec 62:321–329

Zimmerman-Phillips S, Murad C. (1999). Programming features of the CLARION multi-strategy cochlear implant. Ann Otol Rhinol Laryngol Suppl 177:17–21

Zue V. (1985). The use of speech knowledge in automatic speech recognition. Proc IEEE 73:1602–1615

18

Advantages of Binaural Hearing

Camille C. Dunn,

William Yost,

William G. Noble,

Richard S. Tyler, and

Shelley A. Witt

The human auditory system possesses an amazing ability to hear sounds with two ears and to combine the two signals into one to be processed by the brain. This is called binaural processing. This chapter discusses the cues that our auditory system uses to recognize sounds and to separate them into different sound sources, and how listeners with hearing aids and cochlear implants use these cues to enable binaural hearing.

It should be noted that most of this discussion on how the auditory system processes sounds is based on findings generally tested in a controlled laboratory environment. Therefore, we try to generalize our discussion to how the auditory system may work in a noncontrolled environment (i.e., a local restaurant).

◆ Advantages of Binaural Hearing in Normal Hearing Listeners

Through studies of normal-hearing listeners, we have come to better understand the advantages of hearing with two ears. The ability to determine the location of a sound source is an important function performed by the auditory system. It allows one to know where objects in our world are located. The fact that the auditory system can locate the position of various sound sources aids a listener in sorting out different sound sources in a complex acoustic environment. That is, binaural processing may aid in detecting and attending to target sound sources, such as speech, in a background of competing sound sources (noise).

Because sound does not have a physical dimension in space, locating a sound source requires some form of neural computation by the auditory system. Binaural processing is one such computation that allows the auditory system to determine the location of sound in the horizontal or azimuth plane (the left–right dimension) (**Fig. 18–1**). This computation is based on the interaction of sound with the body (e.g., the head) of the listener or objects in the listener's environment. A sound source can be localized in space based on the characteristics of the sound produced by the source. A sound source on one side of a listener arrives at the ear closer to the source before it arrives at the ear farther from the source. This difference in arrival

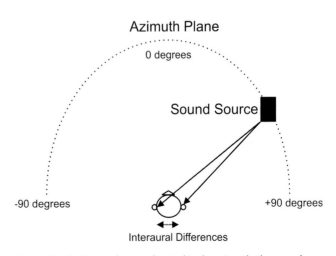

Figure 18–1 A sound source located in the azimuth plane produces interaural differences of time and level at the listener's ears.

time is called interaural time difference (ITD). The level (loudness) of the sound at the ear nearer the source is also greater than that at the ear farther from the source, generating an interaural level difference (ILD). The binaural auditory system computes these two interaural differences (ITD and ILD) determine the azimuthal location of the sound source. For example, if the ITD and the ILD are zero, then the source is directly in front of the listener, or at some point in the plane bisecting the body vertically. If the ITD and ILD are large, then the sound source's location is toward one ear or the other.

As will be explained later in the chapter, the ITD is a useful binaural cue only at low frequencies. Thus, above about 1000 to 2000 Hz, the cue used for azimuthal sound localization is the ILD. Between about 700 Hz and 1200 Hz, both the ILD and the ITD provide useful binaural information about azimuthal sound source location. And below about 800 Hz, only the ITD can be used to locate a sound source. The fact that ILDs provide azimuthal information for high-frequency sounds and ITDs provide azimuthal information for low-frequency sounds is referred to as the duplex theory of sound localization (Stevens and Newman, 1936).

Head Shadow Effect

The relative amount of information provided by an ITD or an ILD concerning the azimuthal location of a sound source depends on the frequency of the sound. The ILD is primarily produced by the fact that sound is diffracted around the head. As such, the head produces an "acoustic shadow" at the ear farther from the sound source. That is, the sound arriving at the ear farther from the source is attenuated relative to the sound arriving at the ear nearer the source. This attenuation difference is due to diffraction of sound around the head. The amount of attenuation caused by the head shadow depends on the sound's wavelength. In general, a sound shadow is produced when the wavelength of sound is shorter than the size of the object (e.g., the head) producing the shadow. The smaller the sound's wavelength is relative to the size of the object, the greater the shadow and the larger the ILD. Wavelength is inversely proportional to sound frequency. High frequencies have short wavelengths and produce large ILDs. The average human head produces about a 2-dB ILD at 1000 Hz, and as much as a 20-dB ILD at 6300 Hz (Kuhn, 1987). Below about 500 Hz, the ILD is 1 dB or less and is not detectable by the auditory system.

The head shadow provides a potentially useful advantage for detecting a target signal such as speech that is spatially separated from competing sound sources (noise). For example, if the competing sound source is on the side of the head opposite the target signal, then the noise will be attenuated relative to the level of the signal due to the head shadow. The ability to use the higher level of the sound at the ear closer to the sound source to improve signal detection is not a direct function of binaural processing, but is the physical consequence of sound diffraction around an object such as the human head. This chapter discusses how binaural processing of the sounds from spatially separated signal and competing sources can aid in the detection and intelligibility of a signal relative to competing sound sources.

Binaural Squelch

In addition to the ability to use the neurally computed ITD and ILD to localize a sound source, ITDs and ILDs can be used to "squelch" information provided by a spatially separated competing sound source to aid in the detection of a target signal. The ability to detect a target sound at one location in the presence of sounds at other locations is also referred to as the "cocktail party" effect, as explained below.

The ITD is a cue that is limited to sounds with frequencies below about 800 Hz. A sound with a frequency of 800 Hz has a period of 1.25 milliseconds, and a half period of 0.625 milliseconds. The time it takes sound to travel from one side of the head to the other is about 0.625 milliseconds. For sounds with frequencies below 800 Hz (half periods of 0.625 milliseconds or shorter) that are located opposite one ear, each peak of the sound wave will always arrive at the ear closer to the sound source before it reaches the ear farther from the sound source. Therefore, binaural processing of this interaural time difference would indicate that the sound source is opposite the ear closer to the sound source. If the period of the sound is shorter than about 0.625 milliseconds (frequency higher than 800 Hz), then for all peaks of the waveform except the first peak, the peaks arriving at the ear farther from the sound source may occur before those arriving at the ear closer to the sound source, producing a confusing pattern of interaural time differences. Thus, only sounds with low frequencies can produce an unambiguous ITD for indicating the location of the sound source.

Another kind of ambiguity associated with ILDs and ITDs is the *cone of confusion*. For a stationary listener, a sound at, for example, 45 degrees to the right and in front produces interaural differences nearly identical with those for a sound 45 degrees to the right and behind. All sources on the surface of an imaginary cone, having a slope of 45 degrees, an apex at the center of the head, and an axis that coincides with the line through the two ears (the interaural axis) provide the same, or nearly the same, interaural differences. This geometric principle holds for any location displaced from the body's vertical midline. Various other cues, including monaural outer ear spectral features (Shaw, 1982), interaural disparities in such spectra (Searle et al, 1975), and, more robustly, even very slight movement of the listener's head (Perrett & Noble, 1997), serve to overcome this ambiguity.

Binaural Summation

Sounds that are presented to both ears are up to 3 dB more audible than sounds presented to only one ear [assuming the level of the sound at the two ears is about the same (Wegel and Lane, 1924)]. In many situations, the perceived loudness of sounds presented to both ears is greater than that presented to only one ear. This perceived binaural loudness difference varies from no loudness differences up to as much as 10 dB (a doubling of loudness) depending on the stimulus conditions (Fletcher and Munson, 1933). Thus, sounds presented bilaterally appear to add together in some fashion and this is referred to as binaural summation. But as will be explained below regarding the masking-level difference (MLD), binaural presentation of a target signal plus a competing sound source presented identically to both ears does not yield lower masked thresholds as compared with conditions in which the signal and maskers are presented to only one ear.

Localization

In our natural listening environments, listeners perceive sounds emanating from all directions. In a clinical setting, sounds are generally presented to listeners from loudspeakers or through headphones. Sounds presented from loudspeakers or sounds produced by natural sources produce ITDs and ILDs based on the interactions between the sound and the head as explained earlier. Sounds presented over headphones can be manipulated so that the sound arriving at one headphone is earlier and more intense than that arriving at the other headphone, creating ITDs and ILDs. For many stimulus conditions, the perception of the sound's location differs depending on whether or not it was produced by a loudspeaker (or natural sound sources) or by headphones. Thus, the term *localization* is used to refer to sounds produced by loudspeakers or by natural sound sources, and the term *lateralization* is used to refer to conditions in which sounds are delivered to the ears via headphones.

Azimuthal sound localization for listeners with normal hearing is best at frequencies below about 800 Hz and above about 2000 Hz. Azimuthal sound localization is the worst between 800 and 2000 Hz. These differences are attributed to the duplex theory of sound localization as explained earlier. The threshold ability to discriminate a change in the location of a sound source is referred to as the minimal audible angle (MAA) (Mills, 1972). The MAA is smallest (~1 degree) when the sound source is directly in front of the listener and poorest when the sound source is opposite one ear or the other [the MAA is about 5 to 9 degrees (Mills, 1972)]. The fact that MAA is best for sounds directly in front of a listener means that it is often crucial to control for head movements in studying binaural processing so that listeners do not move their heads to take advantage of the small MAA for sounds located directly in front. The average error in azimuthal location of a broadband sound source (e.g., a broad-band noise or an acoustic transient) for listeners with normal hearing is about 5 degrees (Wightman and Kistler, 1989). Sounds, especially narrow-band sounds such as tones, produced in reverberant spaces are more difficult to accurately localize than sounds produced in echo-free spaces (Hartmann, 1983).

Lateralization

When sounds are presented over headphones, the ITD and ILD values can be carefully controlled and manipulated. Such headphone-produced sounds are generally perceived as being lateralized inside of the head rather than out in actual space. Changes in ITD or ILD produce the perception of sounds located at different places along an imaginary line running inside the head from one ear to the other ear. Large ITDs and ILDs place the sound's perceived lateral location toward one or the other ear. Thus there is a strong correlation between the relationship of ITD and ILD to the perceived location of an actual source and that for the relationship of ITD and ILD to the perceived lateralized location of sounds produced over headphones.

Listeners with normal hearing can discriminate a difference of about 10 microseconds of ITD and about 0.5 to 1.0 dB of ILD, although ITD discrimination is frequency dependent (Yost and Dye, 1991), whereas ILD discrimination is relatively frequency independent (Yost and Dye, 1991). The just noticeable difference in ITD is best at frequencies below 500 Hz and above 750 Hz and worst around 600 Hz; and cannot be measured above about 1200 Hz due the reasons stated above. The fact that binaural processing of ITD cues operates on a scale of 10s of microseconds suggests that the binaural system is extremely sensitive to the temporal fine structure of the sound waveform arriving at the two ears.

"Cocktail Party" Problem

Colin Cherry (1953) argued that one of the cues that listeners could use to attend to one sound source (e.g., one person speaking) at a noisy cocktail party is the fact that different sound source positions are perceived as being at different locations. Thus, sound localization could be used to solve the "cocktail party" problem. Today the cocktail party problem is often referred to as auditory scene analysis (Bregman, 1990), and sound source location is one cue that can be used to analyze an auditory scene.

The MLD produced when a masker is generated with a different set of ITDs or ILDs than the signal is often cited as evidence for the use of binaural processing as a way to sort out an auditory scene or to solve the cocktail party problem (Green and Yost, 1975). The MLD is usually obtained in headphone conditions in which a signal is added to a masker, such that the signal is presented with one set of ITDs and/or ILDs and the masker with a different set. For instance, the masker (M) may be presented the same to both ears (M_0, ITD = 0 and ILD = 0) and the signal (S) presented to one ear out of phase to that presented to the other ear (S_π). This M_0S_π condition yields a masked threshold for detecting the signal that can be 15 dB lower than the masked threshold in the M_0S_0 condition, when the masker and signal are both presented with no interaural differences. In addition, the M_0S_0 masked thresholds are the same as those obtained when the masker and signal are presented monaurally (m) to the same ear (M_mS_m). The fact that the S_π signal is added to the M_0 masker means that nonzero ILDs and ITDs are produced and, as such, the signal-plus-masker is located off of midline, whereas the M_0S_0 condition stimulus is located at midline. Presumably, binaural processing of the interaural differences yields the increased detectability of the signal in the M_0S_π condition (Durlach and Colburn, 1978).

A similar improvement in detection occurs when a signal is presented from a loudspeaker at one location and a masker from a loudspeaker located at a different location. The signal can be as much as 10 dB more detectable when the signal and masker sound sources are separated in space (Bronkhorst, 2000), although the signal detection advantage of spatial separation is significantly reduced in reverberant spaces (Plomp and Mimpen, 1981). Spatially separating a signal source from an interfering masker source can also improve the intelligibility of the signal (Bronkhorst, 2000). The bulk of the effect is likely due to differences in head shadow (Bronkhorst & Plomp, 1989).

Precedence Effect

In reflective spaces like rooms (but even outdoors where the ground can be a significant reflective surface), each reflected sound wave is coming to the listener from a different place giving a perception that a sound source were at the location of the reflection. However, despite the many reflections that occur in most acoustic environments, these reflections, although close in level and in time to the sound arriving at the ears from the originating sound source, do not significantly alter the perceptual fidelity and the spatial location of the originating sound source. The sound from the originating sound source always arrives at the ears of a listener before that of any reflection, because a reflected waveform has to travel a longer path. Thus, the fact that such reflections do not appear to alter the sound localization of the originating source implies that the first arriving sound from the originating source takes "precedence" over that arriving from any reflections (Blauert, 1997).

The effects of precedence (Litovsky et al, 1999) include fusion (in most reflective environments, a single sound is perceived rather than a sound with echoes), localization dominance (the location of the perceived sound source is at or near that of the originating sound source, not at the location of any reflection), and discrimination suppression (the ability of the auditory system to discriminate spatial changes in the reflections is suppressed relative to that for the originating source). These effects of precedence occur when the reflections are about 5 to 50 milliseconds later than the originating sound depending on the reverberant conditions and the type of originating sound source. It is presumed that binaural processing plays a role in suppressing the spatial information coming from the later arriving reflections, and is responsible for the effects of precedence.

Summary

The ability to understand sound using two normally functioning ears allows listeners to hear more effectively in noisy environments and locate the directionality of sound. The normally functioning auditory system can effectively detect differences in timing and level differences between the two ears. The ILD and ITD can be used to squelch competing sounds, attend to an ear with a better signal-to-noise ratio, locate the directionality of a sound, or analyze an auditory scene. Listeners with normal hearing in only one ear (and some hearing in the other ear) can suffer significantly in their ability to localize sound sources in the azimuthal plane. This is especially true if the sound is composed of low frequencies, where localization depends on binaural processing of ITD cues. It may be possible for such listeners to gain some ability to process sounds in noisy environments and in sound localization by using their

"better ear" to take advantage of the head shadow. However, they might not demonstrate a large benefit from binaural processing, such that possibly occurs for binaural squelch.

◆ Advantages of Binaural Hearing in Listeners with Hearing Aids

A common assumption among clinicians and researchers involved with hearing aid fittings is that two hearing aids must offer an advantage over one hearing aid, the one exception being unilateral hearing loss. Speech hearing in noise and localization are two areas in which advantages of wearing two hearing aids are expected.

Speech Hearing in Noise

The advantage of better speech understanding in the presence of noise for bilateral hearing aid fittings derives from the same principles explained earlier, especially the head shadow and squelch effects. [Following a point argued previously (Noble & Byrne, 1991), the terms *unilateral* and *bilateral* are used to refer to fitting profiles, thereby making no assumptions about whether wearing one hearing aid precludes *binaural* hearing or wearing two confers it, neither of which will automatically be the case.] It is relatively straightforward to provide conditions in a laboratory that demonstrate the advantage of a bilateral hearing aid fit. If someone with hearing loss in both ears is presented with a target signal such as speech on one side of the head and a competing signal such as noise on the other side, a single hearing aid on the side of the noise does the listener a disservice. The head shadow effect reduces the overall level of the speech, whereas the hearing aid amplifies the unshadowed portion of the noise. With hearing aids in both ears, by contrast, the shadowing effect is at least equalized and can provide an advantage depending on the relative location of the target sound versus the competing signal. Furthermore, depending on the profile of the hearing loss, there may be the additional benefit of the interaural comparison that characterizes the phenomenon of binaural squelch.

The typical profile of a sensorineural hearing loss shows increased hearing threshold levels at higher frequencies versus those thresholds at lower frequencies. As discussed earlier in this chapter, the head shadow effect is greater for higher frequency sounds. Because of this, the differences in signal-to-noise ratio between shadowed and unshadowed sides for individuals with typical high-frequency sensorineural hearing loss are less noticeable when unaided than for a normally hearing listener. Binaural squelch, by contrast, is most pronounced for low-frequency sounds, given that low-frequency features of waveforms to the two ears are more readily compared at the level of the central nervous system. Thus, for people with the typical sensorineural profile, it may be less likely that bilateral fitting of hearing aids will promote an advantage over a unilateral fitting in terms of improving central processing

(Dillon, 2001). It may be assumed, however, that bilateral fitting will improve the audibility of higher frequency components of signals sufficiently to return at least some part of the head shadow advantage. Dillon (2001) argues that "bilateral advantage arising from head diffraction will be least for those whose high-frequency hearing loss is only mild and for those whose high-frequency hearing loss is so severe that the high frequencies make no contribution to intelligibility" (p. 381). By implication, for the greater majority of listeners with sensorineural hearing losses, the fitting of bilateral hearing aids will afford this advantage.

In a laboratory-based study (Köbler & Rosenhall, 2002) involving patients with the typical sensorineural profile, a small advantage in speech intelligibility for bilateral fitting was observed. A Swedish report (Arlinger et al, 2003) inquiring into what is known about the effectiveness of hearing aids included comprehensive reviews of literature worldwide. It stated that "laboratory studies [show] two hearing aids can provide better speech comprehension than a single hearing aid." But this report goes on immediately to say, "there is no support from controlled clinical trials to show whether two hearing aids are superior to one" (p. 9). Thus, although laboratory conditions indicate that bilateral fittings should be better than a unilateral fitting in the domain of speech hearing in noise, no good field trial evidence exists to support the proposal. This is a serious gap in our knowledge of the benefits of bilateral hearing aid fittings. It needs to be determined whether bilateral hearing aid fittings actually pay off in making a difference in people's lives. We summarize, at the end of this section, the most recent outcome of an ongoing project, which indicates that researchers and clinicians may not have been looking in the right places to uncover the real benefits of fitting people with two hearing aids.

Localization

The picture is clearer for the domain of localization with regard to the value of bilateral hearing aid fittings. The term *localization* is understood to refer particularly to the directional component (especially in the horizontal plane) of a more general *spatial hearing* function (Blauert, 1983), a function that extends to discrimination of distance and movement. The dependence of the directional component of spatial hearing on an effective binaural system was spelled out earlier. The evidence in favor of bilateral fittings for directional hearing is fairly well established, although the research findings indicate that the benefit may not be universal. Much of the research on hearing aids and sound localization is reviewed in Byrne and Noble (1998). Especially for patients with more severe loss, two hearing aids offer unquestioned advantage over one. This has been shown in performance testing of experienced unilateral and bilateral users (Byrne et al, 1992). The factor of experience is critical, however, as there is abundant evidence that listeners adapt to changes in interaural cues, brought about by changes in such things as hearing aid profile (Byrne & Dirks, 1996). The implication is that initial performance with two hearing aids, for someone who has been used to

wearing only one, might be worse, but that performance improves as the listener adapts to the new profile.

For patients with milder hearing loss, the performance picture is less clearly in favor of bilateral hearing aid fittings. Byrne et al. (1992) found that for average losses (over 0.5, 1, 2, and 4 kHz) up to 40 dB, no performance difference in horizontal plane localization was observed between experienced listeners aided unilaterally versus those aided bilaterally. In this study, signals were presented at the listener's most comfortable level. It is understood, however, that if the level of a target signal were to be reduced to the point where it was inaudible in the unaided ear, such similarity of performance between unilaterally and bilaterally aided listeners would no longer be observed. Nonetheless, in a study based on self-assessment of spatial hearing (Noble et al, 1995), two groups of experienced unilateral and bilateral users, closely matched for degree of hearing loss, rated their aided ability as equally improved over their unaided. The average losses of the two groups were 45 dB. If the performance data noted above are reliable, rated ability aided should be better for a bilateral than a unilateral sample with more severe levels of hearing loss.

One clinical group that shows particularly strong localization benefit following bilateral hearing aid fitting is those with predominantly bilateral conductive hearing loss. Unaided, such patients reveal severe performance decrements (Häusler et al, 1983; Noble et al, 1994). The likeliest explanation for this is loss of acoustic isolation between the cochleae, taking the form of a greater proportion of sound energy reaching both cochleae virtually simultaneously, that is, via the skull, hence negating interaural differences (Zurek, 1986). Aided bilaterally, many with this form of hearing disorder show marked improvement in localization (Byrne et al, 1995), presumably because there is an increase in air conduction energy, hence some recovery of cochlear isolation. It follows from the acoustics of bilateral conductive hearing loss that only bilateral aiding can have this beneficial effect.

New Findings About Bilateral Hearing Aid Fittings

A project dedicated to examining a broad range of binaural hearing functions has begun with the development of a self-assessment scale, derived in part from previous work reported on by Noble et al (1995). The resulting questionnaire is titled the Speech, Spatial and Qualities of Hearing Scale (SSQ) (Gatehouse & Noble, 2004). The SSQ covers an extensive range of speech hearing contexts. Some of the content covered includes circumstances of one-to-one and group conversation in quiet and noise; a range of contexts calling for divided and rapidly switching attention; various aspects of the distance and movement as well as directional components of spatial hearing; and a set of questions addressing segregation, clarity, naturalness, and recognition of everyday sounds, together with items on listening effort.

The SSQ includes questions addressing speech hearing contexts that are challenging even in the case of normal hearing, for example, being able to follow one speech stream while at the same time ignoring another, following two speech streams simultaneously, and following conversation in a group where speakers switch rapidly. Adding movement discrimination to the coverage of spatial hearing is also a new inclusion. Each of these features is nonetheless argued to be common in effective functioning in the everyday world, a point we will return to.

The SSQ was applied as an interview to a large sample of first-time clients at a hearing rehabilitation clinic. Independently (i.e., in advance of the initial appointment at the clinic, and with no prior knowledge they would be interviewed), these clients completed a short questionnaire inquiring about *handicaps* (i.e., social limitations and emotional problems stemming directly from their hearing impairment). The aim was to find out which elements of the range of *disabilities* in the speech, spatial, and quality domains would best predict the social/emotional handicaps that stem from them. It emerged that "identification, attention and effort problems, as well as spatial hearing problems, feature prominently in the disability-handicap relationship, along with certain features of speech hearing. The results implicate aspects of temporal and spatial dynamics of hearing disability in the experience of handicap" (Gatehouse & Noble, 2004, p. 85).

A further examination of these data (Noble & Gatehouse, 2004a), separately for patients with interaurally more asymmetric hearing loss, showed that the dynamic spatial and more demanding attentional aspects of hearing were particularly associated with handicap in that particular group. By contrast, in patients with more symmetrical hearing loss, all aspects of disability were correlated with the handicap experience. This finding gave a strong indication about what might be expected from unilateral versus bilateral hearing aid fittings.

In a subsequent application, the SSQ was administered to patients newly fit with one versus two hearing aids, after 6 months of use with their device(s) (Noble & Gatehouse, 2004b). It emerged that, compared with those unaided, two aids do not seem to provide any further noticeable benefit over one hearing aid in the traditional speech hearing domains, namely, one-on-one and group conversation in quiet and in noise. Rather, it is in the more substantially demanding contexts of following two speech streams, or suppressing one to follow another, or rapidly switching attention among speakers, that bilateral fitting demonstrates leverage in reducing disability. In the spatial domain, although the directional component shows a moderate benefit from bilateral over unilateral fitting, it is with the more dynamic elements of distance and movement discrimination that two aids demonstrate more evident benefit. Finally, bilateral fitting (not unexpectedly) confers a notable benefit over unilateral in permitting greater ease of listening. This is to be expected on the basis of the fact that the more demanding contexts are less disabling with two aids, hence the effort needed to cope in these demanding contexts is less extreme.

It seems fair to say that being able to better handle difficult and challenging communication tasks, and being able to better orient and navigate in the dynamic audible world, enhances a sense of competency and reduces the sense of being socially restricted and emotionally distressed. It still remains to develop performance measures that will allow

more precise investigation of the domains of hearing served by binaural function. In the meantime, it is clear that new arenas have been uncovered in which bilateral hearing aid fittings confer their real benefit, and these merit further study and analysis.

Summary

Laboratory studies and a recent subjective questionnaire have demonstrated the benefits of wearing bilateral hearing aids over wearing only one hearing aid. The benefits include improved dynamic localization abilities, particularly distance and movement discrimination, and better management of demanding conversational situations such as following two speech streams, suppressing one speech stream to follow another, or rapidly switching attention among speakers. It may be predicted that someone with hearing losses (HLs) in both ears in excess of about 40 dB HL over 0.5 to 4 kHz will be more likely to experience these sorts of benefits when using two hearing aids. In less demanding contexts, however, it may be harder to distinguish the benefit of two over one aid. That said, the real-world dynamics and demanding communicative contexts confront people with hearing loss no less than anyone else.

◆ Advantages of Binaural Hearing in Listeners with Cochlear Implants

Individuals who utilize a cochlear implant fall into many different patient profiles. For the purposes of this chapter, we focus on people implanted with a standard long array who fall into the following three categories: patients implanted unilaterally who do not wear amplification in the contralateral nonimplanted ear [cochlear implant (CI) only]; patients implanted unilaterally who wear amplification in the contralateral nonimplanted ear [CI and a hearing aid (HA), denoted as CI + HA]; and patients implanted bilaterally who wear a cochlear implant in each ear (CI + CI).

The CI-only patients do not benefit from most of the advantages of hearing with two ears that were discussed earlier in this chapter. Patients who have only one cochlear implant and do not use amplification in the contralateral ear are not hearing with two ears and will only have the potential to benefit from the head shadow effect. As previously discussed, the head shadow effect is a result of a physical phenomenon rather than due to binaural processing. Unilateral (CI-only) patients have only a 50% chance of benefiting from the head shadow effect because they only have one hearing device to potentially face away from a noise source.

Individuals who wear a cochlear implant and a hearing aid in the nonimplanted contralateral ear have the potential to use binaural processing by utilizing both the electrical signal from the cochlear implant and the acoustic signal from the hearing aid. In general, the cochlear implant serves as the more dominant ear because often the hearing aid alone provides very little benefit. Typically, the hearing aid serves to complement the information received by the cochlear implant. Most CI + HA listeners comment that regardless of the benefit they feel they are receiving from their hearing aid, wearing the hearing aid gives them a more balanced or "full" feeling.

Individuals implanted bilaterally with two cochlear implants have shown promising results with regard to advantages in better speech perception in noise and localization. Perhaps because both ears are being stimulated similarly (i.e., electrically), the ears are able to fuse information providing for many binaural advantages.

Speech Hearing in Noise

The binaural advantages most commonly studied for CI + HA or CI + CI listeners in laboratory conditions are the head shadow effect, binaural summation, binaural squelch, and localization. Some listeners wearing a cochlear implant and a hearing aid in the contralateral ear are able to better understand speech in noise and to identify sound location. However, because one ear is receiving electrical information and one ear is receiving acoustical information, fusing the two different signals is often difficult. Although listeners wearing a cochlear implant and hearing aid receive more binaural advantages than simply wearing one device alone, binaural advantages are not shown in all situations for all listeners (Dunn et al, 2005). Typically, the cochlear implant and the hearing aid are programmed independently from one another. It seems reasonable to assume that the two ears may be providing the central auditory system with distorted ITDs and ILDs, resulting in misrepresented information. More research needs to be done investigating the appropriate way to coordinate the programming of a cochlear implant and hearing aid to promote fusion of the electrical and acoustical signals.

Bilaterally implanted (CI + CI) listeners receive electrical stimulation from both ears, making it easier for the brain to process and fuse the two signals from each ear. In addition, both cochlear implants are programmed to provide equal loudness and frequency information across the two devices. Although this may not provide precise timing of intraaural electrical stimulation, bilateral coordination of pulsed signals is possible (Tyler et al, in press; van Hoesel & Clark, 1997; van Hoesel & Tyler, 2003).

Adding a second cochlear implant or hearing aid to the contralateral ear enables a listener to take advantage of an ear with a better signal-to-noise ratio resulting in improved speech perception in noise due to the head shadow effect (Gantz et al, 2002; Muller et al, 2002; Tyler, Dunn, Witt, & Preece, 2003; Tyler, Parkinson, Wilson, Witt, Preece, Noble, 2002; Van Hoesel & Tyler, 2003; Van Hoesel et al, 2002). In addition, adding an ear with a poorer signal-to-noise ratio allows the auditory system the opportunity to compare timing, amplitude, and spectral differences, canceling parts of the waveform to provide better speech understanding in noise by use of binaural squelch (Gantz et al, 2002; Muller et al, 2002; Tyler et al, 2002, 2003; Van Hoesel et al, 2002).

Fig. 18–2 shows sentence recognition scores with the speech from the front and noise facing the front and left for two bilateral cochlear implant users. In the noise front condition of **Fig. 18–2**, when the left- and right-only scores

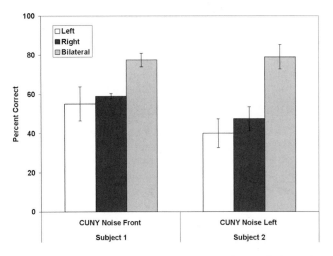

Figure 18–2 Sentence recognition scores with speech from the front and noise facing the front and left for two bilateral cochlear implant users. In the noise-front condition, when comparing the left- and right-only scores to the bilateral score, an advantage is seen for binaural summation. In the noise-left condition, when comparing the left-only score to the bilateral score, an advantage is shown for the bilateral condition indicating a head shadow effect. When comparing the right-only and bilateral scores in the noise-left condition, a bilateral advantage is shown, indicating a binaural squelch effect.

are compared with the bilateral score, an advantage is seen for binaural summation. When the left-only score is compared with the binaural score, the bilateral cochlear implant listeners show that they are able to use the ear with a better signal-to-noise ratio to understand speech more effectively. When comparing the right-only and bilateral scores in the noise left condition, an advantage is also shown for the bilateral condition indicating a binaural squelch effect.

Although the data presented in **Fig. 18–2** represent bilateral advantages in each of the listening conditions, research shows that consistent advantages in each listening condition are often hard to show for a given listener (Dunn et al, 2005). On average, research shows that when listeners with bilateral cochlear implants listen to speech and noise from the front, an advantage is shown with two ears over one. In addition, when an ear with a better signal-to-noise ratio is added, listeners are able to take advantage of the physical effect of head shadow. In contrast, current research shows that when an ear with a poorer signal-to-noise ratio is added, the advantages shown from the binaural processing that must occur from the squelch effect are shown much less than that of the head shadow or binaural summation (Gantz et al, 2002; Muller et al, 2002; Tyler et al, 2002, 2003; Van Hoesel et al, 2002). It is possible, however, that the current measurement tools used to evaluate these benefits are not sensitive enough to show advantages in each condition.

Localization

Laboratory testing of localization reveals that CI + CI listeners are much better at localizing a sound source than CI + HA listeners. Some CI + HA listeners perform as if they are only using one device, whereas some CI + CI listeners can localize almost as well as normal-hearing listeners. This difference in performance across patient types may be due to the fact that CI + HA patients are trying to fuse two very different signals (i.e., electrical and acoustical). As discussed earlier in this chapter, sounds presented from loudspeakers or sounds produced in the natural environment produce ITDs and ILDs based on the interactions between the sound and the head. ITDs are the dominant cue for azimuthal localization in the low frequencies whereas ILDs are the dominant cue for azimuthal localization in the high frequencies. Bilateral cochlear implants are programmed to produce equal loudness across an input frequency spectrum of on average 250 to 6000 Hz in both ears. This provides bilateral cochlear implant listeners with the opportunity to discriminate both level and timing differences across a broad frequency range. Listeners wearing a cochlear implant and hearing aid in opposite ears may only have adequate hearing with their hearing aid in the low frequencies, making ITD the only usable cue for azimuthal localization.

◆ Conclusion

Individuals implanted with only one cochlear implant and who do not utilize a hearing aid on the contralateral ear do not benefit from most of the advantages of hearing with two ears (with the exception of the head shadow effect) discussed earlier in this chapter. Individuals who wear a cochlear implant and a hearing aid in the nonimplanted contralateral ear (CI + HA) have the potential to use binaural processing, fusing together the electrical signal that they are getting from the ear with the cochlear implant and the acoustic signal that they are getting from the hearing aid. However, because the cochlear implant provides the more functional ear, the hearing aid may serve only to complement the information received by the implant.

Individuals implanted bilaterally with two cochlear implants receive similar information to both ears. Because the ears are both stimulated electrically, fusing information between the two ears may be easier than that for listeners wearing a cochlear implant and a hearing aid. Listeners with bilateral cochlear implants show advantages in better speech perception in noise and in localization.

One problem that persists with speech perception and localization in the horizontal plane for listeners with two cochlear implants or a cochlear implant and hearing aid is the potential for difficulty in providing coherent fine-structure information at the two ears. Specifically, interaural phase between the two ears is not likely to be well preserved due to the unpredictable nature of the unsynchronized processor outputs. In the normal-hearing case, time differences as small as 10 microseconds are detectable, whereas the differences provided by two implants or an implant and a hearing aid will be much coarser than this. The extent to which listeners with bilateral cochlear implants and/or hearing aids rely on ITDs to aid in speech perception and localization is yet to be determined. It may be that listeners provided with less than fully coherent timing information will adapt as long as the mismatches remain consistent. However, all efforts should be made to try to ensure that both devices are matched as closely as possible to try to provide coherent fine-timing information.

References

Arlinger S, Brorsson B, Lagerbring C, Leijon A, Rosenhall U, Schersten T. (2003). Hearing Aids for Adults—Benefits and Costs. Stockholm: Swedish Council on Technology Assessment in Health Care

Blauert J. (1983). Spatial Hearing. Cambridge, MA: MIT Press

Blauert J. (1997). Spatial Hearing. Cambridge, MA: MIT Press

Bregman AS. (1990). Auditory Scene Analysis: The Perceptual Organization of Sound. Cambridge, MA: MIT Press

Bronkhorst AW. (2000). The cocktail-party phenomenon: a review of research on speech intelligibility in multiple-talker conditions. Acustica 86:117–128

Bronkhorst AW, Plomp R. (1989). Binaural speech intelligibility in noise for hearing-impaired listeners. J Acoust Soc Am 86:1374–1383

Byrne D, Dirks D. (1996). Effect of acclimatization and deprivation on non-speech auditory abilities. Ear Hear 17:29S–37S

Byrne D, Noble W. (1998). Optimizing sound localization with hearing aids. Trends Amplif 3(2):51–73

Byrne D, Noble W, LePage B. (1992). Effects of long-term bilateral and uni-lateral fitting of different hearing aid types on the ability to locate sounds. J Am Acad Audiol 3:369–382

Byrne B, Noble W, Ter-Horst K. (1995). Effects of hearing aids on localization of sounds by people with sensorineural and conductive/mixed hearing losses. Australian Journal of Audiology 17:79–86

Cherry C. (1953). Some experiments on the recognition of speech with one and with two ears. J Acoust Soc Am 25:975–981

Colburn HS, Durlach NI. (1978). Handbook of Perception, vol (4). New York: Academic Press

Dillon H. (2001). Hearing Aids. Sydney: Boomerang Press; New York: Thieme

Dunn CC, Tyler RS, Witt SA. (2005). Benefit of wearing a hearing aid on the unimplanted ear in adult users of a cochlear implant. J Speech Lang Hear Res 48:668–680

Fletcher H, Munson WA. (1933). Loudness: Its definition, measurement, and calculation. J Acoust Soc Am 75:82–108

Gantz BJ, Tyler RS, Rubinstein JT, et al. (2002). Binaural cochlear implants placed during the same operation. Otol Neurotol 23:169–180

Gatehouse S, Noble W. (2004). The Speech, Spatial and Qualities of Hearing Scale (SSQ). Int J Audiol 43:85–99

Green DM, Yost WA. (1975). Binaural analysis. In Keidel W, Neff WD, eds. Handbook of Sensory Physiology: Hearing (vol 5). New York: Springer-Verlag

Hartmann WM. (1983). Localization of sound in rooms. J Acoust Soc Am 74:1380–1391

Häusler R, Colburn S, Marr E. (1983). Sound localization in subjects with impaired hearing. Spatial-discrimination and interaural-discrimination tests. Acta Otolaryngol Suppl 400:1–62

Köbler S, Rosenhall U. (2002). Horizontal localization and speech intelligibility with bilateral and unilateral hearing aid amplification. Int J Audiol 41:395–400

Kuhn GF. (1987). Physical acoustics and measurements pertaining to directional hearing. In: Yost WA, Gourevitch G, eds. Directional Hearing. New York: Springer-Verlag

Litovsky R, Colburn S, Yost WA, Guzman S. (1999). The Precedence Effect. J Acoust Soc Am 106:1633–1654

Mills AW. (1972). Auditory localization. In: Tobias JV, ed. Foundations of Modern Auditory Theory, vol 2. New York: Academic Press

Muller J, Schon F, Helms J. (2002). Speech understanding in quiet and noise in bilateral users of the MED-EL COMBI 40/40+ cochlear implant system. Ear Hear 23:198–206

Noble W, Byrne D. (1991). Auditory localization under conditions of unilateral fitting of different hearing aid systems. Br J Audiol 25:237–250

Noble W, Byrne D, LePage B. (1994). Effects on sound localization of configuration and type of hearing impairment. J Acoust Soc Am 95:992–1005

Noble W, Gatehouse S. (2004a). Interaural asymmetry of hearing loss, Speech, Spatial and Qualities of Hearing Scale (SSQ) disabilities, and handicap. Int J Audiol 43:100–114

Noble W, Gatehouse S. (2004b). The real benefits of bilateral hearing aid fitting. Paper presented at the International Hearing Aid Research Conference, Lake Tahoe, California

Noble W, Ter-Horst K, Byrne D. (1995). Disabilities and handicaps associated with impaired auditory localization. J Am Acad Audiol 6:129–140

Perrett S, Noble W. (1997). The contribution of head motion cues to localization of low-pass noise. Percept Psychophys 59:1018–1026

Plomp R, Mimpen AM. (1981). Effect of the orientation of the speaker's head and the azimuth of a noise source on the speech reception threshold for sentences. Acustica 48:325–328

Searle CL, Braida LD, Cuddy DR, Davis MF. (1975). Binaural pinna disparity: another auditory localization cue. J Acoust Soc Am 57:448–455

Shaw EAG. (1982). External ear response and sound localization. In: Gatehouse RW, ed. Localization of Sound: Theory and Applications, pp. 30–41. Groton, CT: Amphora

Stevens SS, Newman EB. (1936). The localization of actual sources of sound. Am J Psychol 48:297–306

Tyler RS, Dunn CC, Witt SA, et al. (2006). Soundfield hearing for patients with cochlear implants and hearing aids. In: Cooper, HR and Craddock, LC, (Eds.), Cochlear Implants, A Practical Guide (338–366), London and Philadelphia: Whur Publishers

Tyler R, Parkinson A, Wilson B, Witt S, Preece J, Noble W. (2002). Patients utilizing a hearing aid and a cochlear implant: speech perception and localization. Ear and Hearing 23(2):98–105

Tyler RS, Gantz BJ, Rubinstein JT. (2002). Three-month results with bilateral cochlear implants. Ear Hear 23:80S–89S

Tyler R, Dunn C, Witt S, Preece J. (2003). Update on bilateral cochlear implantation. Curr Opin Otol 11(5)

Van Hoesel RJ, Clark GM. (1997). Psychophysical studies with two binaural cochlear implant subjects. J Acoust Soc Am 102:495–507

Van Hoesel R, Ramsden R, O'Driscoll M. (2002). Sound-direction identification, interaural time delay discrimination, and speech intelligibility advantages in noise for a bilateral cochlear implant user. Ear Hear 23:137–149

Van Hoesel RJ, Tyler RS. (2003). Speech perception, localization, and lateralization with bilateral cochlear implants. J Acoust Soc Am 113:1617–1630

Wegel RL, Lane CE. (1924). The auditory masking of one sound by another and its probable relation to the dynamics of the inner ear. Phys Rev 23:266–285

Wightman FL, Kistler DJ. (1989). Headphone simulation of free-field listening. II: Psychophysical validation. J Acoust Soc Am 1989;85:868–887

Yost WA, Dye R. (1991). Properties of sound localization by humans. In: Altschuler R, Hoffman D, Bobbin R, Clopton B, eds. Neurobiology of Hearing: The Central Nervous System. New York: Raven Press

Zurek PM. (1986). Consequences of conductive auditory impairment for binaural hearing. J Acoust Soc Am 80:466–472

19

Acoustical and Electrical Speech Processing

Bruce J. Gantz,
Christopher W. Turner, and
Kate E. Gfeller

Combining electrical and acoustical speech processing is the newest application of cochlear implant technology. Speech perception performance in quiet with a cochlear implant in postlingually deafened adults and prelingually deafened children has gradually improved over the past 20 years (Gantz et al, 2002; Svirsky et al, 2000; Tomblin et al, 1999). A combination of factors, including improved implant speech processing algorithms, implant design, and importantly the residual hearing of those receiving an implant, has improved performance almost threefold. The average postlingually deafened adult can converse on the telephone and understand almost 50% of monosyllabic words and over 80% of words in sentences. Results continue to be variable for the individual patient. Prelingually deafened children have also benefited from cochlear implant technology. When an implant is stimulated prior to 13 months of age, language development appears to be within normal-hearing language development norms (Tomblin et al, 2005). These results have stimulated an interest in expanding cochlear implants to those with more residual hearing because duration of deafness and residual hearing have been shown to be predictive parameters of performance with an implant (Gantz et al, 1993; Rubinstein et al, 1999). The remarkable word understanding scores obtained by these groups of individuals have enabled those with less than profound deafness to be considered for implantation.

◆ Advantages and Disadvantages of Cochlear Implants: The Role of Acoustic Hearing

The decision to undergo implantation surgery, however, involves some trade-offs, as the patients' residual acoustic hearing is usually no longer usable, and only electric stimulation is available. Residual low-frequency acoustic hearing has some important advantages compared with electrical signal processing available in cochlear implants. Expanding selection criteria for standard cochlear implants to include those with substantial residual low-frequency hearing should be viewed with some caution.

Several factors should be considered before the decision to destroy residual acoustic hearing is undertaken. The electrical signal-processing algorithm that provides important information for speech perception in quiet is reported by users of cochlear implants as "mechanical" or "raspy" when compared with their memories of acoustic hearing. In addition, some report that many of the aesthetic qualities of sound are diminished. This loss of aesthetic quality of sound is most likely related to a decrease in the ability to perceive the pitches of sounds (Gfeller et al, 2002). The loss of pitch perception is primarily a consequence of the limited spectral resolution of current cochlear implants. This does not, however, appear to be a limitation for understanding speech in quiet for the most successful implant users (Fishman et al, 1998). Understanding speech in background noise requires spectral resolution even finer than that required for understanding speech in quiet (Fu et al, 1998). Even the most successful implant users only realize perhaps six to eight channels of distinct "place-frequency" information across the entire spectral range, and this deficit in spectral resolution has a direct negative consequence on the implant user's ability to understand speech in background noise (Friesen et al, 2001).

With regard to music, implant recipients using conventional long electrode implants typically have shown much poorer performance than normal-hearing persons on several pitch-related tasks, including detecting pitch change (frequency difference limens), perception of direction of pitch change (higher or lower), and discrimination of brief pitch patterns. Cochlear implant (CI) recipients using conventional long electrodes almost always require considerably larger frequency differences than normal-hearing adults for detecting pitch change (frequency difference limens) as well as the direction of a pitch change (i.e., whether the second pitch of a pair of notes is higher or lower than the first) (Fishman et al, 1998; Gfeller et al, 2002).

Poor pitch resolution has a detrimental effect on the aesthetic quality of musical sounds, and it also impedes the CI user's ability to do a very basic listening task that normal-hearing people tend to take for granted—the ability to recognize familiar melodies such as "Happy Birthday," "The Star Spangled Banner," holiday songs, and spiritually significant songs when no lyrics are provided. Melody recognition requires the listener to hear a sequence of pitches and accurately perceive the direction of pitch change (higher or lower) as well as the magnitude of each pitch change. Because melodies are made up of sequential pitch patterns, poor perception of pitch, as is common for CI recipients who use the conventional long electrode, has negative implications for this perceptual task (Friesen et al, 2001; Fu et al, 1998; Gfeller et al, 1991, 2002; Pijl & Schwartz, 1995). In short, because acoustic hearing has an important role in pitch resolution, and those hearing tasks facilitated by accurate pitch perception, such as understanding speech in noise, the loss of residual hearing is an important clinical consideration when determining the most appropriate options for patients with severe hearing losses.

The loss of residual acoustic hearing during implantation is the result of a combination of factors including the technique used to create the cochleostomy as well as the size of cochleostomy performed. In addition, the diameter, stiffness, and length of standard intracochlear electrodes may induce substantial intracochlear damage to the basilar membrane and cochlear hair cells as they advance around the upper basilar turn during insertion. This damage is likely caused by forces against the outer cochlear wall during the insertion (Roland, 2005).

◆ Development of Cochlear Implants that Combine Residual Low-Frequency Acoustic Hearing with High-Frequency Electric Speech Processing

In early 1995 we began to explore the possibility of placing a shortened small-diameter electrode into the scala tympani in an attempt to combine residual low-frequency acoustic hearing with high-frequency electrical speech processing of the cochlear implant. Animal research by Shepherd and his colleagues had demonstrated that electrodes placed in cats with residual hearing resulted in damage adjacent to the electrode, whereas the apical organ of Corti remained undisturbed. Low-frequency acoustic hearing was preserved in these animals (Ni et al, 1992; Xu et al, 1997). It was our intent to develop a limited electrode that could be placed in the basal turn of the scala tympani without inducing damage by advancing around the upper basilar turn. The Cochlear Corporation (Sydney, Australia) built the first

electrodes that were 6 mm in length and had a 0.2 × 0.4 mm diameter. The implant had a short 6 mm, six-channel electrode and a secondary reserve standard length (24 mm) electrode containing 16 active electrodes. The reserve electrode was to be used if the short electrode induced a profound deafness without providing significant speech perception. This electrode was placed in the mastoid during the surgery.

The concept of hearing preservation and cochlear implantation was presented at the National Institutes of Health–National Institute on Deafness and Other Communication Disorders (NIH-NIDCD) 10th anniversary meeting in Bethesda, Maryland in October 1998 (Gantz, 1998). In early 1999, the first clinical subject was implanted with the device. Subsequently, two others also received the 6-mm electrode. All three subjects reported that the percept was very high pitched and one thought it was unpleasant. These results were presented at the 5th International Conference on Cochlear Implants in Miami in February 2000 (Gantz and Turner, 2000). A small but significant increase in speech understanding was observed from the addition of the electrical stimulation. The electric speech processing sound was perceived as very high pitched and unpleasant to some. The most important finding of this initial trial was that residual acoustic speech perception and pure tone audiometric testing were unchanged from preoperative levels. Because of the unpleasant pitch percept, it was decided to lengthen the electrode and move the active electrodes into an area in the cochlea closer to a frequency of about 2500 to 3500 Hz according to the Greenwood place frequency map (Greenwood, 1990). The 10-mm electrode was developed with the same diameter dimensions (0.2 × 0.4 mm) as the 6-mm design. The active electrodes were placed toward the apical end (**Fig. 19–3**). Results with the 10-mm (Iowa/Nucleus Hybrid Cochlear Implant; Cochlear Corporation, Sydney, Australia) have been published (Gantz and Turner, 2003). Volunteers implanted with this device have usable acoustic hearing up to 750 Hz, and the electrical stimulation provides the patient with high-frequency speech information (1500–6000 Hz). Thus, these subjects perceive sound via a combined acoustic and electric (A + E) mode. They report that the aesthetic qualities of sound is preserved, they enjoy music, and they exhibit better speech recognition in background noise (Turner et al, 2004).

◆ Surgical Technique for Implanting Iowa/Nucleus Hybrid Implant

The Iowa/Nucleus Hybrid Implant was designed to limit damage to the scala media. The intracochlear electrode has a reduced diameter of 0.2 × 0.4 mm. Unique features of the electrode include a Dacron collar to limit the intracochlear placement to 10 mm and a titanium marker to orient the electrode contacts, thus ensuring the correct alignment of the electrodes adjacent to the modiolus. The length of the electrode was limited to 10 mm to prevent injury to the ascending basal turn of the cochlea and prevent the

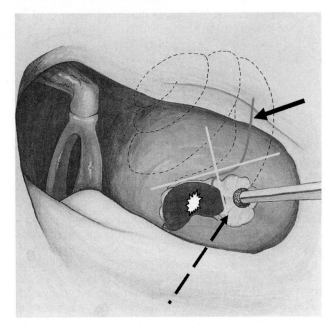

Figure 19–1 Position of cochleostomy in the inferior-posterior quadrant of a box created by drawing a line at the superior margin of the round window and a perpendicular line at the inferior margin of the round window (dashed line). Basilar membrane position (solid arrow), round window membrane (star).

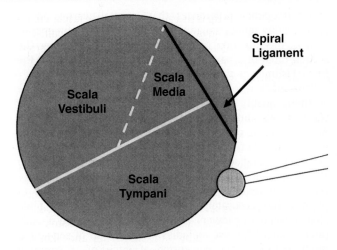

Figure 19–2 The cochlea is oriented in the temporal bone such that the basal turn is tipped anterior-superior with the helicotrema deep to the tensor tympani muscle. The black vertical line indicates the approximate position of the spiral ligament. The cochleostomy should be placed inferior to the spiral ligament to prevent damage to the basilar membrane.

electrode from curling on itself on insertion. A mastoidectomy is done, the bony seat is created for the electronic package, and the facial recess is opened similarly to implantation of a standard cochlear implant. The bony overhang of the round window niche is removed with a 1.8-mm diamond burr exposing the round window membrane.

The strategy for creating the cochleostomy and entering the scala tympani should involve surgical detail similar to performing a "drill-out" stapes for otosclerosis. Bleeding must be controlled and suction must be avoided once the inner ear is opened. The cochleostomy is created anterior-inferior to the round window. To standardize the placement of the cochleostomy, it is suggested that the cochleostomy be placed in the anterior-inferior quadrant of a box created by drawing a line at the superior margin of the round window and one that crosses perpendicular at the inferior aspect of the round window (**Fig. 19–1**).

Creation of the cochleostomy is begun in the inferior portion of the quadrant, slowly saucerizing the otic capsule bone with a 1-mm diamond burr. Approaching the scala tympani from a caudal direction ensures that the cochleostomy will be inferior to the equator of the scala and thus avoiding the basilar membrane, and spiral ligament (**Fig. 19–2**). It should be remembered that the basal turn of the cochlea is oriented oblique in the temporal bone with the helicotrema usually positioned deep to the tensor tympani muscle, and the ascending basilar turn can be deep to the level of the internal carotid artery. As bone is slowly removed over the scala tympani, the lumen will appear as bluish or a faint gray hue. If the cochleostomy is too far superior, adjacent to the spiral ligament, a whitish color will be evident. Drilling inferior will permit entrance into the scala tympani.

A 0.5-mm diamond burr is used to penetrate the final layer of bone, but the endosteum of the scala tympani is left intact (**Fig. 19–3**). The implant is secured in the seat and sutured in place with 4-0 nylon suture. During creation of the mastoid an overhang of the cortex at the tegmen mastoideum is developed; 1-mm holes are drilled in the cortical overhang to secure the electrode with a 4-0 nylon suture before it is placed in the cochlea. This suture helps to stabilize the orientation of the electrode contacts toward the modiolus, and ensures that the electrode is secure within the scala tympani. Prior to placement of the electrode a 1.5 × 1.5 mm piece of temporalis fascia is obtained and pressed in a fascia press. A needle is used to pierce the fascia in the

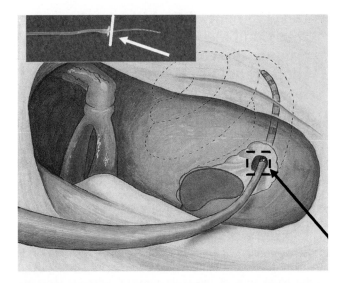

Figure 19–3 The electrode is passed through a fascia washer and is placed against the Dacron collar (white arrow). The fascia washer seals the cochleostomy site (dotted line box, black arrow).

center. The electrode tip is threaded through the fascia, creating a washer that is advanced against the Dacron cuff. The fascia seals the cochleostomy when the electrode is inserted into the scala tympani. The endosteum is opened using a 0.2-mm right-angle hook. The tip of the electrode is guided into the cochleostomy using a needle-tipped instrument at the Dacron collar and an electrode guiding "claw" instrument. The electrode must be directed parallel to the posterior canal wall to ensure the electrode is directed into the basal turn of the cochlea. The electrode is then slowly advanced into the scala tympani. A slow insertion (over a 30- to 45-second period) will limit the intracochlear trauma and allow displacement of perilymph. The electrode is positioned with slight anterior pressure to ensure the electrode is held tightly in the cochlea, and the tegmen mastoideum suture is secured. The subperiosteal tissues and skin are closed in layers.

Twenty volunteers have participated in this research at the University of Iowa as of this writing. The first three Iowa subjects received a 6-mm electrode and 17 were implanted with the 10-mm electrode. Twenty additional subjects have been implanted at participating research centers by seven different surgeons. The 10-mm electrode subjects are enrolled in a Food and Drug Administration (FDA) multicenter clinical trial. The criteria for selection include postlingual hearing impairment, CNC word list understanding between 1% and 50% with an appropriately fit hearing aid in the worse ear and 60% or worse in the better hearing ear. The criteria for inclusion also include pure-tone audiogram thresholds conforming to the limits shown in **Fig. 19–4**. A modification of the original FDA clinical trial was begun in June 2005. The criteria for inclusion were modified to include up to 60% CNC word understanding in the implant ear and up to 80% CNC word understanding in the better hearing ear. **Fig. 19–4** demonstrates the expanded criteria and inclusion of those 15 years of age and older and those with normal pure tone frequency responses from 125 to 1500 Hz.

◆ Results of Hybrid Implants

Subjects were tested in a sound field with their implant alone, hearing aid + implant (hybrid condition), and hearings aids binaurally + implant (combined condition). A recorded version of the CNC word recognition test was administered to the Iowa and participating center subjects (Ni et al, 1992; Peterson and Lehiste, 1962). The 10-mm Iowa Hybrid recipients also were tested using a closed-set spondee word list presented in multitalker background noise (Gantz et al, 1993; Turner et al, 2004). The music perception task demonstrates the ability to recognize in open-set conditions some melodies that are well known within American culture presented in a pitch range of 131 to 1048 Hz. A description of this test, and the outcomes for normal-hearing adults and CI recipients of conventional long electrodes appear in Gfeller et al, 2002.

The method of performing the cochleostomy and insertion of a 6- or 10-mm electrode described above has enabled the preservation of acoustic hearing at 1 month postoperatively in all 40 volunteers undergoing the procedure by multiple surgeons. One subject developed a recurrent cytomegalovirus infection 3 months postoperatively, resulting in total loss of acoustic hearing in the implant ear. Some acoustic hearing has returned at 6 months. A second patient at a participating center experienced a 30-dB pure hearing drop following an episode of pneumonia 3 months postoperatively. A pure tone drop of 9.5 dB across the frequencies between 125 and 1000 Hz was noted for the group presently being tracked for an FDA investigation (**Fig. 19–5**). The range of change was 0 to 30 dB. Another important finding is the preservation of acoustic discrimination. At 1-month postoperative the acoustic CNC word score under headphones is similar to the preoperative level as shown in **Table 19–1** for our first nine subjects.

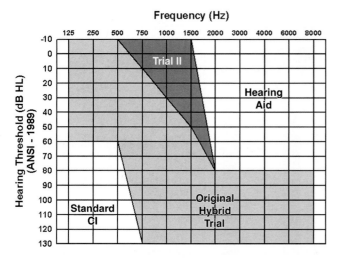

Figure 19–4 New audiometric profile for Iowa/Nucleus Hybrid FDA trial II. Original inclusion criteria shown in light gray. Expansion of criteria for trial II dark gray.

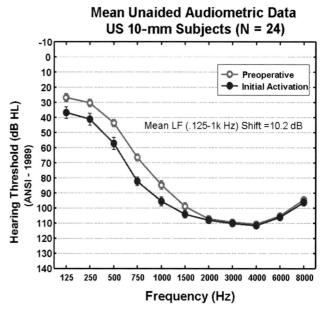

Figure 19–5 Mean unaided pure tone audiometric results for 21 subjects implanted with the 10-mm electrode.

Table 19–1   Preoperative and Postoperative Monosyllabic Word Scores (CNC) Percent Correct Sound Only with a Hearing Aid in the Implanted Ear for the Short Electrode (SE) Subjects with the 6-mm and 10-mm Electrode Implants

	SE1 6 mm	SE2 6 mm	SE3 6 mm	SE4 (PF) 10 mm	SE5 (DZ) 10 mm	SE6 (JB) 10 mm	SE7 (LK) 10 mm	SE8 (ES) 10 mm	SE9 (AP) 10 mm
Preop CNC	9%	10%	15%	16%	10%	25%	23%	15%	26%
Postimplant CNC	8%	10%	20%	14%	8%	29%	20%	16%	24%

Note: Level of presentation was 40 dB above threshold.

The remainder of the subjects have also maintained acoustic speech perception similar to preoperative levels.

Preliminary results from those reaching the 6-month experience interval in FDA study ($n = 11$) are shown in **Fig. 19–6**. Monosyllabic word understanding at 3 months and 6 months compared with the preoperative binaural hearing aid condition demonstrate substantial improvement in 10 of the 11 subjects. Longer-term monosyllabic word understanding scores for the subjects implanted at Iowa using the implant only, implant plus hearing aid, and implant plus binaural hearing aids compared with the pre-implant scores with hearing aids are shown in **Fig. 19–7**. The average score for this group is 79% in the best-aided condition. Some do better without a hearing aid in the implanted ear as they believe that the hearing aid blocks residual low-frequency hearing. It appears that the gains in word understanding in those who have had their devices for up to 3 years remains.

An important finding when acoustic and electrical stimulation is combined was the improved performance for recognizing speech in a noisy background as compared with traditional cochlear implant patients. The background was a two-talker babble signal. Eight of the Iowa patients implanted with the 10-mm electrode have been tested to determine the signal-to-noise (S/N) ratio required for 50% correct recognition of spondees. For comparison purposes, the same measure was obtained for a group of 20 traditional long-electrode patients (who were chosen so that their group speech recognition scores in quiet matched those of the eight A+E patients), as well as 10 mild-to-moderate hearing loss patients (some of whom wore hearing aids) and also a group of eight normal-hearing subjects. A lower S/N ratio indicates better performance. The babble background is a situation that commonly yields complaints from all hearing-impaired patients, and the data of **Fig. 19–8** indicate that normal-hearing listeners can do quite well in this situation. It is easily seen that the A+E approach yields an improvement over the traditional implant (which performs the poorest of all groups), and that the preservation of residual hearing can help implant patients using A+E to nearly equal the level of performance of mild-to-moderate hearing loss patients.

Standard cochlear implant recipients report difficulty recognizing music and familiar melodies (Gfeller et al, 2002). This group of short electrode implant users is substantially more accurate than recipients of standard cochlear implants in melody recognition, pure tone frequency discrimination, and timbre ratings for the low frequencies.

In the open-set test of familiar melody recognition, normal-hearing adults ($n = 17$) achieved a mean score of 87.1% correct, whereas the mean score for 27 recipients of long electrodes [Nucleus 22, Nucleus 24, and Clarion users; Advanced Combination Encoder (ACE), Spectral Peak (SPEAK), continuous interleaved sampling (CIS), and simultaneous

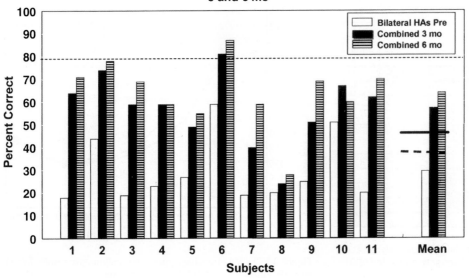

Figure 19–6 The 10-mm-electrode subjects in FDA feasibility trial 3 months (black bar) and 6 months (dashed bar) compared with their preoperative hearing with two hearing aids (white bar). The mean scores are found at the right. Average performance for a group of standard length electrode subjects with the traditional Nucleus CI-24 implant are represented by the dashed line (3 months) and solid line (6 months).

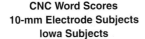

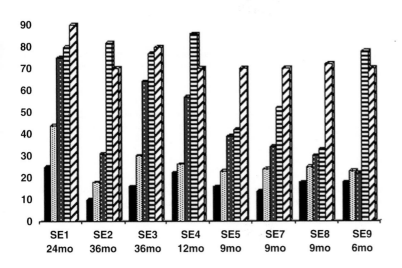

■ HA Pre Imp

▦ HA AU Pre

▩ CI Only

⊟ CI + HA Ips

▨ CI + HA AU

Figure 19–7 Long-term results on monosyllabic CNC word score test for Iowa subjects with 10-mm electrodes. Solid black bar represents the preoperative hearing in the implant ear, stippled bar indicates preoperative performance with two hearing aids, black with white dotted bar is performance in the implant only condition, horizontal bar indicates hearing aid plus implant, and slanted bar is hearing aids binaural plus implant performance.

analog strategy (SAS) speech processing strategies] was 30.7% correct (**Fig. 19–9**). There were no significant differences among the long electrode recipients as a function of either device or strategy. In contrast, the mean score for familiar melody recognition for five short-electrode recipients 1 year after the hook-up was 80.1% correct. In summary, the hybrid short-electrode subjects were significantly more accurate than traditional long electrode implant recipients in the pitch-based task of familiar melody recognition. The A+E strategy, where residual acoustic hearing up to 750 to 1000 Hz is preserved, allows the fundamental frequencies of many melodies to be perceived via the residual acoustic

hearing, where significant advantages in pitch perception exist as compared with electric hearing.

◆ Conclusion

Preservation of residual low-frequency hearing with the addition of electrical speech processing has substantially improved the speech perception abilities and hearing in noise of this group of volunteers. Music appreciation and quality of sound has also been maintained. This is not a trivial consideration, given the ubiquitous nature of music in our society, as well as the fact that implant recipients report enjoyment of music as their most important wish after improved speech perception (Gfeller et al, 2002). The importance of preserving residual low-frequency acoustic hearing cannot be underestimated, in view of the observation that the added benefit of hearing in noise and quality of music is a result of the residual acoustic hearing in this population. This residual hearing provides finer spectral resolution than what is possible from the present cochlear implant speech-processing algorithms. The 10-mm electrode has been successful in preserving hearing and providing sufficient additional high-frequency information to improve speech perception. A balance among intracochlear trauma, acoustic hearing, and delivery of electrical current has been achieved. It could be argued that a longer electrode may deliver more information; however, if individuals with significant residual hearing are to benefit from this technology, preservation of residual hearing is of paramount consideration. It is interesting that some subjects achieve between 60% and 70% CNC word recognition with a six-channel 10-mm electrode using electrical speech processing without a hearing aid. The risk/benefit performance ratio of combined electrical and acoustical stimulation is just beginning to be explored. In addition to pure tone hearing preservation in this group of

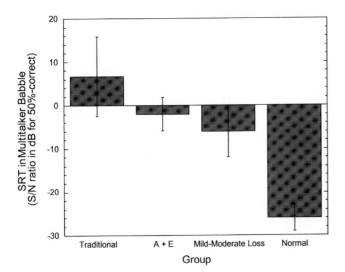

Figure 19–8 The spondee recognition threshold (S/N ratio in dB required for 50%-correct recognition in a multitalker background) for four groups of patients. The error bars represent plus and minus 1 standard deviation about the mean. Traditional, subjects using standard length electrode; A+E, subjects using electro-acoustical stimulation; Mild–Moderate Loss, subjects using hearing aids; Normal, normal hearing subjects.

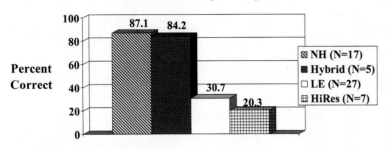

Figure 19–9 Familiar melody recognition task for normal hearing adults (NH), Hybrid electrode patients (SE), standard length electrode subjects (LE), and a group of subjects using Clarion 90K high-resolution speech processing (HiResolution). The results on this task for the 10-mm Hybrid electrode subjects are similar to those of normal-hearing individuals and significantly better than the standard electrode or high-resolution speech processing.

individuals, the acoustic speech perception has been preserved. This is an important finding, and is probably the reason why the subjects are doing well in noise and appreciate music.

A+E processing improved speech perception in noise by 9 dB signal-to-noise ratio (compared with long electrode subjects). To put this improvement in signal-to-noise ratio in perspective, Eddington et al (1997) have demonstrated that a 5-dB improvement in signal-to-noise ratio is comparable to an approximate 30 to 40% improvement in Hearing in Noise Test (HINT) sentence scores. Although the improvement for speech in noise does not bring the implant patient to normal hearing levels, it represents a large advance toward that goal. The speech in noise results for this group of severely hearing-impaired individuals using the A+E approach are nearly as good as those for mild-to-moderate hearing loss patients. Remember that for these individuals, hearing aid technology was unable to improve their speech recognition to acceptable levels in quiet or in noise. It will be interesting to see if those with more moderate hearing losses can realize similar improvements in noise using the electroacoustical stimulation paradigm.

Preservation of any residual hearing must be a goal of all future cochlear implant surgeries. Implant surgeons should adopt surgical strategies to limit intracochlear damage. The ability to enter the inner ear and place a 10-mm electrode opens many possibilities for future therapies. Cochlear implant manufacturers must recognize the importance of inner ear preservation in all individuals undergoing cochlear implantation, and should adjust the design of intracochlear electrodes to accommodate this concept. When considering hearing preservation and future implant designs, the importance of preserving acoustic speech perception must be taken into account as well as pure tone level. This research also demonstrates the need to improve low-frequency fine spectral perception for cochlear implant recipients who do not have residual acoustic hearing to provide more enjoyment of music as well as hearing in noise.

Acknowledgments

This work is supported (in part) by research grants 2 P50 DC00242 and 1 R01 DC 000377 from the National Institute on Deafness and Other Communication Disorders of the National Institutes of Health; grant RR00059 from the General Clinical Research Centers Program; National Center for Research Resources (NCRR), National Institutes of Health; the Iowa Lions Sight and Hearing Foundation; and the Cochlear Corporation, which developed a cochlear implant to our specifications, providing initial devices at no cost, and sharing data from their ongoing clinical trial with the Hybrid implant.

The authors would like to acknowledge the principal investigators who have accrued subjects in the Hybrid Implant clinical trial: Charles Luetje, Kansas City Ear Institute; Noel Cohen, MD, and J Thomas Roland, MD, New York University; William Luxford, MD, House Ear Institute; Joseph Roberson, MD, California Ear Institute; Peter Roland, MD, University of Texas, Dallas; and Richard Miyamoto, MD, Indiana University.

References

Eddington DK, Rabinowitz WR, Tierney J, et al. (1997). Speech processors for auditory prostheses. In: 8th Quarterly Progress Report NIDCD (Contract N)1–62100. Bethesda, MD: National Institute on Deafness and Other Communication Disorders

Fishman KE, Shannon RV, Slattery WH. (1998). Speech recognition as a function of the number of electrodes used in the SPEAK cochlear implant strategy. J Speech Hear Res 40:1201–1215

Friesen L, Shannon RV, Baskent D, Wang X. (2001). Speech recognition in noise as a function of the number of spectral channels: comparison of acoustic hearing and cochlear implants. J Acoust Soc Am 110:1150–1163

Fu Q-J, Shannon RV, Wang X. (1998). Effects of noise and spectral resolution on vowel and consonant recognition: acoustic and electric hearing. J Acoust Soc Am 104:3586–3596

Gantz B. (1998). Cochlear Implant Research: Past, Present, Future–Premises, Promises and Realities. NIDCD 10th Anniversary Celebration, Bethesda, MD, October 2

Gantz B, Turner C. (2000). Electronic Signal Processing for the Moderately Hearing Impaired, CI 2000. The 6th International Cochlear Implant Conference, Miami, February 3–5

Gantz BJ, Turner CW. (2003). Combining acoustic and electric hearing. Laryngoscope 113:1726–1730

Gantz BJ, Tyler RS, Rubinstein JT, et al. (2002). Binaural cochlear implants placed during the same operation. Otol Neurotol 23:169–180

Gantz BJ, Woodworth GG, Knutson JF, Abbas PJ, Tyler RS. (1993). Multivariate predictors of audiological success with multichannel cochlear implants. Ann Otol Rhinol Laryngol 102:909–917

Gfeller KE, Turner C, Woodworth G, et al. (2002). Recognition of familiar melodies by adult cochlear implant recipients and normal hearing adults. Cochlear Implants International 3:29–53

Gfeller K, Lansing CR. (1991). Melodic, rhythmic, and timbral perception of adult cochlear implant users. J Speech Hear Res 34:916–920

Greenwood DD. (1990). A cochlear frequency position function for several species—29 years later. J Acoust Soc Am 1990;87:2592–2605

Ni D, Shepherd RK, Seldon HL, Xu SA, Clark GM, Millard RE. (1992). Cochlear pathology following chronic electrical stimulation of the auditory nerve, I: normal hearing kittens. Hear Res 62:62–81

Peterson FE, Lehiste I. (1962). Revised CNC lists for auditory tests. J Speech Hear Disord 27:62–70

Pijl S, Schwartz D. (1995). Melody recognition and musical interval perception by deaf subjects stimulated with electrical pulse trains through single cochlear implant electrodes. J Acoust Soc Am 98:886–895

Roland JT. (2005). A model for cochlear implant electrode insertion and force evaluation: results with a new electrode design and insertion technique. Laryngoscope 115:1325–1339

Rubinstein JT, Parkinson WS, Tyler RS, Gantz BJ. (1999). Residual speech recognition and cochlear implant performance: Effects of implantation criteria. Am J Otol 20:445–452

Svirsky MA, Robbins AM, Iler Kirk KI, Pisoni DB, Miyamoto RT. (2000). Language development in profoundly deaf children with cochlear implants. Psychol Sci 11:153–158

Tomblin JB, Barker BA, Spencer LJ, Zhang X, Gantz BJ. (2005). The effect of age at cochlear implant initial stimulation on expressive language growth in infants and toddlers. J Speech Lang Hear Res 48:853–867

Tomblin JB, Spencer L, Flock S, Tyler R, Gantz B. (1999). A comparison of language achievement in children with cochlear implants and children using hearing aids. J Speech Lang Hear Res 42:497–509

Turner CW, Gantz BJ, Vidal C, Behrens A, Henry BA. (2004). Speech recognition in noise for cochlear implant listeners: benefits of residual acoustic hearing. J Acoust Soc Am 115:1729–1735Xu S, Shephard RK, Millard RE, Clark GM. (1992). Chronic stimulation of the auditory nerve at high stimulation rates: a Physiological and histopathological study. Hear Res 105: 1–29

Xu S, Shephard RK, Millard RE, Clark GM. (1997). Chronic Stimulation of the auditory nerve at high stimulation rates: a physiological and histopathological study. Hear Res 105:1–29

20

Auditory Brainstem Implants

Eric G. St. Clair,
John G. Golfinos, and
J. Thomas Roland Jr.

The auditory brainstem implant (ABI) was developed in 1979 at the House Ear Institute (Los Angeles, CA) for patients deafened by the bilateral vestibular schwannomas of neurofibromatosis type 2 (NF2). Patients with NF2 typically are left without functioning cochlear nerves bilaterally, either as a result of surgery or of the tumors themselves, and thus derive no benefit from cochlear implants. The ABI was designed to effectively bypass this disconnection and directly stimulate the cochlear nucleus in the brainstem in response to auditory stimuli.

◆ History of Development of Auditory Brainstem Implants

Neurofibromatosis type 2 (formerly "central neurofibromatosis") was first described by Wishart in 1822 and is characterized by bilateral acoustic neuromas, multiple meningiomas, spinal ependymomas, and postcapsular cataracts. Inheritance is autosomal dominant through a gene on chromosome 22 (Miyamoto et al, 1990) though 50% of all cases represent sporadic mutations and the incidence is 1 in 40,000 births (Otto et al, 2000). The Gardner and Wishart forms of NF2 represent subtypes of lesser and greater severity respectively. The more severe form tends to present at a younger age and with more widespread central nervous system (CNS) tumors. Unlike unilateral acoustic neuromas, which typically are well encapsulated, the tumors of NF2 tend to diffusely infiltrate adjacent nerves (Brackmann et al, 1993). Patients with NF2 commonly end up with total hearing loss by the time they are in their 20s or 30s (Ramsden et al, 2005).

The bilateral acoustic neuromas (or more accurately "vestibular schwannomas") of NF2 tend to damage both the vestibular and cochlear components of the eighth cranial nerve (Kanowitz et al, 2004). These nerves are generally sacrificed at surgery; thus, patients with NF2 are not candidates for conventional cochlear implants as these devices require an intact cochlear nerve. The ABI was designed to bypass this disconnection by directly stimulating the cochlear nucleus in the brainstem. Through the pioneering work of Drs. House and Hitselberger, the first ABI device was implanted in a human recipient in 1979.

The hardware design of the ABI is similar to that of a cochlear implant, except that the target is the cochlear nucleus within the brainstem rather than the scala tympani within the cochlea. As with a cochlear implant there are both external and internal components. Externally, a modified hearing aid receives auditory analog signals and transmits them to a miniaturized speech processor. The speech processor analyzes, filters, and digitizes the signals and then sends them to the transmitting coil. The transmitting coil in turn sends the coded signals as radio signals to the implant under the skin. Internally, the ABI delivers electrical signals to the array of platinum electrodes on the cochlear nucleus on the dorsolateral surface of the brainstem. The resulting information regarding intensity and pitch can then be relayed within the central auditory system as sound (Otto et al, 2002): "The sound processing unit (speech processor) requires appropriate programming and must be fitted to individual users. Programming speech processors involves psychophysical assessment of electrically induced auditory percepts, including threshold, comfort level, and pitch. These measures are programmed into the processor and used to control the amplitude and the sequential patterns of stimulation. In multichannel auditory implants, different sites of stimulation can generate different pitch percepts for the listener. Changes in frequency spectrum of sound can therefore be coded by appropriate changes in the patterns of electrode activation." The speech processor and individual electrodes essentially take over the role of the cochlea as a spectrum analyzer, decomposing complex sounds into their frequency components (Kuchta et al, 2004; Otto et al, 2002; Schwartz et al, 2003).

The original design by House and Hitselberger was a simple pair of ball electrodes implanted into the substance of the cochlear nucleus of a single patient. The cochlear nucleus was chosen as the site of implantation both because it is the first neuronal junction in the auditory pathway beyond the cochlear nerve and because it is relatively accessible at surgery. Two years after this first implantation, the electrode was noted to have migrated, resulting in loss of auditory sensation and the development of lower extremity paresthesias. The ABI was subsequently replaced by a new implant designed for surface placement over the cochlear nucleus. This new single-channel ABI was made of two platinum plates on a Dacron mesh carrier (the mesh facilitated development of a fibrous capsule around the implant that impeded migration). It remains functional to this day. Subsequent developments in silicon backing, Dacron mesh, and nonelastic wires have improved "conformal adherence" to the brainstem surface. Postmortem studies by Otto's group confirmed ingrowth of connective tissue into the fabric mesh electrode carrier. Potential damage to surrounding neural structures is minimized by use of a charge-balanced biphasic waveform and by ensuring that charge density does not exceed 20 microcoulomb per square centimeter per phase (Brackmann et al, 1993; Kovacs et al, 2000; McElveen et al, 1985; Otto 2000; Otto et al, 2002).

By 1991, the number of electrodes in the standard ABI was increased to three. The most important aspect of this development was the finding that sound frequency (pitch) varies with electrode location. Furthermore, studies of cochlear implants had demonstrated better speech recognition as a result of spectral (frequency) information with multichannel devices. Subsequently, in 1995, Laszig and colleagues developed the first multichannel ABI consisting of an array of eight platinum disk electrodes in 1991. A multicenter clinical trial of a multichannel ABI began in the United States in 1994. The ABI in current use in the United States is a multichannel implant with 21 electrodes arranged in three rows. The array is small enough to fit within the confines of the lateral recess but large enough such that the individual electrodes do not exceed the critical values of charge density that could damage neural tissue. As many of these patients will require magnetic resonance imaging (MRI) follow-up for tumors of NF2, the receiver-stimulator portion contains a removable magnet. Postoperatively, the patient's pitch perception can be adjusted by manipulating the sites of electrode stimulation. However, at least one recent study found that beyond a critical number—perhaps seven—there is limited usefulness in the increased number of electrodes. The principal limitation of the surface electrode array of the ABI is the tonotopic organization of the cochlear nucleus itself. This tonotopic organization is perpendicular to the surface of the brainstem, thus

limiting the utility of the surface electrode array. A penetrating electrode array is under development to better access this three-dimensional tonotopic organization of the cochlear nucleus. Rauschecker and Shannon (2002) believe that advances in neuroimaging (e.g., functional MRI) and stereotactic neurosurgical techniques will allow better access to small, deep brainstem structures and thus better tonotopic representation by a penetrating electrode. Of note, Colletti et al (2005) believe that the tonotopic mismatch between electrode and nucleus (and thus the limited number of electrodes that can be used) is not an issue in nontumor ABI recipients as they lack the significant anatomic and functional distortion of brainstem structures (Brackmann et al, 1993; Kanowitz et al, 2004; Koch et al, 2005; Kuchta et al, 2004; McCreery et al, 1990; Otto et al, 2000).

◆ Indications for Auditory Brainstem Implants

The ABI was first developed for patients with deafness resulting from the bilateral acoustic neuromas of NF2. Histologic studies demonstrated that these tumors, although usually arising from the vestibular component of the eighth nerve, typically invade rather than compress the nerve to the point of being nonfunctional (Miyamoto et al, 1990). Without a functioning cochlear nerve (whether from the tumor itself or from the subsequent transection at surgery) these patients were not candidates for cochlear implantation.

In the U.S., the criteria for implantation are (1) age greater than 12 years old, (2) English speaking, (3) highly motivated to participate and comply with protocol follow-up, (4) reasonable expectations, (5) bilateral vestibular schwannomas of NF2, and (6) psychologically stable (Kanowitz et al, 2004; Otto et al, 2002). Previous irradiation of acoustic neuromas does not preclude ABI placement but in at least one series was hypothesized to have accounted for delayed deterioration of ABI utility (Grayeli et al, 2003; Laszig et al, 1995).

More recently at centers outside the United States, ABIs have been implanted in patients without NF2 but who are similarly unable to undergo cochlear implantation. These indications have included cochlear ossification (a common complication of meningitis), severe auditory neuropathy (a multiform disorder characterized by cochlear nerve degeneration and subsequent sensorineural hearing loss, with word recognition reduced out of proportion to pure tone threshold), trauma/cochlear nerve avulsion, cochlear nerve aplasia, and severe cochlear malformation. Notably, these patients typically do not have the extensive distortion of brainstem anatomy that is commonly associated with the often large tumors of NF2 patients. This lack of distortion facilitates placement of the ABI in the nontumor patients (Colletti et al, 2002, 2004, 2005; Grayeli et al, 2003; Kuchta et al, 2004).

The use of the ABI in nontumor patients has meant implantation in progressively younger patients. Colletti et al (2005) have implanted ABIs in nontumor, congenitally deafened patients as young as 14 months old. Ramsden et al (2005) state, "The auditory pathway requires stimulation with sound in the first few years of life if it is going to be programmed for future speech perception and consequent language production.... By the age of four years, and certainly by the age of six years, the auditory pathways are losing their plasticity and poorer long-term outcomes are to be expected."

The importance of early stimulation of the auditory system was also demonstrated in a recent report of two patients with congenital deafness in one ear and the subsequent development of a vestibular schwannoma in the other ear. Both patients failed initial attempts at placing a cochlear implant on the congenitally deafened side once the contralateral vestibular schwannoma was discovered. Ramsden et al (2005) hypothesized that the lack of stimulation of the first-order auditory neuron had left the spiral ganglion cells unable to effectively transmit auditory signals. Alternatively, or additionally, there may have been a loss of cell bodies in the cochlear nucleus as a result of lack of ipsilateral stimulation. They point out that in rodent studies, removal of the cochlea before day 12 (when hearing begins) results in death of neurons in the cochlear nucleus. Both patients subsequently underwent placement of an ABI on the side of tumor removal.

◆ Surgical Procedure for Auditory Brainstem Implants

Initially, ABIs were implanted after the removal of the second vestibular schwannoma in a patient with NF2. More recently, it has become relatively common to place the ABI following resection of the first tumor, although benefit from the device will not be noted until removal of the contralateral tumor. Brackmann et al (1993) outlined three reasons for implanting the ABI at first side tumor resection in NF2: (1) to afford the patient experience with the device prior to losing all hearing; (2) to decrease anatomic distortion at the time of implantation; and (3) to retain the option of implanting on the contralateral side should initial implantation prove unsuccessful. Regardless of whether the ABI is placed after removal of the first or second tumor, it is almost always implanted at the first operation on a given side. Implantation at reoperation is extremely difficult as a result of fibrosis in the area of previous resection (Grant et al, 2000). More recently, the U.S. Food and Drug Administration (FDA) has granted permission for implantation in patients with previous bilateral tumor resections.

Historically, the implantation of the ABI has been achieved through a standard translabyrinthine approach (Grayeli et al, 2003; Kanowitz et al, 2004; Kuchta et al, 2004; Otto et al, 2002). The proposed advantages of this approach include direct access to the lateral recess of the fourth ventricle and the surface of the cochlear nucleus complex, minimal cerebellar retraction, early identification of the facial nerve, complete tumor removal from the lateral end of the internal auditory canal, and low rates of morbidity (Otto et al, 2002; Vincent et al, 2002). Although this remains the only approach approved by the FDA, other approaches, including retrosigmoid and subtonsillar, have been used internationally.

Colletti et al (2002) proposed the advantages of a retrosigmoid approach to be: (1) short duration procedure (no extensive drill-out); (2) no risk of intracranial contamination from broaching the mastoid air cells; (3) possible preservation of hearing for some patients, which they propose as the main advantage; and (4) stabilization of the implant by placing the wire in a drilled-out groove in the posterior wall of the petrous temporal bone which may help prevent postimplantation migration. Colletti et al (2005) and Seki et al (2003) advocated subtonsillar placement of the electrode by extending the conventional retrosigmoid craniotomy with foramen magnum opening and C1 laminectomy. They proposed the following advantages of the wider exposure obtained through this subtonsillar (or "cerebello-medullary fissure") approach: (1) it may be better for placing penetrating "depth" electrodes; (2) it is not affected by adhesions from previous surgery, thus making a second operation for ABI feasible; and (3) if necessary, it is possible to do bilateral placement of electrodes by cutting both taenia and then raising both tonsils.

Regardless of the approach used, the goal is to place the electrode array directly on the surface of the cochlear nucleus complex on the dorsolateral surface of the brainstem just rostral to the pontomedullary junction (McElveen et al, 1987). The cochlear nucleus is composed of three subnuclei: the dorsal, superior, and inferior ventral cochlear nuclei. Placement over the dorsal component is believed to result in fewer nonauditory stimuli than over the ventral component (Brackmann et al, 1993; Colletti et al, 2002). Unlike in lower vertebrates, the cochlear nucleus is not visible on gross or microscopic inspection. As such, surface landmarks are essential for correct placement of the ABI. These landmarks include the stump of the transected eighth cranial nerve, the flocculus of the cerebellum, cranial nerves seven and nine, the choroid plexus, and the tenia (the attachment of the tela choroidea to the floor of the lateral recess) of the foramen of Luschka. The dorsal cochlear nucleus lies almost entirely within the lateral recess (foramen of Luschka) of the fourth ventricle; optimal results have been achieved by placing the ABI completely within the lateral recess. This can often be aided by identifying and then transecting the tenia as it overlies the lateral extent of the lateral recess. The tenia crosses the ventral cochlear nucleus (VCN) just medial to the boundary of the VCN and the eighth nerve. Although this relationship is fairly constant, the tenia can be difficult to identify. Identification of the tenia can be aided by finding the apex of the angle between the eighth and ninth cranial nerves (Monsell et al, 1987; Otto et al, 2002; Terr and Edgerton, 1985; Terr et al, 1990; Vincent et al, 2002).

Unfortunately, these anatomic landmarks are often significantly distorted by the often large tumors of patients with NF2. In the minority of patients who do not receive auditory sensation after implantation, anatomic difficulties at surgery have been thought usually to be the cause. In the case of reoperation, gliosis can further impede cochlear nucleus identification. Several electrophysiologic tests, including electrically evoked auditory brainstem responses (EABR), near field potential (NFP), neural response telemetry (NRT), and stimulation with a bipolar probe, can assist in determining the correct location of the cochlear nucleus complex. EABR is a far-field measurement of brainstem activity. Stimulation of the cochlear nucleus in EABR should reveal either mono- or biphasic wave patterns that approximately correlate with waves III and V on traditional ABR tracings. Improper placement of the electrode array can be detected with EABR by subsequent intraoperative cranial nerve stimulation, myogenic responses, vital sign changes, or absent EABR waveforms. NFP is a near field measurement at the cochlear nucleus (Zimmerling et al, 2000). The bipolar probe consists of a circuit board with four gold-plated electrodes that correlate identically with four of the actual ABI electrodes. The electrodes can be stimulated across several electrode pair combinations just like the ABI (Roland et al, 2000). Correct placement in the lateral recess can also be confirmed by noting cerebrospinal fluid (CSF) egress from the foramen of Luschka following a Valsalva maneuver induced by the anesthesiologist. Finally, orienting the electrode array such that the electrodes face medially and superiorly maximizes stimulation of the cochlear nucleus. Intraoperative monitoring of cranial nerves five, seven (orbicularis oris), nine, and ten (ipsilateral pharyngeal muscles) is also essential (Colletti et al, 2002; Colletti et al, 2004; Kanowitz et al, 2004; Kuchta et al, 2004; Laszig et al, 1995; Otto et al, 2000; Toh and Luxford 2002; Vincent et al, 2002; Waring 1992).

Friedland and Wackym (1999) advocated the use of an endoscope to aid in visualizing the lateral recess at surgery. In cadaver studies, the 30-degree endoscope was found to be helpful in translabyrinthine and retrosigmoid approaches to the lateral recess and essential to the middle fossa approach. With the translabyrinthine approach, the endoscope allowed visualization anterior to the flocculus and choroid plexus prior to any retraction. This allowed early visualization of the eight and ninth cranial nerve root entry zones while preserving the delicate tenia. Moreover, the foramen of Luschka can be distinguished from similar structures by direct visualization into its lateral recess with the endoscope. Minimal retraction of the cerebellum and flocculus was also found to be the major advantage of the use of the endoscope with the retrosigmoid approach. The endoscope was found to be essential for the rarely used middle fossa approach, although the risk of injury to the facial nerve was thought to be significant.

◆ Postoperative Care and Complications of Auditory Brainstem Implants

Initial stimulation typically occurs approximately 6 weeks after surgery. Awareness of the consequences of vagal nerve stimulation and significant nonauditory side effects is essential. Bradycardia, motor long tract stimulation, vertigo, throat tightening, and fainting might occur during initial stimulation. For this reason, cardiac monitoring and physician attendance were part of the early protocol. The programming audiologist is always aware of the symptoms and can immediately "program out" untoward stimuli. The speech processor of the ABI is then programmed with respect to various auditory precepts including threshold, loudness, comfort level,

pitch, and reduction of nonauditory sensations. The initial stimulus occurs over a 3-day period lasting several hours per day. The process is generally more complicated than for cochlear implant patients for the reasons outlined by Otto and Staller (1995): (1) presence of nonauditory sensations, (2) the more central locus of stimulation, (3) the uncertainty and irregularity of tonotopic stimulation, and (4) potential central disease from NF2. Moreover, fitting is a dynamic process that requires periodic adjustments to account for small changes in auditory perception over time (Colletti et al, 2002; Kanowitz et al, 2004; Kuchta et al, 2004; McElveen et al, 1985; Otto 2000; Otto et al, 2001; Schwartz et al, 2003).

In multichannel auditory brainstem implants, different sites of electrode stimulation can generate different pitch percepts. Changes in the frequency spectrum of sounds can thus be coded by changes in the patterns of electrode activation. The system is aided by the ability to stimulate between any pair of electrodes on the array (bipolar mode) or by the use of a remote electrode as a ground (monopolar mode). Use of the monopolar mode often allows stimulation at lower current levels and with fewer nonauditory sensations. Pitch scaling and ranking are two procedures used to determine the appropriate tonotopic order of the electrodes. With pitch scaling, electrodes are simulated and patients are asked to assign the sound a "sharpness rating" between one (lowest pitch) and 100 (highest pitch) (Colletti et al, 2002, 2005; Otto et al, 1998). With pitch ranking, two electrodes are stimulated in succession and the patient is asked to determine which sound has the higher pitch. Based on these tests, an appropriate tonotopic order of the electrodes can be determined. Unlike in cochlear implants where tonotopic order is fairly constant from patient to patient, tonotopic order in ABIs can be highly variable across patients. In Coletti's group, the most medial and caudal electrodes tended to elicit higher frequencies. Otto et al similarly found higher frequencies associated with the more medial electrodes, whereas Vincent et al found that in three of five testable patients low frequencies were found dorsally and high frequencies were found ventrally. According to Kuchta et al (2004), however, the appropriate ranking of the pitch was of greater importance than the absolute number of electrodes used. Furthermore, according to Otto et al (1995), the ability to pitch rank is believed to correlate with improved speech recognition. The ability to pitch scale and rank may develop over time and should be tested at each follow-up even if the patient is unable to do this on initial tuning (Vincent et al, 2002).

The Nucleus ABI 22 (Cochlear Corporation, Sydney, Australia) (eight electrodes) uses the spectral peak (SPEAK) speech processing strategy. The Nucleus ABI 24 (21 electrodes) accommodates SPEAK as well as Advanced Combination Encoder (ACE) and continuous interleaved sampling (CIS) encoding strategies. "The SPEAK strategy delivers the signal at … 250–300 pulses/sec and selects the number and location of the electrodes to be stimulated depending on the intensity and frequency of the incoming signal. The CIS strategy presents high fixed rates of stimulation (600 to 1800 pulses/sec) to a small number of channels. The ACE strategy combines the advantages of both SPEAK and CIS strategies by using a high rate of stimulation with dynamic electrode selection and a large number of available electrodes" (Colletti et al, 2005).

A typical postimplantation evaluation protocol was described by Coletti et al (2005). Following initial activation at 6 weeks postimplantation, the patient is evaluated at 1 month, 6 months, 1 year, and then annually thereafter. The perception tests include: (1) recognition of environmental sounds, (2) the closed-set vowel confusion test, (3) the closed-set consonant confusion test, (4) the closed-set word recognition test, (5) the open-set sentence recognition test, and (6) the speech-tracking test.

The primary postoperative complications are CSF leak, implant migration, and nonauditory stimuli. CSF leaks are treated with approximately 5 days of lumbar CSF diversion. Rarely is reoperation and leak repair necessary. Otto et al (2002) reported CSF leaks in two of 61 patients (3.3%). This percentage is comparable to those from other translabyrinthine craniotomies and was not directly attributable to electrode implantation. Roland's group (Kanowitz et al, 2004) reported this complication in two of 18 (11%) patients. Implant migration or aberrant placement of the ABI at surgery can result in an increased number of nonauditory sensations. As discussed earlier, developments in silicon backing, Dacron mesh, and nonelastic wires have improved "conformal adherence" to the brainstem surface and thus decreased the complications of postsurgery implant migration (Kovacs et al, 2000). In the series reported by Kuchta et al (2004), only one of 61 patients "lost" more than one electrode over time.

Nonauditory stimuli develop in up to 42% of users (Otto et al, 1998, 2001, 2002; Vincent et al, 2002) and thus warrant special consideration. Nonauditory stimuli are almost always located ipsilateral to the side of implantation. The most common nonauditory sensations are dizziness and ipsilateral "tingling" (Colletti et al, 2005; Otto et al, 2001, 2004). Other sensations include "jittering" of the visual field (flocculus of the cerebellum), muscle twitches (cranial nerves VII and IX), and contralateral "tingling." These side effects are usually considered to be minimal by the patient and often are rectifiable with adjustment of (usually increasing) the duration of the stimulus or by selecting a different ground electrode. In one series, reduction of nonauditory sensations was achieved by reducing the rate of stimulation; no effect was noted by changing stimulus duration (Vincent et al, 2002) Additionally, nonauditory sensations often decrease over time (Colletti et al, 2005; Kanowitz et al, 2004; Otto et al, 1998, 2002) whereas 9% of patients develop persistent nonauditory sensations (Otto et al, 2004).

These nonauditory stimuli appear to be related to placement low in, and with protrusion from, the lateral recess (Shannon et al, 1993). This aberrant placement allows current spread outside of the cochlear nucleus, potentially stimulating other cranial nerves, the flocculus of the cerebellum, the inferior cerebellar peduncle, and the spinothalamic tract. Keeping the electrode within the confines of the lateral recess would prevent this inappropriate stimulation (Otto et al, 2002). Nonauditory stimuli also tend to be associated with stimulation of the most medial and lateral electrodes (Otto et al, 2002; Toh and Luxford, 2002).

Rauschecker and Shannon (2002) believe that advances in neuroimaging (e.g., functional MRI) and stereotactic neurosurgical techniques will allow better access to small, deep brainstem structures and thus better tonotopic representation by a penetrating electrode.

◆ Results of Auditory Brainstem Implants

The effectiveness of the ABI over the past 25 years has been well studied. A typical follow-up protocol involves testing the patient every 3 months for the first year after the initial stimulation and then annually thereafter. A multi-institutional study in the United States found that overall 81% of implantees received auditory sensations. Results are similar to those of single-channel cochlear implants. The ABI appears to function best as a "lip-reading enhancer" and as a tool for detecting and differentiating different environmental sounds. With regard to the former, it is particularly useful in determining the rhythm, stress, timing, and intensity of speech. When combined with lip-reading cues, 93% of patients demonstrate improved sentence understanding at 3 to 6 months. Sound discrimination and identification are possible, but significant open-set word recognition is rare. In general, speech perception performance and subjective sound quality are better with the patients who received multichannel devices than in the original 25 patients who received single-channel implants (Brackmann et al, 1993; Colletti et al, 2004; Laszig et al, 1995; Lenarz et al, 2002; Otto et al, 2000, 2001, 2002; Ramsden et al, 2005; Roland et al, 2000; Schwartz et al, 2003; Toh and Luxford, 2002; Vincent et al, 2002).

One important finding is that patients gradually improve in their use of the ABI over time, with one study finding increasing benefit as late as 8 years after implantation (Otto et al, 2002; Schwartz et al, 2003; Toh et al, 2002). Additionally, a patient's subjective evaluation of the ABI is generally higher than would be predicted by objective audiometric data (Lenarz et al, 2002). Testing of auditory sensation with visual cues improves the most over time, though auditory testing alone shows significant improvement as well. As a control, vision-only testing tends to stay stable over time (Otto et al, 2000).

Counseling, multidisciplinary rehabilitation, and auditory training are important postoperative adjuncts for all ABI recipients. Kanowitz et al (2004), Lenarz et al (2002), and Otto et al (2004, 2002) found that preoperative counseling with regard to personal motivation, reasonable expectations, and family support was of particular importance in teenage patients. This counseling should stress several points: (1) some patients do not receive auditory sensations; (2) the ABI does not provide normal sound quality; (3) most ABI patients do not achieve open-set speech recognition; (4) regular follow-ups are required for speech processor optimization; and (5) it will take time and experience to develop maximum benefit from the ABI.

Otto et al (2002) reported their results in 61 patients implanted with an eight electrode ABI for NF2. Six of 61 (9.8%) patients did not report useful auditory sensations, though one of these patients subsequently derived benefits from a contralaterally placed ABI. The authors found that their patients often were initially disappointed with the "muffled" sounds from the new ABI. However, most patients ultimately reported significant improvement in sound quality and performance following a period of adaptation and learning. Motivation and persistence, particularly in the first 3 months postimplantation, were noted to be of particular importance for long-term improvement.

The Sound Effects Recognition Test (SERT) test for environmental sound discrimination was at or above the 50% correct level for most of the 61 patients. As with other tested parameters of ABI function, scores on this test improved with experience. On Monosyllable Trochee Spondee Test (MTS) testing, 87% of patients scored above chance on closed-set word identification and 98% scored above chance on syllable stress identification. The Northwestern University Children's Perception of Speech (NU-CHIPS) test is a closed-set sound-only test wherein the patient must choose the correct word from a list of four rhyming monosyllable words. On this test 84% of ABI recipients in this series scored significantly above chance.

Scores on vowel and consonant recognition were overall less impressive, although a few patients were able to perform at high levels. Moreover, the investigators found that to achieve sound-only speech recognition, the patient's performance on the vowel and consonant tests has to approach 50%. A small but significant number of ABI patients were subsequently able to demonstrate some level of sound-only sentence recognition on the City University of New York (CUNY) sentence test.

Regular experience with the ABI is important for continued improvement. Regular users of the ABI with more than 2 years' experience generally performed better on all speech perception tests than those with less experience. Additionally, MTS scores continued to improve as late as 8 years postimplantation. Some patients eventually developed some degree of open set speech recognition.

Otto et al (2000) found that 85% of patients receive some sort of auditory sensation. Lenarz et al (2002) found that all of their patients were able to differentiate speech from environmental sounds. Additionally, in that group 73% of patients were able to differentiate between adult's and children's voices, 64% were able to distinguish men's and women's voices, and 82% found the ABI to be "very useful" in differentiating environmental sounds (e.g., ringing telephone and barking dog). Two of the 11 regular ABI users developed "open-set" abilities and are able to converse on the telephone. The device appears to work best in quiet settings and when listening to a familiar voice; however, according to Lenarz et al (2002), 90% of patients found the device useful even with an unfamiliar voice.

Vincent et al (2002, 2000) reported their results with a 15-electrode device developed in France. Overall, 12 of 14 patients (86%) were able to achieve auditory sensations from their device. Eleven of 14 patients (79%) received auditory sensations at initial testing after translabyrinthine approach to device placement. One of these patients subsequently lost auditory sensation after 2 weeks. Three patients who underwent a retrosigmoid approach did not have auditory sensations at initial testing. Two of these patients were subsequently able to achieve auditory sensation after reoperation via a translabyrinthine approach.

On reoperation, the electrode array was noted to be protruding from the lateral recess in both of these patients.

In Vincent's group, nonauditory sensation occurred in five of the 12 testable patients (42%) and involved 12 electrodes (6.7%). The side effects included "dizziness" (67% of the nonauditory sensations), tingling of the arm or shoulder (17% of nonauditory sensations), and "facial stimulation" (16% of nonauditory sensations). In only one patient did auditory and nonauditory sensations ("dizziness") emanate from the same electrodes. In this case the nonauditory sensation was eliminated by lowering the stimulation frequency. Changing the duration of stimulation had no effect on nonauditory side effects.

Twelve patients in Vincent's group were able to detect the presence of environmental sound and on average scored 63% (range 0 to 100%) on open-set recognition of environmental sound. All patients with normal vision demonstrated improved lip-reading in sound plus vision mode when compared with vision alone. Three of nine patients (33%) scored at least 15% on sound only mode. One patient was able to converse on the telephone with people familiar to her.

Kanowitz et al (2004) reported that 17 of 18 (94%) patients had some auditory sensation at initial device stimulation. However, at 6-month follow-up one patient reported facial nerve twitching with loud noise stimulation. A subsequent computed tomography (CT) scan demonstrated that the electrode paddle had shifted to a more lateral position. Eleven of 18 patients use their ABIs daily for an average of 9.6 hours per day. Patients with the Nucleus 22 (eight electrode) implant demonstrated scores significantly greater than chance on MTS Word, MTS Stress, and NU-CHIPS (word recognition) testing. However, at subsequent follow-up, only the scores on MTS Word and MTS Stress demonstrated improvement. Patients with the Nucleus 24 (21 electrode) device similarly showed scores on MTS Word, MTS Stress, and NU-CHIPS that were significantly better than chance. The scores in the Nucleus 24 patients were considerably higher in all tests but, owing to large standard deviations, not significantly so. Neither device demonstrated open-set speech discrimination with the Central Institute for the Deaf (CID) sentence test. One of 18 patients (5.6%) developed a CSF leak. No patients limited their use because of nonauditory side effects.

Colletti et al (2005) reported their results with both tumor (NF2) and nontumor ABI recipients. In their study, all 29 patients (20 adults and nine children) received auditory sensations. At 1 year, the average adult closed-set auditory alone word recognition score was 86% (improved from 56.6% at 6 months) in nontumor patients and 24.5% (improved from 19.3%) in tumor patients. The average adult auditory alone sentence recognition score at 1 year was 63% (improved from 35% at 6 months) in nontumor patients and 12.1% (improved from 9.1%) in tumor patients. By 1 year, seven nontumor adult patients and three tumor adult patients were able to achieve some speech-tracking (improved from three and one patients at 6 months, respectively). The better results in the nontumor patients are hypothesized to be related to the significant anatomic and functional distortion caused by tumors compressing the brainstem. The authors further report that progress in children takes place "at an almost exponential rate" in the first few months after activation.

Colletti et al (2004) also reported their results in three adults and two children implanting an ABI as a "salvage" procedure after unsuccessful cochlear implantation. The adults all suffered from complete cochlear ossification. One child was diagnosed with bilateral cochlear nerve aplasia and the other with auditory neuropathy. All three adults had been unable to achieve word/sentence discrimination with a cochlear implant. Two of the adult ABI recipients were subsequently able to achieve some degree of both speech tracking and open-set (auditory only) sentence recognition. The third adult was able to detect 100% of environmental sounds, and discriminate 80% of and identify 40% of two- or three-syllable words. The two children had achieved no hearing ability with the cochlear implant but were able to detect sounds and words as early as 2 months after ABI activation.

Grayeli et al (2003), in a case report of a patient deafened by pneumococcal meningitis, similarly found that "the overall performances of ABI are similar to, and in some cases better than, those reported for cochlear implants in totally ossified cochleae."

◆ Conclusion

Because of the pioneering work of Drs. House and Hitselberger, about 200 patients have received auditory brainstem implants. These modified cochlear implants allow more proximal stimulation of the auditory system for patients without functioning cochlear nerves. Although originally developed exclusively for patients with neurofibromatosis type 2, ABIs have more recently been implanted for several other causes of bilateral hearing loss. Appropriate placement of the ABI within the confines of the lateral recess of the fourth ventricle allows the best stimulation of the cochlear nucleus complex in the brainstem and decreases nonauditory sensations. The device works best as a lip-reading enhancer, although a small minority of patients achieves some level of open-set speech recognition. Improved access to the tonotopic gradient of the cochlear nucleus, perhaps through the development of a penetrating electrode array, may lead to improvements in ABI sound quality.

References

Brackmann DE, Hitselberger WE, Nelson RA, et al. (1993). Auditory brainstem implant: I. Issues in surgical implantation. Otolaryngol Head Neck Surg 108:624–633

Colletti V, Carner M, Miorelli V, Guida M, Colletti L, Fiorino F. (2004). Cochlear implant failure: Is an auditory brainstem implant the answer? Acta Otolaryngol 124:353–357

Colletti V, Carner M, Miorelli V, Guida M, Colletti L, Fiorino F. (2005). Auditory brainstem implant: new frontiers in adults and children. Otolaryngol Head Neck Surg 133:126–138

Colletti V, Fiorino F, Carner M, Miorelli V, Guida M, Colletti L. (2004). Auditory brainstem implant as a salvage treatment after unsuccessful cochlear implantation. Otol Neurotol 25:485–496

Colletti V, Fiorino F, Carner M, Sacchetto L, Miorelli V, Orsi A. (2002). Auditory brainstem implantation: the University of Verona experience. Otolaryngol Head Neck Surg 127:84–96

Colletti V, Fiorino F, Carner M, et al. (2002). Hearing restoration with auditory brainstem implant in three children with cochlear nerve aplasia. Otol Neurotol 23:682–693

Friedland DR, Wackym PA. (1999). Evaluation of surgical approaches to endoscopic auditory brainstem implantation. Laryngoscope 109:175–180

Grant IL, Hall BB, Welling DB. (2000). Cochlear implantation in neurofibromatosis type 2. In: Waltzman SB, Cohen NL, eds. Cochlear Implants, pp. 367–368. New York: Thieme

Grayeli AB, Bouccara D, Kalamarides M, et al. (2003). Auditory brainstem implant in bilateral and completely ossified cochleae. Otol Neurotol 24:79–82

Kanowitz SJ, Shapiro WH, Golfinos JG, Cohen NL, Roland TJ Jr. (2004). Auditory brainstem implantation in patients with neurofibromatosis type 2. Laryngoscope 114:2135–2146

Koch DB, Staller S, Jaax K, Martin E. (2005). Bioengineering solutions for hearing loss and related disorders. Otolaryngol Clin North Am 38:255–272

Kovacs R, Janka M, Hochmair-Desoyer I, Helms J, Roosen K, Hochmair E. (2000). A new electrode design for the stable placing of a brainstem electrode. In: Waltzman SB, Cohen NL, eds. Cochlear Implants, pp. 368–369. New York: Thieme

Kuchta J, Otto SR, Shannon RV, Hitselberger WE, Brackmann DE. (2004). The multichannel auditory brainstem implant: how many electrodes make sense? J Neurosurg 100:16–23

Laszig R, Sollmann WP, Marangos N. (1995). The restoration of hearing in neurofibromatosis type 2. J Laryngol Otol 109:385–389

Lenarz M, Matthies C, Lesinski-Schiedat A, et al. (2002). Auditory brainstem implant part II: subjective assessment of functional outcome. Otol Neurotol 23:694–697

McCreery DB, Agnew WF, Yuen TGH, Bullara L. (1990). Charge density and charge per phase as cofactors in neural injury induced by electrical stimulation. IEEE Trans Biomed Eng 37:996–1001

McElveen JT Jr, Hitselberger WE, House WF. (1987). Surgical accessibility of the cochlear nuclear complex in man: surgical landmarks. Otolaryngol Head Neck Surg 96:135–140

McElveen JT Jr, Hitselberger WE, House WF, Mobley JP, Terr LI. (1985). Electrical stimulation of cochlear nucleus in man. Am J Otol Suppl:88–91.

Miyamoto RT, Campbell RL, Fritsch M, Lochmueller G. (1990). Preservation of hearing in neurofibromatosis 2. Otolaryngol Head Neck Surg 103:619–624

Monsell EM, McElveen JT Jr, Hitselberger WE, House WF. (1987). Surgical approaches to the human cochlear nuclear complex. Am J Otol 8:450–455

Otto SR, Brackmann DE, Hitselberger WE. (2004). Auditory brainstem implantation in 12- to 18-Year Olds. Arch Otolaryngol Head Neck Surg 130:656–659

Otto SR, Brackmann DE, Hitselberger WE, Shannon RV. (2001). Brainstem electronic implants for bilateral anacrusis following surgical removal of cerebellopontine angle lesions. Otolaryngol Clin North Am 34:485–499

Otto SR, Brackmann DE, Hitselberger WE, Shannon RV, Kuchta J. (2002). Multichannel auditory brainstem implant: update on performance in 61 patients. J Neurosurg 96:1063–1071

Otto SR, Ebinger K, Staller SJ. (2000). Clinical trials with the auditory brainstem implant. In: Waltzman SB, Cohen NL, eds. Cochlear Implants, pp. 357–366. New York: Thieme

Otto SR, Shannon RV, Brackmann DE, Hitselberger WE, Staller S, Menapace C. (1998). The multichannel auditory brain stem implant: Performance in twenty patients. Otolaryngol Head Neck Surg 118:291–303

Otto SR, Staller SJ. (1995). Multichannel auditory brain stem implant: case studies comparing fitting strategies and results. Ann Otol Rhinol Laryngol 104(suppl):36–39

Ramsden R, Khwaja S, Green K, O'Driscoll M, Mawman D. (2005). Vestibular schwannoma in the only hearing ear: cochlear implant or auditory brainstem implant? Otol Neurotol 26:261–264

Rauschecker JP, Shannon RV. (2002). Sending sound to the brain. Science 295:1025–1029

Roland JT Jr, Fishman AJ, Cohen NL. (2000). Bipolar stimulating probe for cochlear nucleus localization in auditory brainstem implant surgery. In: Waltzman SB, Cohen NL, eds. Cochlear Implants, pp. 373–377. New York: Thieme

Schwartz MS, Otto SR, Brackmann DE, Hitselberger WE, Shannon RV. (2003). Use of a multichannel auditory brainstem implant for neurofibromatosis type 2. Stereotact Funct Neurosurg 81:110–114

Seki Y, Samejima N, Kumakawa K, Komatsuzaki A. (2003). Subtonsillar placement of auditory brainstem implant. Acta Neurochir Suppl 87:85–87

Shannon RV, Fayad J, Moore J, et al. (1993). Auditory brainstem implant: II. Post surgical issues and performance. Otolaryngol Head Neck Surg 108:634–642

Terr LI, Edgerton BJ. (1985). Three-dimensional reconstruction of the cochlear nuclear complex in humans. Arch Otolaryngol 111:495–501

Terr LI, Fayad J, Hitselberger WE, Zakhary R. (1990). Cochlear nucleus anatomy related to central electro auditory prosthesis implantation. Otolaryngol Head Neck Surg 102:717–721

Toh EH, Luxford WM. (2002). Cochlear and brainstem implantation. Otolaryngol Clin North Am 35:325–342

Vincent C, Lejeune JP, Vaneecloo FM. (2000). The Digisonic auditory brainstem implant: report of the first three cases. In: Waltzman SB, Cohen NL, eds. Cochlear Implants, pp. 369–371. New York: Thieme

Vincent C, Zini C, Gandolfi A, et al. (2002). Results of the MXM Digisonic auditory brainstem implant clinical trials in Europe. Otol Neurotol 23:56–60

Waring MD. (1992). Electrically evoked auditory brainstem response monitoring of auditory brainstem implant integrity during facial nerve tumor surgery. Laryngoscope 102:1293–1295

Zimmerling M, Kovacs R, Janka M, et al. (2000). A new method to find the optimal location for an auditory brainstem electrode on the cochlear nucleus: preliminary results. In: Waltzman SB, Cohen NL, eds. Cochlear Implants, pp. 371–373. New York: Thieme

21

Considerations for Devising a Totally Implantable Cochlear Implant

Noel L. Cohen

Cochlear implants (CIs) have become extremely useful tools in the treatment of severe to profound hearing loss. Not only are modern implants able to provide environmental sounds to even the profoundly deaf, but also in the large majority of cases they are able to provide a significant degree of speech understanding without lip-reading. Although the modern multichannel CI has also become smaller in size, one remaining problem is that it requires external visible equipment during use. This external equipment brings with it problems that are both very concrete, as well as psychological.

External hardware, since it is exposed to the atmosphere as well as to the effects of head movement and gravity, tends to be somewhat unstable and prone to damage. This can take the form of actual damage to the transmitter coil, the speech processor, or whatever cables are included in the device, or there can be direct trauma to the hardware while it is being worn. Broken wires, cables, and transmitter coils are a constant source of annoyance and expense, both for the patient and for the manufacturer. When there is external hardware failure, much work is generated for the implant team, and the patient may be "off the air" for a distressing period of time. Much of the above would be minimized were the device totally implantable.

The necessity of wearing obvious and, in some cases, bulky external equipment calls attention to the patient's hearing impairment. Although many of the implant recipients were accustomed to wearing visible hearing aids prior to implantation, the CI, even with a behind-the-ear (BTE) speech processor, is at least as visible as the largest modern hearing aid. In addition to the cosmetic aspect, some recipients (especially adolescents and those in the public eye) would prefer to be able to conceal their deafness by not having to wear any external hardware to hear. Finally, the CI is typically not worn during sleep, and cannot operate in water or during some types of physical activity.

◆ Fundamental Requirements for Design of Totally Implantable Cochlear Implant

In designing a totally implantable cochlear implant (TICI) several requirements are fundamental. First, the performance of the TICI must be equal to that of a conventional CI. Second, there must, by definition, be no visible hardware during use of the device. Third, there must be no additional risk to the patient, either during the implantation of the device or during extended use of it. Finally, there must be a plan for the long-term use, because as we will see later, battery failure is an inevitable occurrence.

◆ Totally Implantable Cochlear Implant Design

Although the device itself will be concealed beneath the scalp and within the mastoid cavity, middle ear and cochlea, there will be additions to the current components of the contemporary CI. In addition to the magnet and antenna coil, the electronics, and the electrode array, it will be necessary that there be an implanted power supply, rechargeable battery, and microphone and speech processor.

The external hardware would then be used primarily for recharging the battery, but there must also be components to allow remote control of the device, an on/off switch, diagnostics, and, if necessary, a power supply backup. In essence, the TICI will consist of several components: the microphone, the electronics, the electrode array, and the power supply. These can all be integrated into a single titanium and Silastic case, the so-called monobody design. Or the various components may be attached to one another by connectors that would potentially allow replacement of each of the several modules, should that fail or otherwise require replacement. The diagnostics and remote control would have to include an on/off switch (although that could also be incorporated into the implanted device); a battery level indicator; an alarm, should there be impending battery failure or some other problem a volume control and a sensitivity adjustment. This external control must also allow the audiologist to create and change programs, allow the patient and/or parent, to change programs, and permit the use of external devices such as FM and telephone coils. In addition to the above, there might be an audio output from the implanted device that allows the parent or audiologist to check on the sound quality received by the patient.

◆ Challenges for the Totally Implantable Cochlear Implant

Of paramount importance is the necessity for safety. The surgery will necessarily be more complex than conventional CI surgery, but it must not be so difficult that it becomes hazardous. There must also be certainty that the device itself is not going to cause any harm to the patient. Two of the great challenges are the power supply and the design and location of the microphone. The design of the power supply offers a very significant challenge. Currently, there is no infinitely rechargeable battery. It is inevitable that, given even the most advanced current technology, every rechargeable battery will have a finite life. In addition to this fundamental problem, it is important that the battery be as small as possible, that it maintain a charge to allow at least a full day's uninterrupted use between charges, that it has no "memory effect" that would over time diminish the interval between charges, and that it not generate excessive heat during operation. The demands on the power supply for the TICI emphasize the need for effective power management by the entire device, and make it highly desirable that the power requirements of the system keep the drain on the battery as low as possible. In addition to these considerations, the battery must be incapable of permitting an injurious discharge of current. Because battery failure is inevitable, the manufacturer must have a clear strategy for dealing with the consequences. This will be the first instance in which a CI device will be guaranteed to fail rather than being warrantied against failure.

Battery failure options consist of adopting a modular design that would allow the surgical removal of the battery module and connection of a fresh battery module. Although this has been done with cardiac pacemakers, creating a sufficiently small, safe, and surgically feasible connector poses a major challenge. Two other options remain following battery failure: (1) use the TICI as a conventional CI with a conventional external speech processor, microphone, and power supply; perhaps in the future it may be possible to drive the entire device with just an external power source, simplifying the amount of external hardware; (2) surgically remove the TICI and place another TICI. All three of these strategies bring with them advantages and disadvantages. Replacing the first TICI with a second will give the patient the use and enjoyment of all the advantages of the TICI. It also brings with it the possibility of implanting an upgraded model, just as has been done with the present conventional CI. Against this strategy of replacement with a new TICI is the fact that the patient will need a second operation and perhaps several operations as batteries sequentially fail. This strategy also exposes the patient to repeated endocochlear trauma in removing the one electrode and replacing it. Finally, the cost of replacing these highly sophisticated and expensive devices every few years may be prohibitive.

The strategy of replacing the battery pack only brings with it the advantage of a much smaller operation with a lower cost and no additional endocochlear trauma. Against this strategy are the facts that repeated use of a connector brings with it an increased risk of failure. It is well known that connectors exposed to body fluids are notoriously liable to leak. This strategy still requires multiple surgeries, although each of them is less than replacing the entire TICI.

The third option would be to use the failed TICI as a conventional CI. This brings with it the advantages of no additional surgery, no further endocochlear trauma, and no additional cost. Against this strategy is the fact that the patient will have to revert to the use of a conventional CI after having had all of the advantages of the TICI.

It is to be hoped that advances in rechargeable battery and/or connector technology will mitigate these problems, but they continue to pose a serious weakness in the concept of the TICI.

The second major challenge for the design of a TICI is that of the microphone. An attractive site for the location of the microphone would be the external auditory canal. A totally implantable middle ear implant was designed by Zenner et al (2000), in which the titanium microphone was placed through an opening in the posterior wall of the external auditory canal, beneath the intact skin. This would allow it to function much like the tympanic membrane, receiving sound waves through the external auditory canal, and it would be safe from external trauma. Unfortunately, there is a long history of placing hardware deep into the skin of the external auditory canal, with unfortunate results that there has been a large incidence of erosion of these metallic elements through the very thin skin of the external auditory canal. This concept has been expanded by the work of Huttenbrink et al (Huttenbrink, 1997; Huttenbrink et al, 2001).

Other potential sites for the microphone are above and behind the auricle, yet these generally suffer from the disadvantage that they are likely to be deep to hair-bearing skin and exposed to the noise of head wear, hair brushing, or even the sound of hair moving external to the microphone. On the other hand, this location would allow the microphone to be incorporated within the device, rather than having to be a separate module. It is likely that the first experimental uses of the TICI will include such an integrated microphone. Maniglia et al (1999) and Ko et al (2001) devised an ingenious method of using the tympanic membrane itself as the membrane of a microphone by connecting it to an electromechanical system, which in turn could be connected to a CI electrode. This would eliminate the need for a separate microphone with the above-mentioned problems. Unfortunately, this system may be so difficult to place surgically and tune properly that it appears to have been largely abandoned.

◆ Conclusion

The critical requirements of the TICI include the battery, microphone, and safety. These three issues will determine the ultimate utility of what, if successful, will constitute a very real major step in the evolution of the CI. TICI devices are currently in various stages of development at all three major CI manufacturing companies. It remains to be seen how soon these devices will supplant current designs.

References

Huttenbrink KB. (1997). Implantable hearing aids for severe hearing loss. Basic considerations on their use and attempt at technical development (Dresden/Bochum model). HNO 45:742–744

Huttenbrink KB, Zahnert TH, Bornitz M, Hofmann G. (2001). Biomechanical aspects in implantable microphones and hearing aids and development of a concept with a hydroacoustical transmission. Acta Otolaryngol 121:185–189

Ko WH, Zhu WL, Kane M, Maniglia AJ. (2001). Engineering principles applied to implantable otologic devices. Otolaryngol Clin North Am 34:299–314

Maniglia AJ, Abbass H, Azar T, et al. (1999). The middle ear bioelectronic microphone for a totally implantable cochlear hearing device for profound and total hearing loss. Am J Otol 20:602–611

Zenner HP, Leysieffer H, Maassen M, et al. (2000). Human studies of a piezoelectric transducer microphone for a totally implantable electronic hearing device. Am J Otol 21:196–204

Index

Note: Page numbers followed by t and f indicate tables and figures, respectively.